THE
LIMBIC SYSTEM

THE
LIMBIC SYSTEM

Robert L. Isaacson

Department of Psychology
University of Florida
Gainesville, Florida

PLENUM PRESS • NEW YORK AND LONDON

Library of Congress Cataloging in Publication Data

Isaacson, Robert Lee, 1928-
  The limbic system.

  Bibliography: p.
  1. Limbic system. I. Title.
  [DNLM: 1. Limbic system. WL307 173L 1974]
  QP383.2.I82   599'.01'88   74-8298
  ISBN 0-306-30773-1

First Printing — August 1974
Second Printing — May 1976

© 1974 Plenum Press, New York
A Division of Plenum Publishing Corporation
227 West 17th Street, New York, N.Y. 10011

United Kingdom edition published by Plenum Press, London
A Division of Plenum Publishing Company, Ltd.
4a Lower John Street, London W1R 3PD, England

Printed in the United States of America

PREFACE

While this book is intended to be an introduction to the neuroanatomy of the limbic system and to studies of the behavior of animals in which the limbic system is stimulated or damaged, it is primarily intended for advanced students of brain—behavior relationships. I have assumed the reader to have some understanding of the structure of the brain, of basic neurophysiology, and of modern behavioral techniques. It has been written for students in graduate programs in psychobiology, physiological psychology, and the neurosciences, but it also should be of interest to some medical students and to others with catholic interests in the biology of behavior.

In the first chapter, I review the structure of the limbic system and in subsequent chapters consider the behavioral effects of lesions and stimulation of components of the limbic system. Supplement information derived from recording the electrical signals of the brain is included where it seems appropriate. The final chapter presents a perspective of the limbic system related to brain stem mechanisms and the neocortex. Understanding the behavioral contributions of the limbic system presupposes understanding how the limbic system interacts with other systems of the brain.

Even though there is only one chapter overtly devoted to theoretical issues, various biases of mine influence all chapters. Anyone reading the book with a critical attitude will soon be aware of them. I would like to alert the reader to some of them ahead of time.

Simply put: the book is flavored by my own orientation to research and reading. For the past 15 years, I have been involved in research programs which were directed at elucidating the effects of limbic system destruction on behavior in the rat, cat, and rabbit. Therefore, studies using these species and using lesion techniques probably are overly represented. Other biases of mine will be apparent.

In many later chapters, consideration is given to the behavioral correlates of electrical rhythms recorded from various limbic structures. In these chapters, the effects of electrical stimulation of various limbic structures on behavior are also discussed. Yet, while these topics are discussed, much less emphasis is placed on them and on studies using other species with which I am less well acquainted.

My biases, the topics and areas given emphasis, come in part from my own research. This research is based on beliefs pertaining to research strategies. I believe that the most substantial knowledge available about the limbic system comes from the use of stimulation and lesion techniques in rats and cats. There is far less useful information available today arising from work using other techniques and other species. Since a great deal more information is needed before an adequate conceptualization can be achieved, this information must come from careful studies using species like the cat and the rat. These animals are amenable to laboratory experimentation and can be used in sufficient numbers so as to provide this information relatively quickly. If we had to rely on studies using nonhuman primates, our understanding of the behavioral contributions made by the limbic system could be greatly delayed. The rat is a necessary laboratory tool, both for neuroanatomists and for those interested in the behavioral contributions of the limbic system. The cat makes its greatest contribution to neurophysiological research.

The other obvious orientation of the book is the emphasis

placed on understanding the functions of the limbic system as revealed by destruction of its parts. For 30 years and more, investigations have been underway of the behavior of animals which have had some portion of the limbic system destroyed by aspirative or by electrolytic lesions. Seeking to understand a structure by destroying it is a useful technique for the behaviorally oriented neuroscientist, although it has many faults, dangers, and traps for the unwary experimenter. Nevertheless, equally dangerous are the faults and traps awaiting those using other techniques in the neurobehavioral sciences. In reality, the lesion technique is no better or worse than any other, such as recording electrical rhythms or recording from single units. Satisfactory understanding of the limbic system will not come from the studies of animals with lesions of this or that part of the limbic system or from the analysis of single cell activity but from theoretical contributions derived from the use of all available techniques. Theories must be evaluated on the basis of whether they make sense of the facts to be explained. A theory must provide a meaningful and useful synthesis of information derived from any and all techniques.

Even though the book has a large number of references to published work on the limbic system, it is not a truly comprehensive review of the literature. I doubt that a totally comprehensive review of the experimental literature can be done by anyone. Still, I have tried to represent fairly most of the important studies which have influenced present research directions. Nevertheless, some of my colleagues will be offended by not finding their favorite studies in the book. To them I apologize for the oversight. On the other hand, some studies were omitted because I felt that they had not added a great deal to our understanding of the limbic system. I have tried to select articles from the literature which highlight information of the greatest importance for the understanding of the limbic system.

Theories of limbic function have not been emphasized in this book, since I do not think there are any adequate theories of limbic system function. My theory, presented in the last chapter, is offered in an apologetic fashion. At best, it offers only the broadest of outlines for a schema of limbic system function. In almost a playful spirit, it is offered as a potential stimulant to others. In a lecture given at the University of Florida in the spring of 1973, Paul MacLean suggested that scientists did not belong in the laboratory if their work and the generation of ideas were not fun. All of my days in the laboratory have been rewarding. I cannot imagine a more fascinating or more interesting life than struggling to find out how the brain works. Therefore, I hope the reader will evaluate the last chapter with understanding.

But my research and study of the limbic system is motivated by far more than the joy it provides. It is motivated by the belief that learning at least some of the secrets of the nervous system will be of value to mankind. This is not an intangible or abstract motive. Retarded children are very real, as are people with other brain disorders. While much of my present work is directed toward problems of general interest rather than toward retardation specifically, the ultimate goal is to better understand the human condition and to help provide information on which effective therapies and treatments for the brain-damaged can be based.

Accordingly, this is the appropriate time to acknowledge the fact that much of the research summarized in this book, my own included, would not have been possible without the financial support provided by two agencies of the government: the National Institute of Mental Health and the National Science Foundation. The administrators in these agencies who have been advocates and supporters of the peer-review system for the support of biobehavioral sciences have made a real contribution.

Part of the joy which comes from the academic life and the laboratory is the association with young, powerful minds coming to grips with the challenge of science. One of the most pleasant features, therefore, of my academic life has been the opportunity to watch students become accomplished neuro-behavioral scientists. I feel that I have been very lucky to count among my former students so many who have made substantial contributions to man's knowledge of brain and behavior. Therefore, if this book has any group to whom it should be dedicated, it would be to my graduate students, both those who have left the laboratory and those who are presently struggling through the ordeals of graduate education. The present group of students has helped me in the preparation of this book by their thoughts and criticisms. These include Michael L. Woodruff, Ron Baisden,

Barbara Schneiderman, Linda Lanier, Ted Petit, and Tom Lanthorn.

In addition, in the preparation of this book I have benefited from the advice of friends, well known in neurobehavioral fields, who have read portions of the manuscript. These include Dr. Paul MacLean, Dr. Graham Goddard, Dr. Charles Votaw, Dr. Elliot Valenstein, Dr. Joel Lubar, and Dr. Frederick A. King. Most especially, I would like to acknowledge the comments made by my colleagues Drs. Carol Van Hartesveldt and Peter Molnar. Their ideas and research in the area of the limbic system function always have been top flight.

At last, I would like to thank Mrs. Virginia Walker for her help in preparing the manuscript in all of its various revisions. She has tolerated the almost endless changes of the text I have made and without her assistance the book just could not have been completed.

Gainesville, Florida   Robert L. Isaacson

CONTENTS

CHAPTER 1
The Structure of the Limbic System **1**

    The Limbic System in Nonmammals   3
    The Question of Homology   8
    The Hypothalamus   10
        Nuclear Groups   12
        Fiber Systems   13
    The Amygdala   18
        Nuclear Groups   18
        Fiber Systems   19
    The Hippocampus   27
        Layers of the Hippocampus   29
        Subdivisions of the Hippocampus   34
        Layers of the Fascia Dentata   34
        Transitional Zones to the Hippocampus   37
        The Fornix   40
    The Septal Area   45
        Nuclear Groups   46
        Fiber Connections   46

The Mammillary Bodies, the Anterior
Thalamus, and the Cingulate Cortex 50
Limbic System—Midbrain Relations 55

CHAPTER 2
The Hypothalamus 59

Pleasurable Reactions 60
The Location of Pleasure Regions 62
Pain and Punishment 63
The Location of Pain Regions 65
Elicited Behaviors 67
Changes in Elicited Behaviors 68
Self-Stimulation, Arousal and Elicited
Behaviors 71
Relations with the Autonomic Nervous System . . . 74
Lesions of the Lateral Hypothalamus 75
A Modification of the Lateral Hypothalamic
Syndrome 78
Escape Behavior 79
Sensory Neglect 81
Ventromedial Hypothalamic Lesions 82
Selective Lesions in the Hypothalamus 83
Neurochemical Systems 86
The Neurochemistry of Eating 89
The Neurochemistry of Behavioral Suppression . . . 93
The Mammillary Bodies, the Mammillothalamic
Tract, and the Cingulate Cortex 95
Lesions of the Mammillothalamic Tract 95
The Cingulate Cortex: Avoidance Tasks 98
Other Behavioral Contributions of the
Cingulate Cortex 100
Reflections and Summary 103

Chapter 3
The Amygdala 107

General Effects Produced by Amygdala
Stimulation or Lesions 108

Autonomic Effects 108
Orienting and Habituation 110
Emotional Changes 111
Arousal and Social Reactivity 114
Studies of Learning and Memory 117
Aversive Conditioning 117
Response Suppression in Appetitive Tasks . . . 124
Transfer and Transposition 128
Reflections and Summary 131

CHAPTER 4
The Septal Area 133

General Changes Following Septal Lesions 133
Emotionality 133
Water Consumption 136
Social Behavior 138
Activity 139
Changes in Performance on Learning Tasks After
Septal Lesions—Avoidance Behaviors 140
Response Inhibition in Appetitive Tasks 145
Electrical Stimulation of the Septal Area 149
Autonomic Effects Produced by Septal Stimulation . 153
Neurochemical Considerations 154
Reflections and Summary 157

CHAPTER 5
The Hippocampus 161

General Changes Produced by Hippocampal
Damage 161
Locomotor Activity 163
Distractibility 165
Alternation 167
Relations to the Autonomic Nervous System . . 169
Endocrine Relations 170
Studies of Learning and Memory—Avoidance
Conditioning 171
Learning in Appetitive Tasks 175

The DRL Impairment 176
Discrimination Learning 178
Frustration 188
Individual Differences in Learning Studies . . . 192
Perseveration 193
Regional Differences Within the Hippocampus . . . 195
Electrical Rhythms of the Hippocampus 200
The Conditioning of Hippocampal Slow Waves 206
Electrical Seizure Activity 207
Seizures and Memory 209
Behavioral Consequences of Artificial
Epileptogenic Foci 211
Summary and Reflections 214

CHAPTER 6
The Graven Image, Lethe, and the Guru 219

The Triune Brain 220
Animals with Predominantly Protoreptilian
Brains 221
More Complicated Forms of Learning and
Memory 224
The Limbic System and the Paleomammalian
Brain 229
Proactive Interference 232
Inferred Characteristics of the Reptilian Core
Brain 235
The Neocortex: The Guru 239

References 245
Author Index 281
Subject Index 289

Chapter 1

THE STRUCTURE OF THE LIMBIC SYSTEM

The term "limbic system" derives from the concept of a "limbic lobe" presented by the French anatomist Broca, in 1878. The word *limbic* refers to a border, fringe, or hem. Broca used the term "limbic lobe" to designate that brain tissue which surrounds the brain stem and which lies beneath the neocortical mantle. In a gross fashion, this includes the cingulate and hippocampal gyri, as well as the isthmus which connects the two. It also includes the various gyri which surround the olfactory fibers running back from the olfactory bulb and stalk. Within this inner lobe of the brain, the structures are presumed to be organized into two layers. The tissue thought to be phyletically the oldest (allocortex) makes up the inner ring. The outer limbic ring does not resemble either neocortex or allocortex based on study of its cellular structure. It is therefore called transitional cortex or juxtallocortex (next to the allocortex). This approach is of some value as a general conceptual scheme, but it fails to recognize that the inner ring is not a uniform band of tissue. In fact, it is a discrete set of structures which can be identified more or less readily by gross dissection, and it is these structural

1

subunits of the inner ring of the limbic lobe on which our attention will be centered during the remainder of this book.

Broca emphasized two aspects of the limbic lobe: (1) its strong relationships with the olfactory apparatus and (2) its presence as a common denominator among the brains of mammals. The first of these is based on the observation that most of the structures of the limbic lobe receive plentiful projections from the olfactory system in the brains of simple animals, e.g., amphibians and reptiles. As a result, the limbic lobe has been considered as the rhinencephalon, the "smell brain," presumably responsible for analysis of the olfactory environment.

The structures of the inner portions of the limbic lobe are surrounded by transitional cortical tissue. In different regions of the brain, the transitional cortices are given different names, e.g., entorhinal cortex, retrosplenial cortex, periamygdaloid cortex. Understanding of the limbic system must include understanding the activities of both the inner ring of the limbic structures and the outer ring of transitional cortex (juxtallocortex). Most of the information available today is about the inner ring structures of the limbic lobe. Much less is known about the transitional cortex.

Historically, there have been various debates about the particular anatomical structures of the inner brain which "should be" considered as belonging to the limbic system. The nervous system is not easily distributed into categories on the basis of any hard and fast rules. It is possible, in fact, to call a collection of structures a system on some arbitrary basis. The value of a categorizing scheme must be the extent to which it helps us to understand the activities of the brain and its relationship to behavior. For the purposes of this book, I am going to emphasize the role of certain inner core limbic structures and refer to them as the "limbic system." The structures include the hypothalamus, the amygdala, the hippocampus, and the septal area. Some consideration will be given to the cingulate cortex—anterior thalamic relationships.

The justification for this grouping is based on the fact that the hypothalamus has strong interconnections with all of the other regions. From a functional point of view, this classification can be justified by the fact that many, if not all, of the effects produced by stimulation and lesions of the extrahypothalamic limbic structures can be replicated by stimulation or lesions of the hypothalamus.

The Limbic System in Nonmammals

Knowledge of the structure of the limbic system in the amphibian brain can help us to understand the basic organizational plan of the limbic system in mammals. Many of the connections among brain structures in mammalian brain exist in a simpler, more direct form in the salamander. The interrelationships among limbic structures are more difficult to trace in more advanced brains owing in part to the extensive development of the neocortex and the corpus callosum. Their development is correlated with distortions of the fiber pathways of the limbic system.

Probably the most prominent portions of the forebrain of the salamander are the olfactory bulb and rudimentary cerebral hemispheres. These cerebral hemispheres are made up of cells arranged in a more or less laminated fashion, although only a small portion of the hemispheres is considered "general cortex"— the precursor of neocortex. The hemispheres surround diencephalon and basal ganglia. These internal structures were considered by Elliot Smith (1910) to be the heart of a protomammalian brain, and it was around them that higher neural systems were thought to develop in evolution.

The actual structure of the brain of a prototypical mammal can, of course, only be guessed, since there is no way to determine the brain structures of nonexistent animals. Theories of their structures have to be based on inferences drawn from living species available for study. These species are only the recent progeny of earlier animals and are considerably different from their ancestors. Existing animals in all species are the current products of the forces of natural selection acting over thousands of years on genetic materials which have changed through mutations and selective matings.

Therefore, it is surprising that there seems to be considerable uniformity in the interconnections among the structures of the limbic system in all living vertebrates. It is on this basis that

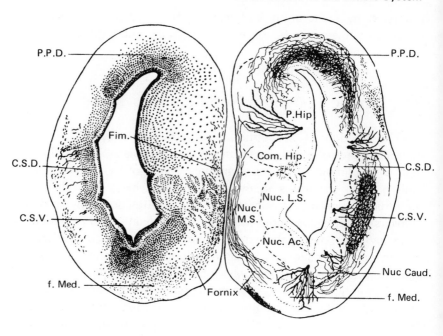

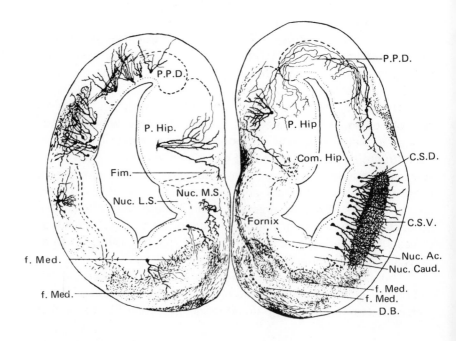

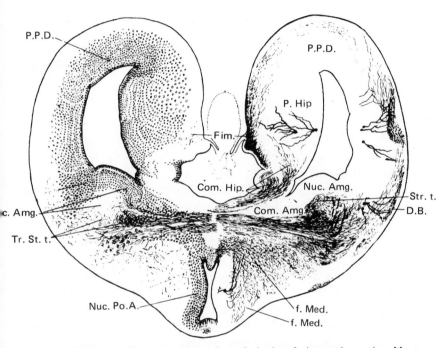

Figure 1. Diagrams of cross-sections through brain of tiger salamander. Most anterior section is at top, most posterior at bottom. Drawings have been simplified to emphasize limbic structures and tracts. Abbreviations: P.P.D., primordial dorsal pallii dorsalis (general cortex); P.Hip., primordium hippocampi; Com.Hip., hippocampal commissure; C.S.D., dorsal part of corpus striatum; C.S.V., ventral part of corpus striatum; Nuc.Caud., caudate nucleus; f.Med., medial forebrain bundle; Nuc.Ac., nucleus accumbens septi; Nuc.M.S., medial septal nucleus; Nuc.L.S., lateral septal nucleus; Fim., fimbria; D.B., diagonal band of Broca; Nuc.Amg., amygdala; Com.Amg., amygdalar commissures; Nuc.Po.A., anterior preoptic nucleus; Str.t., stria terminalis. Figures adapted from Herrick (1948).

many investigators believe that study of the brains of lower animals can provide help in understanding patterns of neural organization of all vertebrates.

Figure 1 shows some figures from Herrick's classic book, *The Brain of the Tiger Salamander* (1948). Large pyramidal cells in the area identified as the hippocampus (P.Hip.) project into the area immediately beneath it, labeled as the septal area (Nuc.L.S. and Nuc.M.S.). Some of these fibers project past these septal areas into regions situated along the base of the brain. This is an area containing fibers of the medial forebrain bundle (f.Med.). Its location can be considered as approximately that of the lateral hypothalamus. The fibers of hippocampal origin extending into the hypothalamus can be thought of as precursors of the fornix system as it is found in animals with more complex brains. The fornix system connects these three areas, which happen to be close to each other in the salamander. These same relationships are found in the more complex brains, even though the hippocampus, septal area, and hypothalamus have become physically separated from each other to a much greater extent.

A conceptual division of the simple salamander forebrain into a mesial division, dealing with the regulation of the internal organs and the autonomic nervous system, and a lateral division, involved with the coordination of somatic activities, has often been proposed. The hippocampus and septal area may be considered as most closely associated with the mesial division. At least a substantial portion of the amygdala develops from the lateral systems concerned with somatic activities. Because of this, it could be classified with the basal ganglia which also are related to the lateral forebrain systems. Yet, the amygdala also lies close to the hypothalamus and has rich interconnections with it. The fibers which interconnect the amygdala with the hypothalamus are maintained in the more complex brains of mammals even though the amygdala is much farther away from the hypothalamus than it is in the salamander. In the mammalian brain, the amygdala and the hippocampus lie next to each other in the temporal regions, yet there are very few fibers interconnecting them. Proximity in the more complicated brain does not assure a large number of interconnecting fibers. However, proximity in the relatively simple brain does seem to assure that strong interconnections will be maintained in the more complicated brain.

In Figure 1, some of the commissural systems of the forebrain have been sketched. Commissures connecting the amygdalae and hippocampi are shown (Com.Amg. and Com.Hip.). The amygdalar commissure is incorporated into the anterior commissure in mammals, whereas the hippocampal commissure maintains itself as a separate system. In more complex brains, such as those of primates, the anterior commissure is mainly a commissural pathway connecting neocortical and limbic structures. The contribution of the fibers of the intermediate olfactory tract which loop from one side of the brain to the other becomes relatively less significant.

The lateral hypothalamic area of the salamander has few, if any, cells in it. It is made up of a dense neuropil consisting of a fine mesh of axons and dendrites. This is the same area through which the fibers of the medial forebrain bundle system pass as they run along the base of the brain. The fibers of the medial forebrain bundle exist in the salamander in the lateral hypothalamic region, just as they do in more complicated brains. The nuclei of the lateral hypothalamus which are found in mammals are thought to be a bed nucleus for the medial forebrain bundle system (Valverde, 1963). Anatomically, the lateral hypothalamic region cannot be dissociated from the medial forebrain bundle. The cells of the lateral hypothalamus live in the midst of a considerable amount of nerve impulse traffic, passing through the medial forebrain bundle.

Many neural systems related to activities of the limbic system are well developed in the salamander. For example, a fiber system running from the habenulae to the ventral tegmentum and the interpeduncular nucleus is very prominent. This fiber system of the habenulae is considered to be analogous to the habenulo-interpeduncular tract, or tractus retroflexus, found in mammalian brains. The habenulointerpeduncular tract should be considered as a discharge pathway from the limbic system, because the habenulae receive fibers from the septal area, the dorsal hippocampus, and the lateral preoptic area of the anterior hypothalamus, among other areas. A neural tract, the stria medullaris, is the most direct pathway between the septal area and the habenulae, but influences from the septal area and the thalamus may also reach the habenulae by other routes, such as by the inferior thalamic peduncle. Some investigators believe that descending limbic system influences converge on both the hypothalamus and the habenulae. The former is thought to represent a ventral relay nucleus and the latter to represent a relay nucleus for more dorsal systems (e.g., Mok and Mogenson, 1972).

The pathways of the limbic system do not become diminished in brains which have great neocortical development. Even though in the brains of animals with a large neocortical development the relative volume of the limbic system structures has become less, the number of axons in the fiber tracts has become greater, both in absolute number and relative to other fiber systems of the brain. In man, for example, there are five times the number of fibers in the fornix as in the optic tracts.

The identification of the habenulointerpeduncular tract in the salamander brain depends on identification of regions which can be considered to be the habenulae and the interpenduncular nucleus. But the "habenulae" and the "interpeduncular nucleus" of the salamander are sometimes identified on the basis of the large fiber tract connecting them. Thus the identification of both pathways and nuclear areas can be circular. The study of comparative anatomy rests on the criteria used to establish anatomical homologies among various species.

The Question of Homology

At this point, it may be worthwhile to consider some general issues related to "homologous" neural structures. What are the criteria by which a nuclear group or fiber system in the brain of one species can be said to be comparable to a nuclear group or fiber system found in the brain of another species? One example might be the habenulointerpeduncular tract. How can a set of fibers identified in the amphibian be homologous to a set found in a more complex mammalian brain? It depends on the identification of an area in front of the tectum as being "homologous" to the highly organized habenular nuclei of the mammalian brain. This identification is based on the large fiber system coming from it and descending into the ventral portion. Thus it is impossible to separate criteria used to identify nuclear and fiber systems. Fiber systems define nuclear areas and nuclear areas define fiber systems—the essence of circular reasoning.

Another possible means for the identification of homologous nuclear areas would be similarities of cytological structure. For example, this approach would imply that a nuclear area densely populated with small cells in the brain of one species ought to be populated with small, densely packed cells in all species. In some cases this criterion may be useful, but it cannot be of general applicability, since many areas of any brain share similar cytoarchitectural characteristics. Two types of criteria can be used together. Nuclear areas could be considered as homologous if they had structural similarities *and* shared similar input and output characteristics. The famous anatomist C. J. Herrick used both types of criteria but considered the similarity of structural anatomy to be most important. His identification of the hippocampus in the brain of the tiger salamander was based on the fact that this area contains pyramidal cells similar to those found in the hippocampus of mammalian brains. In addition, he found the area identified as the hippocampus to be interconnected with the hypothalamus and an area he identified as the septal area on the basis of cytoarchitecture.

Other anatomists believe that the only appropriate criterion for considering brain regions of different species to be homologous is the origin of the cells in these regions. Two brain areas in different species should be considered homologous only if they arise from similar cell groups during development.

Campbell and Hodos (1970) have discussed the various criteria used to establish homologous areas. They conclude that neither the ontogenetic ("common ancestor") criterion nor the anatomical similarity criterion should be used exclusively. They propose that many criteria must be used to establish whether two brain areas of different species are homologous. The experimentally determined fiber connections between areas, the topology and topography of the areas involved, the position of reliable sulci, the origin of the areas in embryonic development, the morphology of the nerve cells, the histochemical composition of the areas, the electrophysiological activity of the areas, and finally the comparability of behavioral changes found after lesions or stimulation of the areas all must be taken into consideration. Each of these is a "soft criterion" for the establishment of homologous brain areas. It is only when all, or many, of them converge on a similar conclusion that the areas should be considered as "homologous."

Given these consideration, the many similarities which have been described in the organization of limbic areas in salamanders and mammals become less certain. Only a few criteria have been used to identify the septal area, hippocampus, amygdala, etc., in the nonmammalian vertebrate brain. Even if the identifications of homologous areas in amphibians have been correct, their interconnections only approximate those found in other species. They provide information only about the general pattern of interconnections among limbic regions and tell nothing about the fine-grain patterns of interconnections which are the hallmark of a particular species. Thus the evolutionary approach is a vague and uncertain guide to understanding the anatomy of the limbic system. The serious student of comparative anatomy must study the specific patterns of limbic interconnections found in particular species.

At the same time, however, there can be a progression in understanding from the general to the specific. While each species does have its unusual modifications of limbic system anatomy, there is a basic plan which appears in the mammals and which was foreshadowed in the amphibian and reptile brains. In the next sections, the patterns of limbic system organization revealed in the mammalian brain will be presented with some comments as to variations of pattern found in certain species where appropriate.

The Hypothalamus

For many years, the hypothalamus has been known as that region of the forebrain most concerned with the regulation of the internal organs. In fact, it has been called the "head ganglion" of the autonomic nervous system. In addition, it has the neural and vascular capability to regulate the secretion of various hormones produced or stored in the hypophysis. Consequently, the hypothalamus has been the target of research relating the brain to endocrine activities.

However, it is now well established that the hypothalamus is also concerned with regulation of somatic activities. In addition, it can alter the level of neural activity in widespread areas of the forebrain. Its effects are exerted both forward into limbic structures and neocortex and backward into midbrain, brain stem, and spinal cord.

The hypothalamus is the most ventral structural "unit" of the diencephalon. Other major diencephalic components are the dorsal thalamus, the ventral thalamus, and the epithalamus.* It is a bilaterally symmetrical structure, being divided into left and right halves by the third ventricle. The hypothalamic sulcus, an indentation of the walls of the ventricle, is used as a landmark to divide the hypothalamus and the thalamus. At its rostral extreme, the hypothalamus merges with the preoptic area. It is called "preoptic" because it is rostral to the optic chiasm. There is no clear boundary between these regions, and consequently the separation is made on an arbitrary basis.† The posterior margin of the hypothalamus is usually considered to be the caudal aspects of the mammillary bodies. Laterally it is limited by various nuclei of the ventral thalamus and in other regions by various fiber tracts.

Looking at the base of the brain, the following landmarks can be seen: the paired or single protuberance (depending on the species) of the mammillary bodies caudally; a raised, longitudinally oriented middle section called the tuber cinerum; a small median eminence, the infundibular stalk and pituitary; and, most rostrally, the optic chiasm.

Throughout the hypothalamus, three zones or regions can be described running from the third ventricle toward the more lateral aspects. These are (1) a periventricular region, (2) a middle or medial zone, and (3) a lateral region. For the most part, cells in the periventricular region are small and lie in rows adjacent

---

* This descriptive summary follows the approach proposed by Crosby *et al.* (1962).
† Some authors consider the preoptic area to be a component of the hypothalamus, and the term "prothalamus" has been used to include the preoptic area and the anterior hypothalamus.

to the ventricular lining. The periventricular nucleus (also called the arcuate nucleus) is a columnar arrangement of cells in the periventricular gray extending from the infundibular region to in back of the ventromedial nucleus. It is found along the base of the third ventricle. It is thought not to have a glia cell barrier separating it from the ependymal lining of the ventricle.

Nuclear Groups

Most of the nuclei of the hypothalamus lie within the medial region of the hypothalamus. The supraoptic and paraventricular nuclei are the most rostral of the medial nuclei. The supraoptic nuclei are found at the lateral margins of the optic tract. The paraventricular nuclei lie just outside of the periventricular region and are near the top and sides of the third ventricle. Fibers from these nuclei extend to the neural lobe of the pituitary gland. In some species, including the rat, a suprachiasmatic nucleus has been described which, as the name implies, is found above the optic chiasm.

The anterior hypothalamic area is a region beginning behind the preoptic area and extending past the infundibular and middle regions of the hypothalamus. It has small, relatively evenly distributed cells which are richly interconnected with the forebrain and thalamic areas.

The ventromedial nuclei are found in the ventral parts of the medial hypothalamus. This nucleus contains large cells, although they are not as large as the large cells of the paraventricular nucleus. Proceeding caudally from its origin, the nucleus grows rapidly in size and comes to occupy most of the ventral regions of the hypothalamus. The dorsomedial nuclei become visible above the ventromedial nuclei. In the rat, the ventromedial nuclei are more prominent than the dorsomedial but both may be seen without difficulty. The dorsomedial nuclei are less prominent in primates than in most nonprimate mammals.

In some regions of the hypothalamus, the columns of the fornix are surrounded by cells which are called the perifornical nucleus. Above and extending caudally over the dorsomedial nuclei is the posterior hypothalamic area. More anteriorly, this region is continuous with the dorsal hypothalamic area.

Primates have paired mammillary bodies, but the rat has

only a single eminence at the posterior aspect of the hypothalamus. The medial mammillary nuclei are the largest of the mammillary complex. Some fibers of the medial forebrain bundle pass between the medial and the lateral nuclei, thus producing one obvious anatomical distinction between them. Fibers from the fornix also richly penetrate the region. The supramammillary commissure contains fibers of the fornix and the medial forebrain bundle which cross from one side to the other, although fibers from the red nuclei and several tegmental nuclei also pass in this commissure.

Behind the medial mammillary nuclei is the most posterior portion of the hypothalamus, sometimes called the posterior mammillary nucleus. Just rostral to the mammillary nuclei are the dorsal and ventral premammillary nuclei, which are considered to be "bed nuclei" for the periventricular system. Further details concerning the mammillary complex can be found later in this chapter. A drawing of the hypothalamic nuclei as they would appear in a sagittal section is shown in Figure 2.

Only a few relatively minor nuclei of the lateral hypothalamus are identified in man. These are the tuberomammillary, the mammilloinfundibular, and the lateral tuberal nuclei. The cells in the first two nuclei are identified on the basis of their staining characteristics. Their cells are found in clusters in the posterior reaches of the hypothalamus. The lateral tuberal nuclei are found as columns of cells through the ventral aspects of the hypothalamus. At least some of these cells have fibers which reach to infundibular stalk.

Fiber Systems

The hypothalamus resembles a crossroad of fibers from forebrain and hindbrain regions. The impulses traveling over these fibers may act to establish a balance of activities in different hypothalamic regions. As is being more and more recognized, the *balance* of activities reaching any particular nuclear region is of great importance and may be more important than the total amount of neural input received. It is likely that the balance of activities received by a nuclear area over fibers using different transmitter systems is of significance, too.

Many of the fiber systems related to the hypothalamus are

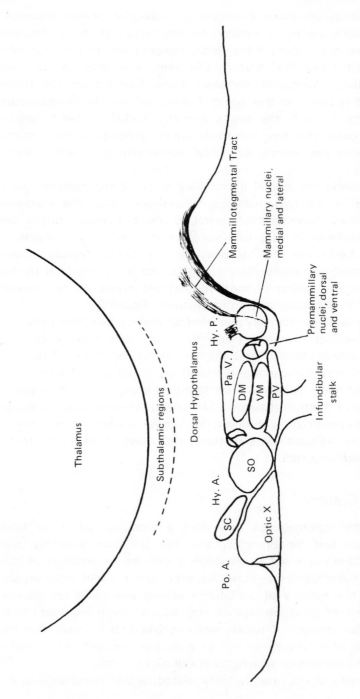

Figure 2. Schematic representation of hypothalamic nuclei as they extend in longitudinal view of diencephalon. Abbreviations: Po.A., anterior preoptic area; SC, suprachiasmatic nuclei; SO, supraoptic nuclei; DM, dorsomedial nucleus; VM, ventromedial nucleus; Pa.V., paraventricular nucleus; PV, periventricular nucleus; Hy.A., anterior hypothalamus; Hy.P., posterior hypothalamus.

poorly myelinated and difficult to study. In addition, there are many sources of artifact in experimental histological studies, which makes the knowledge of the relationship of the hypothalamus to other areas less than completely certain.

The preoptic area has strong connections with the anterior hypothalamus. This could be anticipated from the fact that there is no clear boundary between these regions. On the other hand, the preoptic area is considered to be of telencephalic origin while the anterior hypothalamus is a diencephalic region.

A major afferent source of neural input to the hypothalamus arrives over the mammillary peduncles. Some fibers originate in the "dorsal visceral gray" in the primate brain. This region of the midbrain is concerned with information about tastes. Some fibers ascending in the medial lemnisci leave the lemnisci in the midbrain and turn into the mammillary peduncle. There are many fascicles in the mammillary peduncle, some from tegmental nuclei and others from the brain stem reticular formation. Some fibers of the mammillary peduncle may also arise from the substantia nigra. As the mammillary peduncle approaches the diencephalon, it exchanges fibers with various nuclei in the anterior midbrain region. The fibers of the mammillary peduncle are thought to terminate in the lateral mammillary nucleus and the anterior portions of the medial mammillary nucleus in the cat.

The medial forebrain bundle courses through the lateral hypothalamic area connecting structures of the medial aspects of the hemispheres with preoptic, hypothalamic, and midbrain regions. The terminology describing the relationship is such that some authors prefer to say that the medial forebrain bundle ends in the hypothalamus and that further interconnections with the midbrain are by means of the anterior and posterior hypothalamotegmental tracts.

The anterior hypothalamotegmental tract interconnects the preoptic area and the anterior hypothalamus with the tegmentum, particularly the region ventral to the red nucleus. As this tract travels along the ventromedial aspect of the medial forebrain bundle, it collects fibers from the ventromedial nucleus, the periventricular nucleus, and the posterior hypothalamus. The posterior hypothalamotegmental tract arises mainly from the ventromedial nucleus and reaches to areas above the red nucleus. Thus the red nucleus is surrounded, top and bottom, by fibers from the posterior and anterior hypothalamotegmental tracts. The point is, however, that the hypothalamus by means of these components of the medial forebrain bundle has ample interactions with various tegmental and midbrain regions. The general plan of the medial forebrain bundle is that it is a fiber system which provides the neural means for intercommunication of the medial forebrain (e.g., parolfactory areas, septal area, hippocampus, amygdala, preoptic area, hypothalamus) with the midbrain. What is surprising, perhaps, is that the hypothalamic and limbic fibers do not extend caudally beyond the midbrain.

The fornix provides a major source of input into the preoptic areas, the anterior and lateral hypothalamus, and especially the mammillary bodies. While the hippocampus is often thought to be the major source of such fibers, fornix fibers do arise from the septal area, the anterior subcallosal areas, the cingulate cortex, and the transitional, periamygdaloid cortex of the temporal lobe (and perhaps the amygdala) as well. Some axons of the fornix go past the hypothalamus, enter the supramammillary decussations, and reach the midbrain tegmentum. It should be noted that there is some evidence of a specialized distribution of fibers from the hippocampus into the hypothalamus. The superior region of the hippocampus (see p. 34*ff*) projects mainly to the mammillary complex, while the inferior region projects to preoptic and anterior hypothalamus as well as the septal and diagonal band regions (Raisman *et al.*, 1966).

Afferents from the amygdala reach the hypothalamus over two major routes: (1) the stria terminalis and (2) the ventral amygdalofugal fibers. Fibers from the amygdala reach the preoptic region, the anterior hypothalamus, and the outer rim of the ventromedial nucleus. The fibers coming into the hypothalamus arise from the pyriform cortex and the olfactory tubercule as well as from the amygdala itself.

Other fibers reach the hypothalamus from the habenulae (over stria medullaris) and from the globus pallidus over the pallidohypothalarnic tract. This fiber bundle is thought to reach the ventromedial nuclei.

Some regions of the frontal neocortex are also thought to project to the hypothalamus. Lesions of the orbitofrontal cortex in primates have produced degeneration in the paraventricular and the ventromedial nuclei. A more widespread pattern of projection has been reported when the propagation of strychnine-induced spike discharges has been studied.

Very fine fibers are found in the periventricular zones of the hypothalamus. These fibers run both vertically along the edges of the third ventricle and longitudinally throughout the system. Some of the vertically oriented fibers run from the periventricular zone and leave the hypothalamus to reach the dorsal thalamus. Some of the fibers running in a rostral–caudal direction gather into more or less discrete fiber bundles at the aqueduct. Caudal to this region, they continue to the Edinger–Westphal nuclei and to the tectal region. These fibers are known as the dorsal longitudinal fasciculi. These tracts have two main branches which interconnect with different regions of the midbrain and brain stem. A medial bundle interconnects with the nuclei of the raphe, nearby tegmental nuclei, and other medial nuclear groups in the brain stem and medulla. A lateral portion interconnects with other tegmental nuclei and the salivatory nuclei.

The mammillothalamic tracts are predominantly efferent. They contain fibers from the mammillary complex going to the anterior nuclei of the thalamus. These are discussed in greater detail below.

The tracts reaching the hypothalamus, and beyond, from midbrain and brain stem areas are important routes by which catecholamine- and serotonin-containing fibers reach forebrain areas, as indicated by formaldehyde-induced fluorescent techniques (Anden *et al.*, 1966). There is also a suggestion that fibers of the medial forebrain bundle play a role in governing synthesis of presumptive transmitters in neocortex independently of their role in "transmitting" materials along their axons (Heller, 1972).

It is likely that there are several separate systems of catecholaminergic fibers ascending from the brain stem. One is a dorsal pathway running from the locus coeruleus reaching the cerebral cortex and the hippocampus. The second is a ventral pathway from the reticular formation going to the hypothalamus (Fuxe *et al.*, 1970). A serotonergic system originates in the nuclei of the raphe and ascends in the medial forebrain bundle. Their forebrain distribution parallels that of the adrenergic system.

The Amygdala

"The amygdala" is the name of a collection of nuclei found in the anterior portions of the temporal lobes in the brains of primates. Its cellular composition makes the nuclear group "stand out" from surrounding cortical areas when appropriately stained and viewed microscopically. In general shape the nuclear complex resembles an almond, hence its name. *Amygdala* is the Greek word for almond.

The amygdalar nuclei are found in different locations in different animals. In marsupials they are in the floor of the temporal horn of the lateral ventricles, but in most mammals the nuclei lie forward of the temporal tip of the horn of the lateral ventricles.

Nuclear Groups

Many subdivisions have been made of the amygdalar nuclei. The subdivision of the amygdala into nuclear groups has produced counts of from five to 22 in various species and by various authors. However, the two major nuclear divisions are the corticomedial division and basolateral division (Johnston, 1923).

The corticomedial complex is generally thought to be comprised of the cortical, medial, and central nuclei as well as the nucleus of the lateral olfactory tract. The basolateral complex is considered to be made up of the lateral, basal, and accessory basal nuclei. The corticomedial complex is found more medially located in the brain and is closely related to fibers from "olfactory structures" carried over the lateral olfactory tracts. The basolateral division is thought to have a strong association with neocortical systems, and it is the most pronounced nuclear group of the amygdala in the human.*

The cytoarchitecture of the amygdala has presented various problems to anatomists, including the question as to how many nuclear groups (and subgroups) should be identified. Different

---

* There are reasons for considering the cortical nucleus to be a true cortical formation, related to the pyriform cortex, rather than a nucleus of the amygdalar complex (see Valverde, 1965; DeOlmos, 1972).

histological techniques produce different groupings of cells, and workers in different countries base their analyses on different anatomical traditions. For example, Koikegami (1963) identifies more subunits of the amygdala than is common among American investigators. An enlightening discussion of the cytoarchitecture of the amygdala can be found in Hall (1972), who discusses the different criteria used by various authors in making subdivisions within the amygdalar complex. Drawings of the amygdalar nuclei as they are found in the rat are shown in Figure 3.

One of the problems arising from attempts to describe the nuclear systems of the amygdala is that the nuclear masses are not homogeneous with regard to size or shape of the cells as revealed in Golgi-impregnated material. For example, the amygdalar complex contains three types of cells: stellate cells, pyramidal (type) cells, and modified pyramidal cells. The lateral, basal, and cortical groups all have cells with similar shapes, as do the medial aspects of the cortical nucleus and the anterior amygdalar area. The lateral nucleus contains very small cells not found in other nuclei. Also, all of the cells in a particular amygdalar nucleus fail to exhibit a uniform appearance when subjected to various neurochemical stains. The lateral nucleus shows a greater density of acetylcholinesterase in the ventromedial area than in the dorsolateral extreme. It should be emphasized, however, that there are wide species differences in the amount of acetylcholinesterase staining which occurs in any particular amygdalar nucleus (see Hall, 1972).

Fiber Systems

The fiber connections of the amygdala are less than perfectly understood, but two main efferent systems are recognized. These are the stria terminalis and the ventrofugal bundles (ventral amygdalofugal pathways). Fibers of amygdalar origin pass to more anterior regions of the forebrain, primarily the preoptic and ventromedial areas of the hypothalamus, over the stria terminalis. The stria terminalis probably arises predominantly from the corticomedial division of the amygdala, although the basolateral nuclei also contribute some fibers to it. The ventral amygdalofugal pathways to the hypothalamus are thought to arise from both nuclear divisions, but many fibers in this

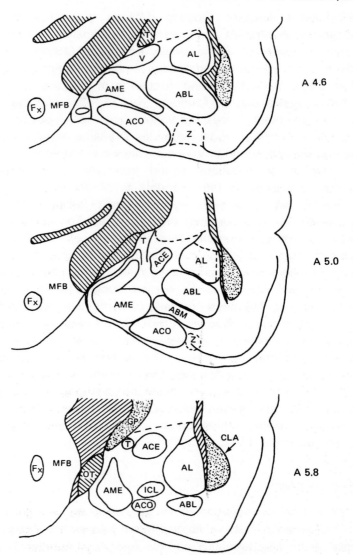

Figure 3. Drawings of major amygdalar nuclei in rat. The letters and numbers to the right of each figure represent the anterior–posterior coordinates of the deGroot atlas from which the drawing was made. Abbreviations of amygdalar nuclei: AL, lateral nucleus; ABL, basal nucleus, lateral part; ABM, basal nucleus, medial part; AME, medial nucleus; ACO, cortical nucleus; ACE, central nucleus; T, stria terminalis; V, ventricle; GP, globus pallidus; CLA, claustrum; Z, transitional zone; ICL, intercalated nucleus; Fx, fornix; MFB, medial forebrain bundle. Redrawn from deGroot (1959).

pathway arise from periamygdaloid cortex rather than from the amygdala itself in many species including the rat. The contributions of fibers from the basolateral nuclei have been established only in primates (e.g., Nauta, 1961). At least in the rat, and perhaps in other species as well, the stria terminalis is the major efferent pathway to telencephalic and diencephalic structures from the amygdala.

The fibers in the stria terminalis from the amygdala reach the hypothalamus and preoptic areas, some coursing in front of and others behind the anterior commissure. There are at least three components to the stria terminalis: dorsal, ventral, and commissural. According to DeOlmos (1972), the dorsal component sends fibers to the bed nucleus of the stria terminalis, the basal part of the lateral septal nucleus, the posterior—medial part of nucleus accumbens septi, the olfactory tubercule, portions of the anterior olfactory nucleus, the granular layer of the accessory bulb, the medial preoptic area, the area around the ventromedial nucleus of the hypothalamus, and an area just ahead of the mammillary nuclei. The ventral component distributes to the bed nucleus of the stria terminalis, the junction of the preoptic area and the hypothalamus, the central core of the ventromedial nucleus of the hypothalamus, and the premammillary area. The commissural component connects the amygdalae of the two hemispheres through the anterior commissure as does a small portion of the dorsal component of the stria terminalis. A diagrammatic representation of these projections is found in Figure 4. An illustration of the terminations of fibers from the stria terminalis around the ventromedial nucleus of the hypothalamus is shown in Figure 5. In some species, other fibers reach the septal area, the habenulae (over stria medullaris), and other brain regions. This apparent redundancy in the termination of the fiber systems seems to be a commonplace in the limbic system. For example, fibers from both the stria terminalis and the ventral amygdalofugal fibers end in the lateral preoptic areas.

The distribution of fibers originating in the amygdala and reaching forebrain sites over the ventral pathways has been difficult to establish owing to the difficulty of producing lesions restricted to the amygdalar nuclei. When lesions are made in the amygdala, there is always incidental damage to periamyg-

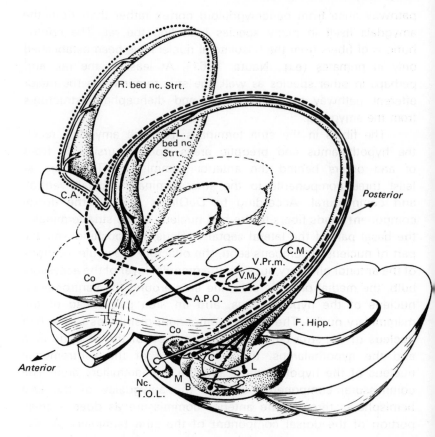

Figure 4A. Schematic representation of stria terminalis system (dorsal amygdalofugal pathway).

daloid cortex and an interruption of fibers passing through the amygdalar complex. Therefore, it is difficult to establish the contribution of the amyglalar groups per se as opposed to fibers originating outside of the amygdala. From the studies of DeOlmos (1972), short fibers of the ventral system reach from various nuclei of the amygdala to the claustrum and to the posterior part of the anterior olfactory nucleus. Fibers also interconnect the several nuclear groups, and others extend toward the prepyriform, pyriform, and entorhinal cortex. Some fibers reach to the subiculum. A rostral segment of the ventral fibers forms a more or less compact bundle containing axons of cells located

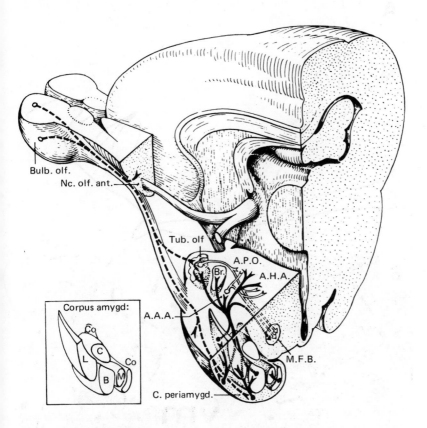

Figure 4B. Ventral amygdalofugal pathways. Abbreviations: R., right; L., left; bed nc.Str.t., bed nucleus of stria terminalis; C.M., mammillary bodies; V.M., ventromedial nucleus of hypothalamus; V.Pr.m., ventral region of premammillary region; Co., cortical nucleus; A.P.O., preoptic area; C, central nucleus of amygdala; Nc.T.O.L., nucleus of the lateral olfactory tract; L, lateral nucleus of amygdala; C.A., anterior commissure; M, medial nucleus of amygdala; B, basal nucleus of amygdala; Br., diagonal band of Broca; A.H.A., anterior area of hypothalamus; A.A.A., anterior amygdalar area; Tub.olf., olfactory tubercule; Bulb olf., olfactory bulb; C.periamygd., periamygdaloid cortex; M.F.B., medial forebrain bundle; F.Hipp., hippocampus. From Lammers (1972).

in the pyriform cortex and in the basolateral group. This tract courses between the central and lateral nuclei and forms a part of the "longitudinal association bundle" of Johnston (1923). At its rostral extreme, the fiber systems turn medially to go toward the substantia innominata and terminate in the bed nucleus

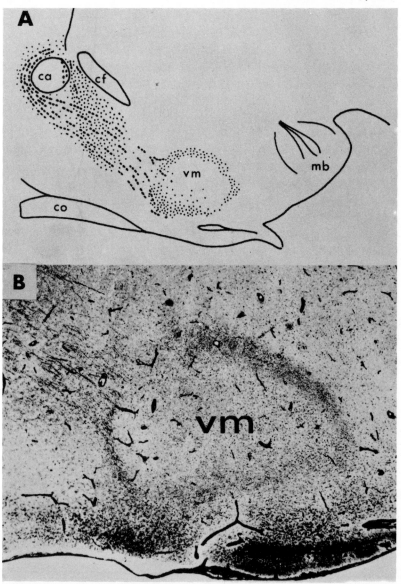

Figure 5.(A) course and distribution of terminations of stria terminalis fibers around ventromedial nucleus of hypothalamus. (B) Low-power photomicrograph of sagittal section of hypothalamus in region of ventromedial nucleus. Material stained by Fink–Heimer method (II). Abbreviations: ca, anterior commissure; cf, columns of fornix; mb, mammillary bodies; co, optic chiasm; vm, ventromedial nucleus of hypothalamus. From Heimer and Nauta (1969). Reproduced with permission of authors and Elsevier, Amsterdam.

of the stria terminalis. Other fibers in this rostral, compact pathway go to the ventral portions of the caudate–putamen complex, nucleus accumbens septi, and to the olfactory tubercule. Some fibers reach the anterior olfactory nucleus and area paragenualis 25. Fibers in the compact bundle reach the lateral preoptic area, the nucleus of the horizontal limb of the diagonal band, and some can be traced into the medial forebrain bundle.

In addition to the compact, rostral component of the ventral amygdalofugal fibers, there is a diffuse projection of fibers in this pathway. Some of the small fibers in this group take origin in the nuclei of the amygdala, but other small fibers and most of the large fibers probably originate in the pyriform cortex. These latter fibers extend to the precommissural and supra-commissural hippocampus, but, as mentioned above, these thick fibers probably are not of amygdalar origin. These fibers also contribute to the stria medullaris, the lateral hypothalamus, the dorsomedial and ventromedial nuclei of the thalamus, and the lateral habenulae. A component of small fibers, perhaps of amygdalar origin, reaches the ventrolateral hypothalamus.

Of interest is the fact that the amygdala lesions which produce the greatest degeneration in the medial forebrain bundle and lateral hypothalamus are those of the anterior aspects of the central amygdalar nucleus. Lesions of the pyriform cortex or the basolateral complex produce much less degeneration. Apparently, most of the fibers in the ventral bundles originate in the anterior two-thirds of the amygdalar complex.

There is a great deal of overlap in the distribution of fibers from the ventral amygdalofugal fiber system and those from the stria terminalis. However, the fact that one component of the limbic system projects to another area over two (or more) different routes does not necessarily imply redundancy in the system. In the case of the amygdala, it is likely that each of the various components has its own special pattern of projections in the hypothalamus. This may imply different routes of regulatory control, and perhaps different types of control, by different cell groups of the amygdala.

In the cat and monkey, projections from the amygdala reach the posterior aspects of the dorsomedial nucleus of the thalamus. This is of significance because of the strong interconnections between the dorsomedial nucleus and the lateral and orbital frontal cortex. In primates, influences from the amygdala can also reach the prefrontal neocortical areas by another route as well, i.e., the uncinate fasciculus which runs between the anterior temporal lobe and the prefrontal areas.

Another area which receives fibers from the stria terminalis system is the ventral septal area. Some fibers from the amygdala come over the stria terminalis to turn caudally at the level of the septal area to run through stria medullaris to the habenular complex. As was mentioned above, the habenulointerpeduncular tract originates in the habenular complex and projects to ventral tegmental areas. While the fibers reaching from the amygdala to the habenulae via the stria medullaris are extremely long, there are even longer ones in the stria terminalis. One example is the commissural fibers originating in the amygdala which follow the stria terminalis to the level of the anterior commissure and cross to the other side of the brain before terminating in the contralateral amygdala.

There are further complications of the stria terminalis system. These include fibers which leave the stria terminalis at its most rostral extent and turn into the fornix. These fibers terminate in the septal area much like other fibers in the fornix which arise from the hippocampus.

The projections from the amygdala over the ventral bundles reach many areas. These include the caudal aspects of orbito-frontal cortex in the monkey. This led Nauta (1962) to conclude that the amygdala, or part of it, is one portion of a rather wide-spread neural system which includes the magnocellular region of the dorsomedial thalamic nucleus and the orbitofrontal cortex. In addition, connections between the orbitofrontal cortex and the amygdala in the rostral aspects of the temporal cortex are made via the uncinate fasciculus. Cells in the inferotemporal cortex have been shown to project directly into the amygdalar complex.

Both the medial forebrain bundle and the system of the habenulointerpecuncular tract provide means for conveying impulses from amygdala and other limbic areas to the midbrain tegmentum and central gray. Some fibers from these systems also spread out into the region of the mesencephalic reticular formation. There is the possibility of direct connections between the amygdala and midbrain reticular formation as well, although these have been demonstrated only in electrophysiological studies. Even if direct connections do not exist, there is ample opportunity for the regulation of the reticular formation by the amygdala through indirect connections.

Afferents to the amygdala arise from several sources. These include fibers from the olfactory bulb which terminate in the corticomedial division in many, if not all, species. Axons from cells in the transitional cortex of the pyriform cortex reach the basolateral group. Afferent fibers also arise from many of those regions receiving efferents from the amygdala, including several nuclei of the thalamus (Powell and Cowan, 1954), the hypothalamus (Cowan *et al.*, 1965), and from the prefrontal cortex.

The Hippocampus

One of the problems faced by the student of the limbic system anatomy is just what is meant by the term "hippocampus". Those concerned with human anatomy often use the term to mean all of the tissue making up the hippocampal gyrus. This use of the term is too broad, since it includes too many neural tissues of a diverse nature. A more useful approach is to use the term to refer to the structures within the hippocampal formation which have simple laminar composition, which share certain inputs and outputs, and which are closely interconnected: the fascia dentata and Ammon's horn. The latter is also called the "hippocampus major" or the "hippocampus proper." In this book, "hippocampus" will be used to designate *either* the unit comprised of the hippocampus (proper) and the fascia dentata (or dentate gyrus) *or* only the "hippocampus proper." Hopefully, the context will provide information about which usage is intended. For example, the latter usage will be used when considering relationships between the hippocampus (proper) and the dentate gyrus. Another term, the "hippocampal formation," is sometimes used to designate the hippocampus (proper), the dentate gyrus, and the subiculum.

A diagram of the hippocampus and dentate gyrus as they

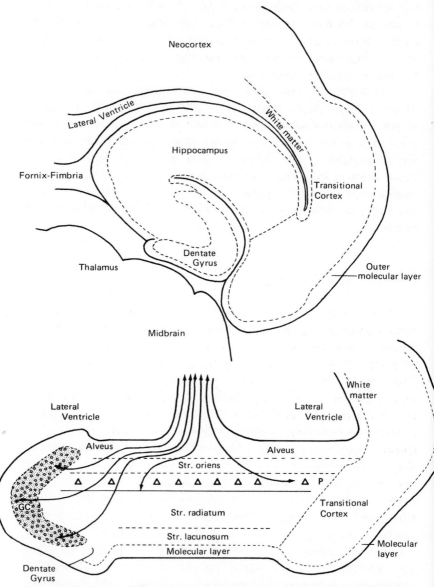

Figure 6.(A) Sketch of hippocampal formation as seen in horizontal section made through right hemisphere of rat brain. (B) Sketch of "unfolded" hippocampal formation. This drawing shows similarity of alveus to deep white matter of nonlimbic cortex and continuity of molecular layer of hippocampus with outer molecular layer of hemispheres. Traditional layers of hippocampus are labeled. Abbreviations: Str., stratum; P, stratum of pyramidal cells; GC, granule cells of dentate gyrus.

would be seen in a horizontal section of the right hemisphere in a rodent brain is shown in Figure 6A. This diagram is oversimplified, of course, and only tries to convey an "overview" of the principal subdivisions and the general configuration of cells in different regions. As can be seen in this figure, the hippocampus and the dentate gyrus appear to be interlocked gyri. It should be noted also that the outer surface of the neocortex (see Figure 6B) continues around to the hippocampal fissure and subsequently along around the edge of this fissure until the fornix—fimbria complex is reached. Thus the leftmost edge of the hippocampus and dentate gyrus in this figure represents the most medial aspects of the structure. Inside of this medial edge is the diencephalon or brain stem, depending on the height in the brain at which the section is made. The point is that the most medial aspects of the hippocampus and the dentate gyrus are really their "outer surface" and the most lateral aspects are comparable to the deeper layers of neocortex. The deepest major layer of the hippocampus would be the alveus, while the "deepest" layers of the dentate gyrus would be the fiber complex found at the junction of the hippocampus and dentate through which the axons enter and leave the dentate gyrus.

Layers of the Hippocampus

Although the hippocampus and dentate gyrus are often said to be primitive because they have fewer layers of cells than does the neocortex, a recent translation of a book on the hippocampus by Ramon y Cajal (1968) indicates that this great anatomist accepted a seven-layered conceptualization of the structures, which reveal marked similarity to other cortex, including the neocortex. The following represents a brief summary of the descriptions provided by Ramon y Cajal of the layers found in the hippocampus.

1. Stratum Moleculare
The outermost zone of the hippocampus and the dentate gyrus (which are continuous with each other) is called the stratum moleculare. It contains many nerve fibers but relatively few cells. At least some fibers run horizontally in the molecular zones

and probably these are long dendritic processes of the pyramidal cells. Other fibers in this zone are probably axons entering the hippocampus from the subiculum. The few cells found in this zone give rise to fibers running parallel to the direction of the molecular layer for short distances.

2. Stratum Lacunosum

The stratum lacunosum consists of many irregularly spaced cells and rather a large number of fibers. The axons of the cells that Ramon y Cajal was able to follow in his Golgi impregnations came from the cell and turned horizontally running through the stratum lacunosum for some distance. Some fibers ended in this layer, while others ascended into the molecular layer. Ramon y Cajal was not sure whether fibers from cells reached to the alveus beneath or not, although fibers were observed running between the stratum lacunosum and the alveus. He was inclined to believe that these fibers were afferent to cells in this layer.

Large bundles of parallel fibers run through the stratum lacunosum. They arise from the "inferior" region of the hippocampus and reach to the subiculum. Some of these fibers are collaterals from pyramidal cells, some turning upward from the alveus to do so. Other fibers ascend directly from the point at which they branch off the vertical aspect of the axon. Other fibers of unkown origin enter the stratum lacunosum from the white matter (alveus) beneath and send both to the pyramidal layer and the cells in the stratum lacunosum, while others send their axons directly to the stratum lacunosum.

3. Stratum Radiatum

The stratum radiatum lies between the stratum lacunosum and the pyramidal cell layer below. It is less densely populated by cells than the stratum lacunosum and contains many bushy dendritic arborizations of the pyramidal cells beneath it. It also contains many fiber systems coursing through it from various points of origin which make contact with the dendrites of the pyramidal cells. Ramon y Cajal believed that the layers designated as stratum moleculare, stratum lacunosum, and stratum radiatum together were comparable to the outermost layer, the molecular layer (layer one) of the neocortex.

4. Pyramidal Layer

The large pyramidal cells of the hippocampus are found in the pyramidal layer below the stratum radiatum. In many animals, the pyramidal cells are closely packed. There may be three or four tightly packed rows of cells in the pyramidal layer with the outer cells being somewhat smaller than the inner cells. Ramon y Cajal noted the suggestion made earlier by Schaffer that the large and small pyramidal cells found in the neocortex in different layers (3 and 5) have become collapsed into a single layer in the hippocampus. However, the usefulness of this view is suspect since the pyramidal cells of the hippocampus are markedly different from pyramidal cells of the neocortex. In the hippocampus, the pyramidal cells have tufted dendritic arborizations extending both toward the surface (toward the stratum moleculare) and toward the deeper regions (the alveus). For this reason, the pyramidal cells of the hippocampus are often called "double pyramids." The pyramidal cells of the neocortex are marked by a single extensive dendritic arborization directed toward the surface of the brain (the apical dendrites). Herrick (1926) pointed out that double pyramidal cells are characteristic of neurons in the reptilian cortex, and he felt that this indicated that the hippocampal tissue of mammals is probably the neural inheritance from primitive ancestors.

Axons from the pyramidal cells descend toward the alveus, giving off some collaterals along the way. Some fibers reach the alveus and continue forward in the fornix to reach other regions of the telencephalon or diencephalon. Some axons bifurcate in the alveus. One branch apparently exits through the fornix, while the other goes in a "decidedly different" direction. Thus there are two main systems of descending collateral systems which arise from pyramidal cells of the fourth layer: (a) those which arise just below the pyramidal layer (in the stratum oriens) and run for a short distance before terminating in this layer and (b) others which arise from bifurcations in the alveus and whose collateral runs for some distance in the alveus.

There are many types of collateral fibers given off from cells in all layers of the hippocampus. These collaterals ascend and descend to different layers while bifurcating frequently. In the inferior region of the hippocampus, especially thick collaterals arise from the axons of pyramidal cells which come off a descending axon in the stratum oriens. The main portion of the axon continues to the alveus, while the collateral branch continues in stratum oriens for some distance. From either of these parts of the axon, branches turn toward the stratum lacunosum. These fibers were described by Karl Schaffer toward the end of the nineteenth century and have been called "Schaffer collaterals." They are thought to provide the main route by which pyramidal cells of the inferior region of the hippocampus (CA3 and CA4) influence activities of the pyramidal neurons in the superior region. The original Golgi studies of these fibers showed the Schaffer collaterals to follow a tortuous course from the stratum oriens to the stratum lacunosum, giving branches off into the stratum oriens and stratum radiatum. In the stratum lacunosum-moleculare, the fibers continued to the region superior. These early studies were done in very young animals, and there is reason to believe that in older animals the Schaffer collaterals reach the superior region through the stratum radiatum and stratum oriens (Hjorth-Simonsen, 1973).

5. Stratum Oriens

The stratum oriens lies below the pyramidal cells and above the white matter of the alveus. Many of the cells appearing in this region resemble cells found in the deeper layers of the neocortex. This layer is often divided into two subregions: (a) an inferior subzone bordering the alveus and (b) a superior subzone lying beneath the line of pyramidal cells. Cells of the inferior regions are predominantly oriented parallel to the fibers of the alveus, although some axonal processes have been traced upward into the pyramidal cell layer. Cells in the superior subzone are densely packed and of several types. This is also the region into which the deep tufts of the double pyramidal cells are directed. There are some large cells in this zone whose axons turn upward and reach the molecular layer. Axons of other large cells in this region turn toward the superficial layers, go beyond the pyramidal layer into the stratum radiatum, and then arch back toward the pyramidal cell layer and terminate in the pyramidal layer or even back in the stratum oriens. Collaterals of these axons course through the stratum radiatum and run parallel to the fibers of the alveus, sometimes turning downward to reach the pyramidal cells in other areas.

6. Alveus

For the most part, the alveus is composed of white matter, i.e., axons arising from pyramidal cells deeper within the hippocampus and from other regions. There are some polymorphic cells in it which are thought to be displaced from the stratum oriens.

7. Epithelial Zone

The hippocampus lies inside the lateral ventricle, and separating it from the ventricle is a layer of epithelial cells. Ordinarily, this layer would not be considered a part of the neural organization of the hippocampus and consequently not one of the "layers" of the structure, but Ramon y Cajal found that processes of these cells reached into the hippocampus, to terminate in the stratum oriens in very young animals. In older animals, these fibers terminated in the alveus.

The description of these seven layers of the hippocampus presented by Ramon y Cajal is somewhat misleading, since in describing the neocortex the underlying white matter and its epithelial zones (in areas bordering the lateral ventricles) are not considered as cortical layers. Furthermore, as noted before, layers 1, 2, and 3 are considered together as being homologous to the molecular layer of the neocortex. Therefore, it may be proper to combine various layers described by Ramon y Cajal in order to provide a simple summary of the cell layers of the hippocampus.

> Ramon y Cajal layers 1, 2, and 3 = Hippocampal layer 1
> Ramon y Cajal layer 4 = Hippocampal layer 2 (Pyramids)
> Ramon y Cajal layer 5 = Hippocampal layer 3

The main differences between this cortical arrangement and that of the neocortex would be in the fact that the neocortex has two pyramidal cell layers (layers 3 and 5) and a granule cell layer (layer 4) interposed between these two pyramidal cell layers. In addition, the appearance of the pyramidal cells in the neocortex and hippocampus is quite different, being "single" in the former and "double" in the latter.

Subdivisions of the Hippocampus

Probably the easiest way to consider the subdivisions of the hippocampus is to distinguish two major sections: a superior and an inferior section. The superior section is a zone beginning with a compact layer of pyramidal cells and extending to the point where this layer becomes less compact. This is the boundary between the superior and the inferior regions. As can be seen in Figure 7, the inferior part of the hippocampus lies "ahead" of (rostral to) the superior region and extends throughout the frontal convexity of the hippocampus. The hippocampus was further subdivided into "fields" by the anatomist Lorente de No. These are designated by the letters "CA" (meaning cornu ammonis) and numerals from 1 to 4. The superior part of hippocampus would correspond to CA1. Most of the inferior region would be CA3, with a small region between CA1 and CA3 being designated CA2. CA4 is also a small area more or less distinct from CA3 which appears just before the transition from the hippocampus proper to the dentate gyrus. Some investigators believe that the CA2 region is not a distinct area of the hippocampus based on the examination of histological materials from adult animals. However, Angevine (1970) has shown that the cells in area CA2 are formed at different times in the development of the organism than are cells in CA1 and CA3. This would suggest that they should be recognized as a distinctive neural component in the hippocampus. For most purposes, however, the division of the hippocampus into inferior and superior sectors is sufficient.

Layers of the Fascia Dentata

Ramon y Cajal considered the fascia dentata to be simple three-layered cortex imposed on the end of the molecular layer of the hippocampus proper. It has a molecular zone, a granule cell zone, and a zone of polymorphic cells.

There are only a few neurons with very short processes in the molecular layer, with the exception of a few misplaced

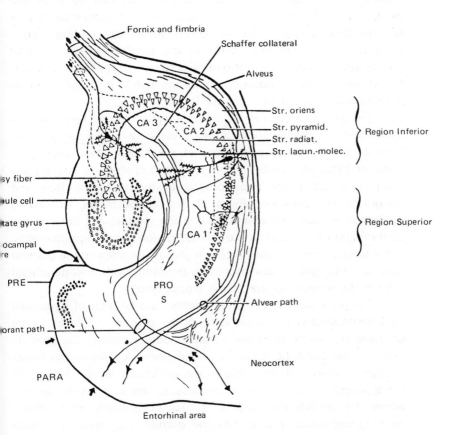

Figure 7. Schematic drawing illustrating superior and inferior divisions of hippocampus and divisions into CA fields. Abbreviations: Str. oriens, stratum oriens;
Str. pyramid., stratum pyramidale; Str. radiat.: stratum radiatum; Str. lacun.-Molec.:
stratum lacunosum-moleculare; PRO, prosubiculum; S, subiculum; PRE, presubiculum; PARA, parasubiculum. Drawing adapted from Brodal (1969). Reproduced by permission of author and Oxford University Press.

granule cells from the layer beneath. The granule cell layer
consists of densely packed cells in several layers. These cells
resemble pyramidal cells of the hippocampus proper to some
extent, but they also have some special characteristics. They
have little protoplasm in their cell bodies and very few basal
dendrites. Most of the dendritic arborizations reach out into the
molecular zone of the dentate fascia. The axons from cells in the

granule cells descend into the polymorphic cell zone of the dentate and, further, into the molecular and pyramidal layers of the hippocampus proper. Often these descending axons bifurcate, with branches going to the nearby granule cells of the dentate and to cells in the inferior region of the hippocampus. Collaterals of these descending axons reach into the layer of polymorphic cells in the dentate fascia.

The axons of cells in the dentate gyrus have a dense, mossy appearance as they wander above and below the pyramidal cell layer of the hippocampus. Most of the fibers travel above the zone of pyramidal cells in the stratum radiatum of the hippo-campus. These fibers end abruptly at the transition from the inferior to the superior region of the hippocampus. According to Ramon y Cajal, the axons leaving the granule cell layer of the dentate end exclusively in the inferior region of the hippocampus. None goes as deep as the fimbria or alveus. As a result, the granule cells are thought to communicate primarily with the pyramidal cells in the inferior region of the hippocampus.

The polymorphic cell layer begins with an area of pyramidal cells embedded in the lower parts of the granule cell layer. Some of these pyramidal cells are actually lodged among the granule cells. Radial dendritic processes subdivide in or above the layers of granule cells and terminate in the molecular layer. These cells have several basilar dendritic processes, and their axons ascend above the granule cell layer to course horizontally above them, sending collaterals down into the granule cell layer. The final termination of these axons is in the granule cell layer. Some axons run among the granule cell layer itself. Other axons from cells in the polymorphic cell layer descend to enter the alveus.

Below the pyramidal cells at the edge of the granule cell layers are several types of nerve cells scattered in an irregular manner through the polymorphic cell zone. Some of these send fibers back up into the granule cell zone, others have axons which descend into the alveus, and still others have short axons which remain in the polymorphic zone. The last type is a short-axon stellate type of cell. It should be noted that, to reach the alveus, the fibers from the dentate gyrus must pass through the pyramidal cell layer, and other layers, of the hippocampus proper.

At the bottom of the fascia dentata are stellate and horizontal fusiform cells. Cells in this region have axons which reach along the border of the polymorphic cell zone, as well as ones which ascend and descend. Some fibers reach the alveus and others go to the granular cell region of the dentate.

Transitional Zones to the Hippocampus

The transition between the cortex and the hippocampus begins with the entorhinal cortex.* The anatomical designation of the entorhinal cortex is based on a plexus of nerve fibers which are found in layers 2 and 3 of the cortex. This is illustrated in Figure 8. This plexus marks the limits of the entorhinal cortex. At the inner edge of the entorhinal cortex is the parasubiculum. Inside the parasubiculum is an area called the presubiculum. It is marked by a dense fiber plexus and by a layer of granular cells. The next area leading to the hippocampus is the subiculum itself. The cells in this region do not have a laminated appearance, but are scattered in an apparently unsystematic fashion throughout a wide area. The beginning of the hippocampus is marked by the appearance of the densely packed pyramidal cell layer which is the beginning of the region superior. Near the dorsal aspects of the hippocampus, a triangular area is found inserted between the parasubiculum and the presubiculum. This area is called "area entorhinalis e" in the rat. It is practically devoid of fibers. It becomes smaller and finally disappears as the hippocampal formation is followed ventrally.

The main types of fiber input to the hippocampus from the entorhinal region which can be noted are the perforant path, the alveus pathway, and the psalterium. The last of these is a commissural system connecting the hippocampal formations of each hemisphere. Fibers entering the hippocampus from the psalterium mix with fibers in the fimbria before their final termination in the hippocampus. The perforant path enters the hippocampus from the entorhinal region, crosses the hippocampal fissure, and reaches the molecular layer (broadly defined) of the hippocampus and the dentate gyrus. The fibers in the per-

---

* The following description is based on anatomical studies of the rat hippocampal complex (e.g., Blackstad, 1956; White, 1959).

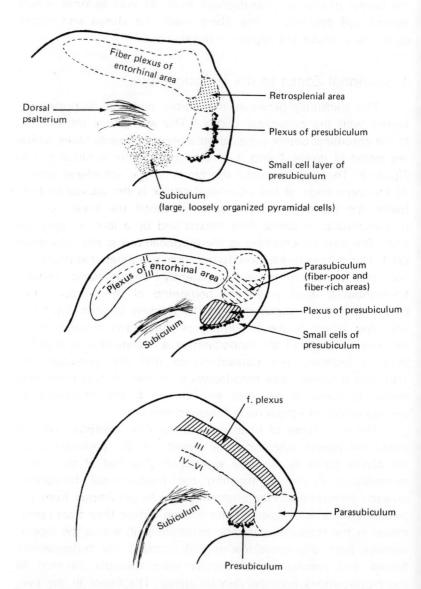

Figure 8. Highly simplified, schematic drawings of transitional regions outside of hippocampus in rat. The three drawings represent sections made through upper, middle, and lower parts of entorhinal and parasubicular areas. Modified from Blackstad (1956, Fig. 5, p. 427).

forant path make contact with the apical arborizations of dendrites of pyramidal cells in all areas of the hippocampus and the dentate (Blackstad, 1958).

The fibers reaching the hippocampus over the psalterium are from the contralateral hippocampus. Such fibers reach the superior sector, making contact with the apical dendrites near the cell body and with the basilar dendrites. In addition, fibers from the contralateral entorhinal cortex reach the granule cells in the fascia dentata. These fibers make contact nearer the cell body than do the ipsilateral afferents from the entorhinal cortex to the same cells which arrive over the perforant path. Thus there is a spatial distribution of terminations on the dendrites of cells in the hippocampus and the dentate gyrus based on the ipsilateral or contralateral sources of the fibers. In general, the distal portions of the dendrites receive ipsilateral input over the perforant path while the proximal portions of the dendrites receive input from commissural, contralateral fibers. The origin of the perforant path seems to lie in the middle regions of the entorhinal cortex.

However, Hjorth-Simonsen and Jeune (1972) have described the termination of the perforant pathway in the rat to be in the middle regions of the molecular layer of the dentate gyrus and the region lacunosum-moleculare, near the stratum radiatum, in the inferior region of the hippocampus. Terminations were not found in the superior region. It is of some interest that Hjorth-Simonsen and Jeune offer evidence to the effect that the perforant path fibers are neither adrenergic nor cholinergic in nature. Hjorth-Simonsen (1971) has demonstrated fibers from the inferior region to the entorhinal cortex which may be considered to be reciprocals of the perforant pathway fibers. He also has shown that cells in the superior region of the hippocampus project to the subiculum, near the boundary with the presubiculum, by means of fibers which travel in the alveus (Hjorth-Simonsen, 1973). In this study, no fibers were found to reach the inferior region of the hippocampus or the dentate gyrus from the superior region. As mentioned before, the primary projections of the inferior region to the superior region are via the Schaffer collaterals.

The perforant pathway exerts a profound excitatory influence on the hippocampus, both directly on the cells in the region inferior (CA3) (Gloor et al., 1963) and indirectly by the activation of the granule cells of the dentate gyrus whose axons also activate these same neurons over the mossy fiber system (Andersen et al., 1966).

A marked enhancement of synaptic efficiency in the superior region of the hippocampus which lasts for hours can be produced by tetanic stimulation of fibers in the perforant path (Lömo, 1970, 1971; Bliss and Lömo, 1970). Cells in the inferior region of the hippocampus activate cells in the superior region via the axon collaterals which were described by Schaffer.

The Fornix

One emphasis in research on the distribution of fibers to and from the hippocampus involves those fibers which course through the fimbria and continue into the fornix system. In addition to commissural fibers, this system contains fibers which interconnect the hippocampus with the septal area and with lateral preoptic and hypothalamic areas. Fibers to and from the medial forebrain bundle also pass through this system. Between the hippocampus and the hypothalamus, the fornix can be considered to have two components: (1) postcommissural and (2) precommissural. The "postcommissural" fornix system is made up of fibers from the hippocampal formation which do not enter the septal area but continue beyond it, passing behind the anterior commissure. At this point, they turn caudally to go through the lateral hypothalamic areas to reach the lateral aspects of the medial mammillary nucleus at the posterior end of the hypothalamus. Some fibers from the hippocampus also reach the other parts of the mammillary complex, although the greatest number of terminations is found in the medial mammillary nucleus. Some fibers branch off the fornix as it passes along the base of the brain to distribute to the lateral hypothalamic areas, the medial forebrain bundle, the lateral preoptic area, and in some species medial hypothalamic areas as well.

The "precommissural" fornix fibers of hippocampal origin distribute to the septal area, although some of them continue through the septal area without making contact. These are joined

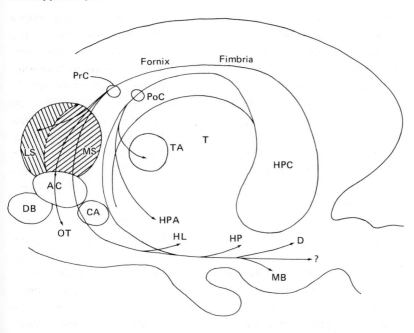

Figure 9. Schematic drawing of distribution of major efferent fornix fibers from hippocampus. Abbreviations: MS, medial septal area; LS, lateral septal area; DB, diagonal band of Broca and its nucleus; OT, olfactory tubercule; AC, nucleus accumbens; TA, anterior nuclear group of thalamus; T, thalamus; HL, lateral hypothalamus; MB, mammillary bodies; D, nucleus of Darkschewitsch; HP, posterior nucleus of hypothalamus; HPA, paraventricular nucleus of hypothalamus; PrC, precommissural fornix; PoC, postcommissural fornix; CA, anterior commissure.

by fibers originating in the septal area to form the precommissural fornix and continue into the same area as described above for the distribution of postcommissural fibers. The fibers from the hippocampus and septal area reaching toward the medial forebrain bundle areas are sometimes known as Zuckerkandl's bundle.

There appear to be different patterns of terminations of fornix fibers arising from cells in the dorsal and ventral hippocampus. These include terminations in the septal area as well as in the diencephalon (Siegel and Tassoni, 1971*a, b*).

The "basic plan" of distribution of fornix fibers found in most mammalian species is shown in Figure 9. For example, in most animals fibers distribute to the central gray of the midbrain through fornix projections which go past the mammillary complex. In certain animals, fibers of the fornix system projects past the mammillary complex and end in the ventral tegmental areas. In the guinea pig, there are significant numbers of fibers which turn dorsally from the medial forebrain bundle system (and perhaps from the fornix) to terminate in the rostral thalamic areas and the lateral thalamic nucleus, as well as the intralaminar nuclear complex. The rat, on the other hand, shows a distribution of fornix fibers to the anteroventral thalamic nucleus which projects to the cingulate cortex and which also receives projections from the mammillary bodies. Also, in the rat there are some fibers which distribute to the medial hypothalamic areas.*

In the cat, fornix fibers project to the intralaminar nucleus of the thalamus; fibers projecting to the lateral thalamic nucleus or to the medial hypothalamic areas have not been reported. The cat is perhaps distinctive because of its massive fornix projections to the central gray of the diencephalon. In the monkey, there are some direct projections from the fornix system to the anteroventral nucleus and the intralaminar complex of the thalamus. The nucleus lateralis dorsalis also receives an abundant supply of fornix fibers. This suggests a strong relationship of the fornix system to the parietal association areas of the neocortex in this animal. In addition, the dorsomedial nucleus of the thalamus receives fibers from the fornix system and from the amygdala. This suggests a dual activation of dorsomedial nucleus by both hippocampal and amygdalar systems and suggests that they may help to regulate activities in the dorsolateral prefrontal cortex in primates.

In terms of projections reaching the midbrain, the greatest number is found in the guinea pig, and only a few, if any, in the rat. These projections are essentially absent in cat and monkey, as well. In the guinea pig, there are at least three sets of fibers which run past the mammillary bodies. There are the fibers which turn to the central gray just behind the mammillary bodies, a set of fibers which reaches the posterior hypothalamic nucleus

---

* Some of these apparent anatomical differences could be due to differences in the extent to which the tissues of the species are susceptible to stain impregnation. Therefore, caution should be exercised in accepting the results unequivocally.

(which is a medially located nucleus behind the mammillary bodies), and a ventral tegmental bundle reaching toward the nucleus of Bechterew. This last bundle turns dorsally into central tegmental areas. In addition, there are branches of the fornix into the subthalamic field "H" of Forel below the medial geniculate nucleus. These fibers are not found in the rat, but have been reported in the monkey. At one time, these tegmental pathways were thought to be of septal origin in the rat, but Nauta now believes that these fibers arise from the hippocampus (perhaps CA1) and go over the corpus callosum in the dorsal fornix (Nauta, 1972). It is likely that the fibers to the tegmental regions arise from several areas and not only from hippocampus or septal area. In the cat, a few fibers of hippocampal origin extend past the mammillary bodies into the midbrain to terminate in the nucleus of Darkschewitsch (Siegel and Tassoni, 1971a).

The hippocampus sends fibers over the fornix system which take a rather extended course. These are the fibers of the dorsal fornix, sometimes called the fornix superior or the fornix longus. These depart from the main body of the fornix and enter the corpus callosum, penetrate it, and turn rostrally over it to the septal area. Then they turn downward into the medial septal area. Some of the supracallosal fibers (also known as the stripes of Lanscisi) do not reach the medial forebrain bundle and the anterior hypothalamus but terminate in the intralaminar nucleus of the thalamus, the anterior nuclei of the thalamus, the habenula, and the mammillary bodies. In rats, at least, the dorsal fornix also projects to the nucleus of Bechterew and other tegmental regions.

In the guinea pig, there are some few fibers from the hippocampus which turn back toward the habenulae from the region of the septal area and join the stria medullaris. Apparently, these fibers to the habenulae arise entirely from the septal area in the rat, cat, and monkey.

Almost certainly there are differences in the areas to which cells in the dorsal and ventral hippocampus project. In the cat, the ventral hippocampus sends fibers to the entire lateral septal area and nucleus accumbens. The dorsal hippocampus and the medial septal area have been reported to be heavily interconnected (Siegel and Tassoni, 1971a, b).

The posterior crux of the ventral hippocampus is reported to project to the midlateral septal area between the projections from the dorsal and ventral hippocampus. Both dorsal and ventral hippocampus project to the nucleus of the diagonal band, anteroventral nucleus, lateral hypothalamus, and the mammillary bodies.

However, there is lack of agreement on the interconnections of the dorsal and ventral hippocampus with the septal area. Ibata et al. (1971) did not find evidence for a difference in the termination of fibers in the hippocampus arising in the septal area. These authors found evidence for a direct pathway from the medial septal area to the apical dendrites of cells throughout the dorsal–ventral extent of the hippocampus. The pattern of degeneration found after the medial septal lesions was much like that found after lesions of hippocampal commissural fibers (Blackstad et al., 1965; Laatsch and Cowan, 1967). The results of Ibata et al. confirmed observations of Raisman (1966) and Genton (1969) which indicate that the terminations of septal fibers are restricted to the inferior region of the hippocampus. However, this study was concerned with fibers reaching the hippocampus from the septal area and not fibers reaching the septal area from the hippocampus. The reciprocity between the septal area and the hippocampus need not be exact, and therefore the results obtained by Ibata et al. are not directly contradictory to those of Siegel and Tassoni.

In a study of the distribution of fibers from the hippocampus in the cat, no differential distribution of septal area terminations was found from subregions of the hippocampus by Siegel and Tassoni (1971a), even though they were looked for specifically. This is in contrast to the results of Raisman et al. (1966), who found that fibers from CA1 (region superior) project to the medial septal area whereas fibers from CA3 and CA4 (region interior) project to the lateral septal areas. From their results, Siegel and Tassoni conclude that cells in the ventral hippocampus have the lateral septal area as their main target area while cells in the dorsal hippocampus have the lateral hypothalamus and the mammillary bodies as their principal targets. In the same study, these authors also found evidence of a pathway from the ventral hippocampus to the pyriform cortex which could be distinguished from terminations of fibers arising in the lateral septal area which reach the same region. These results may be related to previous observations made by Votaw (1959, 1960) which indicated the presence of an efferent fiber system into the transitional cortex outside of the hippocampus both on anatomical and physiological grounds and to the studies of Hjorth-Simonsen discussed above.

While the differences between the results obtained by Siegel and Tassoni and by Raisman *et al.* cannot be resolved at the present time, it must be noted that these groups of researchers have used different species. It is possible that there are qualitative differences in the interconnections and the septal area and the hippocampus of the cat and rat. This problem will be further discussed on p. 49 when considering the septal area.

The Septal Area

The septal area lies in a special position relative to the limbic system and to the rest of the brain. Parts of it stand as unpaired medial structures. All parts receive massive input from a wide variety of limbic regions as well as the hypothalamus. Its influences in other brain regions are as widespread as its sources of incoming neural traffic. Part of the challenge is to discover the ways in which the septal area acts to integrate and regulate the diverse areas with which it is connected.

The septal area is prominent in nonprimate mammals and is an area below the anterior portions of the corpus callosum bounded in front by the anterior hippocampal rudiment* and in back by the hippocampal commissures. The homologous nuclei in primates may be those found in the front of the anterior

---

* The anterior hippocampal rudiment, or precommissural hippocampus, is an area marked by vertical columns of darkly staining pyramidal cells at the inner edges of the hemispheres just below the genu of the corpus callosum. These cells seem to be continous with a very thin band of similar cells which stretch over the top of the corpus callosum, called the induseum griseum. Both the anterior hippocampal rudiment and the induseum griseum are thought to represent displaced pyramidal cells of the hippocampus.

commissure at the base of the brain. The septum pellucidum in man is not homologous to the septal area complex of non-primates. There have been suggestions relating the size of the septal complex with the development of the hippocampus, but this correlation is by no means certain.

Nuclear Groups

The cytoarchitecture of the septal area of the rat reveals homogeneous nuclear areas made up of medium-sized neurons. Despite few differences in cytoarchitecture, it has been divided into various subregions. In the anterior portions of the septal area, near the nucleus of the diagonal band, giant cells are found but only in the medial septal area. These cells project to the hippocampus and undergo degeneration when the fornix is sectioned.

This medial septal nuclear area blends into the parolfactory area, which may be an extension of the olfactory tubercule. Just below the genu of the corpus callosum, the head of the lateral septal nucleus begins. This extends back over the entire length of the septal area. Caudally, the medial septal nucleus becomes smaller and smaller and finally the lateral septal nuclei join together at the midline before it disappears. The medial septal nucleus becomes penetrated by fibers of the fornix which enter the area at an oblique angle. The area between these two bundles of fornix fibers is called the nucleus triangularis septi.

At times, the bed nucleus of the stria terminalis has been considered to be a component of the septal region, although it also could be considered related to the preoptic area. Most often, it is not included in the septal area complex for research purposes. Likewise, the nucleus accumbens septi, surrounding the anterior aspects of the anterior commisure, is usually not thought to be a septal nucleus. The nucleus of the diagonal band of Broca, which lies under the cortex of the olfactory tubercule, is often considered as a part of the septal complex.

Fiber Connections

There is a convergence of fibers from the hypothalamus, the hippocampus, the preoptic area, and the medial forebrain in the medial septal area. Terminals of the different afferent systems end on different portions of the cells in this area. Fibers from the hippocampus tend to reach the axodendritic terminals more than do fibers from the hypothalamus. For example, some 35% of the terminations of fibers from the hippocampus end on dendrites, whereas only 19% of the terminations of fibers from the hypothalamus do so. Very few terminations of fibers from the hippocampus end on the soma of the medial septal area cells, while some 24% of the axosomatic synapses are produced by fibers from the hypothalamus (Raisman, 1969). Only about half of the total number of terminals in the septal area are from either the hippocampus or the hypothalamus. Even though the fibers originating in the hippocampus seldom have axosomatic terminations, they can form such connections. If the normal input to the septal area from the hypothalamus is surgically destroyed, an increase in axosomatic terminals of hippocampal origin will be found after a suitable period of time. Fibers from the hippocampus come to "sprout" and form new synapses on the cells in the septal area deprived of their normal hypothalamic contacts.

Over and beyond the basic interconnections of the septal area with the medial forebrain bundle, the septal area is interconnected with other hypothalamic regions: the supraoptic and periventricular nuclei. These hypothalamic connections are primarily with the medial septal area. It has been suggested that the connections between the septal area and the supraoptic and periventricular systems are important for the regulation of oxytocin release. In addition, the septal area is interconnected with the midbrain central gray, the midline thalamus, the intralaminar nucleus of the thalamus, the anteroventral nuclei of the thalamus, the basal lateral aspects of the amygdala, the mammillary bodies, and the habenulae. The septal area has also been reported to be strongly inter-connected with the cingulate cortex and the orbital frontal cortex in the monkey and the suprasylvian and extosylvian gyri in the cat.

In many species, the habenulae recieve fibers only from the medial aspects of the septal area. There seems to be a topographic relationship between the septal area and the habenulae. The lateral—ventral septal area tends to project to the lateral habenulae and the central gray of the midbrain, whereas cells in the more posterior regions of the septal area distribute fibers to the medial habenulae.

Not all authors agree with these observations, however. Siegel and Tassoni (1971*b*) found degeneration in the stria medullaris and the habenulae only after lesions that involved the most caudal aspects of the septal regions and damaged the columns of the fornix. At least in some species, fibers from the septal area to the habenulae are joined by fibers originating in the hippocampus which deviate from the fornix to turn back to the habenulae, although in rat, cat, and monkey these direct hippocampal–habenular fibers are few or nonexistent.

Not all of the fibers in the stria medullaris originating in the septal area terminate in the habenulae. Some course back through the habenular complex to reach the central gray of the tegmentum, and some continue to the superior colliculi. Other fibers from the septal area reach the inferior colliculi by a ventral system which runs through the internal capsule into tegmental regions and then turn up into the brachium of the inferior colliculus. Thus fibers originating in the septal area reach many midbrain and epithalamic areas.

The projections from the hippocampus into the septal area are probably more complicated than the anatomical studies have yet indicated. For example, the work of Freeman and Patel (1968) indicates that when the dorsal hippocampus is electrically stimulated the response in the septal area can be analyzed to reveal six components. This suggests that there may be as many as six different routes by which information can reach the septal area from the hippocampus. This division of the hippocampal–septal area response is based on electrophysiology, but some anatomical substrate of this complex electrophysiological response remains to be understood. Furthermore, very little in the way of an electrophysiological response can be induced in the septal area by stimulation of the ventral hippocampus.

Powell *et al.* (1968) have shown that stimulation of the ventral hippocampus produces evoked responses in the fibers of the diagonal band and in the nucleus accumbens septi, but not in the septal area proper. They suggest that this implies a ventrofugal fiber system originating in the hippocampus which passes along the ventral aspects of the brain, goes through the diagonal band, and terminates in the nucleus accumbens septi. These results are somewhat surprising on the basis of the projections traced by Siegel and Tassoni (1971a) in the cat from the ventral hippocampus to the lateral septal areas.

Powell and Hoelle (1967) also reported fibers of septal origin in the cat going to the superior colliculi over the stria medullaris, but in addition they described a system of fibers which do not go over the stria medullaris, but through peduncular systems to the brachium of the inferior colliculus. These may be a continuation of fibers described by Whitlock and Nauta (1956) which reach the medial geniculate system.

As mentioned before in connection with the hippocampus, there is some dispute over the fiber relations between the hippocampus and the septal area. In the albino rat, Raisman (1966) found that lesions of the medial septal area produced degeneration in the inferior region of the hippocampus. This pattern of terminal degeneration was found in both dorsal and ventral hippocampus. On the other hand, Siegel and Tassoni (1971b) reported that medial septal lesions produces widespread degeneration only through the dorsal and not the ventral hippocampus in the cat. In their study, lesions of the lateral septal area produced degeneration in the ventral hippocampus, whereas Raisman found no projections to the hippocampus from the lateral septal nuclei (Raisman, 1969). In further contrast, Siegel and Tassoni found degeneration from septal lesions spreading out to the subiculum and adjacent cortex while Raisman did not. Electrophysiological evidence of the projection described by Siegel and Tassoni has been demonstrated in the cat (Coyle, 1969). Similar degeneration to that reported by Siegel and Tassoni has been reported in the rabbit (Cragg, 1965). The reasons for the discrepancies between investigators cannot be due to differences among species since Siegel and Edinger (1973) have found the same pattern of projections from the hippocampus to the septal area as described by Siegel and Tassoni in rats, rabbits, and gerbils. One other possible source of variance between the studies could be the staining techniques used. Raisman used the Nauta—Gygax technique, whereas Siegel and Tassoni used the Fink—Heimer modification of the Nauta method. The latter method is thought to have a greater capacity to stain the smaller fibers and terminals.

The Mammillary Bodies, the Anterior Thalamus, and the Cingulate Cortex

Consideration must be given to the mammillary bodies, the anterior nuclei of the thalamus, and the cingulate cortex for historical reasons, since they were given a prominent place in the theories of the limbic system proposed by Papez (1937). Papez considered the limbic system to be the anatomical basis of the emotions. The influences of the limbic system converging on those of the cingulate cortex were thought to be the two major governing systems acting on the hypothalamus. Papez assumed, as has often been the case, that the cerebral cortex had to participate in activities in order for the human or the animal to experience emotional phenomena. He did not, however, believe that the cingulate cortex, or any other part of the neocortex, need be involved in the mechanisms responsible for the behavioral expression of emotion. It is worthwhile to note this distinction which is often found in the literature between mechanisms responsible for the overt expression of internal events and the experience of the internal events. It may be that the distinction is justified, at least in some conditions, but certainly emotions can be influenced by bodily actions. The major output of the mammillary bodies is directed to the anterior thalamic nuclei over the mammillothalamic tract (tract of Vicq-d'Azyr). From there, fibers arise which project to the cingulate cortex via the thalamocortical radiations. Changes in neural activity arising in the cingulate cortex are thought to pass into the areas bordering the hippocampal formation, and into the hippocampus itself. Papez' circuit is completed when changes in neural activity are sent from the hippocampus to the mammillary bodies by way of the fornix.

In such a system, neural activity representing the emotional processes originating in the neocortex would be passed along into the hippocampus, the fornix, the mammillary bodies, and the anterior nuclei of the thalamus and finally be projected onto the receptive region of the "emotional cortex," i.e., the cingulate cortex. From the cingulate cortex, activity representing emotional processes could pass into the other regions of the cerebral cortex and "add emotional coloring to psychic processes occurring elsewhere." Papez considered that emotional experience could arise in one of two ways, either as a result of "psychic activity" (presumably neocortical activity) or as a result of activities originating in the mammillary bodies.

The cingulate cortex borders and lies directly above the corpus callosum on the medial side of the hemispheres. The gyrus cinguli is sometimes called the gyrus fornicatus. In more complicated brains, it is separated from adjacent cortex by the cingulate sulcus. At its posterior extent, it broadens out into a transitional area called "precuneatus" which curves around the splenium of the corpus callosum. This region merges with the hippocampal gyrus. At its anterior end, it merges with the neocortex around the genu of the corpus callosum and continues forward as subgenual cortex. This region is also called the anterior limbic region by some authors. A fiber bundle designated the cingulum bundle courses through the cingulate cortex.

One of the early approaches to the study of the structure of the cingulate cortex involved the use of strychnine neurono-graphy. In this technique, small amounts of strychnine are applied to neural tissue and intermittent epileptiform activity is produced at the site of application and later at more remote sites to which the fibers of the cells in the affected area project. In the monkey, Pribram and MacLean (1953) found that application of strychnine to any part of the cingulate cortex could induce responses in all other areas of the cingulate system. This suggests rich interconnections among all regions of the cingulate cortex. When strychnine was applied to the posterior cingulate regions, evoked activity could be recorded in the pre-cuneate region and in the posterior hippocampal areas as well. The most predominant responses were found in the subicular areas. Strychnine stimulation of the anterior cingulate regions was found to produce activity in the motor cortex and the pre-frontal and orbitofrontal regions (Dunsmore and Lennox, 1950). Projections to the centrum medianum nucleus of the thalamus and reticular formation have also been found using stimulation techniques (French et al., 1955). These studies, taken together, reveal that the cingulate cortex is richly interconnected with many regions of the brain in some species, and that there is a differentiation of the projection systems found within the cin-gulate cortex.

Subdivision of the medial aspects of the rat's hemisphere

are shown in Figure 10. These subdivisions of the cingulate cortex are based on cytoarchitectural differences among the areas, extensively examined and reported by M. Rose (1929). There are pronounced anatomical and physiological differences between the anterior and posterior portions of the medial cortical regions.

Through studies using experimental degeneration techniques, Domesick (1969, 1972) has been able to follow projections from the anterior cingulate areas to the dorsomedial, antero-medial, and to a lesser extent the ventromedial nuclei of the thalamus. Degeneration was not found in these thalamic areas after lesions in the posterior cingulate regions. Posterior cingulate lesions produced degeneration limited to the anteroventral and laterodorsal (lateral) thalamic nuclei. Degeneration could be found in extrathalamic regions after lesions in the anterior and posterior cingulate areas which included the caudate–putamen region, zona incerta, pretectal area, superior colliculus (lower layers), tegmentum, central gray, and the gray matter of the pons. All regions of the cingulate cortex projected to these areas. A similar pattern of degeneration had been found earlier by Showers (1959) using the Marchi method. No degeneration was found in the mammillary bodies, hypothalamus, septal area, or amygdala after any cingulate lesion.

A schematic summarization of the thalamic projections to and from the cingulate cortex found by Domesick (1972) is presented in Figure 10. An important observation made by Domesick was that small lesions which did not invade the cingulum bundle, i.e., those which were restricted to the gray matter of cingulate cortex, failed to produce any degeneration in the presubicular area. An experimental study of the projections of the cingulate cortex to the hippocampal formation without involvement of the cingulum bundle itself is a difficult, but possible, procedure.

It must also be pointed out that Leonard (1969) has reported that the cortex near the midline of the brain in front of the genu of the corpus callosum receives strong projections from the dorsomedial nucleus of the thalamus. Because of its general position in the rat brain, this cortex could be considered to be part of the anterior cingulate system; however, it would not be so considered if cingulate cortex were defined on the basis of projection received from the thalamus. It receives strong

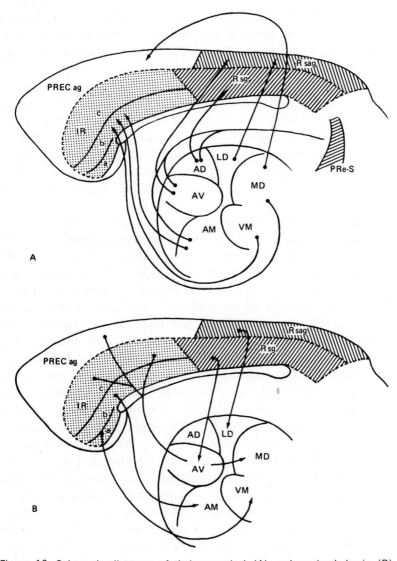

Figure 10. Schematic diagrams of thalamocortical (A) and corticothalamic (B) relations of cingulate cortex of rat. Both area infraradiatae and area retrosplenialis are considered to be cingulate cortex. Relative size of thalamus has been greatly exaggerated relative to cortex. Abbreviations: AD, anterodorsal nucleus of thalamus; AV, anteroventral nucleus of thalamus; AM, anteromedial nucleus of thalamus; LD, laterodorsal nucleus of thalamus; MD, dorsomedial nucleus of thalamus; VM, ventromedial nucleus of thalamus; IR, area infraradiatae; RSg, area retrosplenial granularis; PREC ag, area precentral agranularis; RSag, area retrosplenial agranularis; a, b, and c, subdivisions of area infraradiatae; PRe-S, presubiculum. Drawings based on Domesick (1972).

projections from the dorsomedial nucleus and not from the anterior group. It could be thought of as bearing a similarity to the dorsolateral prefrontal cortex of primates since it receives the dorsomedial projections.

Efferents from the posterior cingulate cortex join the internal capsule and turn in toward the thalamus around the stria terminalis as one component of the lateral thalamic peduncle. Fibers from the anterior regions pierce the cingulum bundle and the corpus callosum to become enclosed in the fiber bundles of the internal capsule which go through the caudate–putamen complex. A few fibers from more caudal cingulate regions join these internal capsule fibers.

The relationship between the cingulate cortex and the cingulum bundle is not easily understood. Domesick (1970) has presented evidence that the cingulum should be considered to be a projection system for thalamic fibers in the rat. In primates, it is likely that the fiber system includes a greater number of fibers contributed from the prefrontal neocortex, and Adey and Meyer (1952) have suggested that there are substantial contributions made to the cingulum bundle from the frontal cortex which terminate in parahippocampal regions. The fiber system described by Domesick leaves the anterior thalamic nuclei, travels forward, and turns to pierce portions of the callosal system. It turns somewhat toward the midline of the brain to become the cingulate fasciculus. This upturning of the thalamocortical fibers occurs at levels anterior to the genu of the corpus callosum. This cingulate bundle sends off fibers along its course, especially into the medial (cingulate) cortex and into the presubicular cortex. In the rat, few, if any, fibers join the cingulum bundle from other cortical areas. As mentioned above, there is evidence that the cingulum bundle does accept fibers from other regions in some species. For example, fibers from the amygdala have been shown to join the cingulum at the pregenual level in the cat and monkey (Lammers and Lohman, 1957; Nauta, 1961). Fuxe et al. (1968) have also found evidence based on the fluorescence of catecholamines that some fibers join the cingulum which have their cells of origin in the brain stem.

The failure to find degeneration in the hypothalamus, septal area, and amygdala after lesions of the cingulate cortex makes it unique among structures of the limbic system. All of the other structures of the limbic system have strong projections to at least one other limbic region and the hypothalamus. The main anatomical basis for the inclusion of the cingulate cortex in the limbic system seems to be its indirect association with the mammillary bodies.

The mammillary bodies are round protuberances found on the ventral surface of the brain. They are often considered to mark the posterior limits of the hypothalamus. In general, the mammillary bodies are divided into two main nuclei: a large medial mammillary nucleus and a small lateral mammillary nucleus. The medial nucleus is in turn divided into two subregions: a large-celled medial portion and a small-celled lateral, or basal, portion. Different authors have made other subdivisions of the lateral nucleus (see Crosby *et al.*, 1962).

The main efferent fibers from the mammillary nuclei are fibers which extend dorsally and at some distance above the mammillary bodies, dividing into a mammillothalamic tract and a mammillotegmental tract. It is uncertain whether or not this division is produced by a bifurcation of axons such that one branch of the axon reaches toward the anterior nucleus of the thalamus and the other toward the tegmentum or whether the axons running in each direction have independent cells of origin. The mammillotegmental portion of the fibers reaches to the dorsal tegmental nucleus. Destruction of the mammillary body produces degeneration in both the dorsal and the ventral tegmental nuclei. It is thought that the degeneration in the ventral tegmental nucleus is produced by degeneration of terminals whose axons arrive over the mammillary peduncle. The mammillopeduncular tract is a small bundle of fibers which runs from the medial mammillary nucleus, and also from the interpeduncular nucleus, to end in the ventral tegmental nucleus.

Limbic System–Midbrain Relations

The limbic system has connections with the midbrain through at least three routes. These are the (1) tractus retroflexus (the habenulointerpeduncular tract), (2) the mammillotegmental tract, and (3) the medial forebrain bundle. These fiber systems distribute into two general areas of the midbrain. One area consists of the central and lateral midbrain regions which receive substantial input from the lateral hypothalamus and from the lateral nucleus of the habenulae. This area of the brain stem system is thought to be an important mechanism for the control of the brain stem recticular formation. A second area is the ventrotegmental areas of Tsai and the interpeduncular nucleus. Fibers from this region and those passing through it turn up to reach the central gray. The neural systems involved with the central gray are of interest since they distribute to such a wide range of areas in the midbrain. Fibers from the central gray fan out in a radial fashion from this area in all directions. It is likely that this most medial system of the neural axis affected by the limbic system exerts profound and continued influences on all of the mechanisms of the brain stem, both those with specific and those with diffuse responsibilities.

The neural chemistry of the medial forebrain bundle is of particular interest to students of the limbic system. It is now clear that the medial forebrain bundle contains fibers transporting norepinephrine and serotonin from cells of the midbrain which reach the entire forebrain. Furthermore, these fibers or other noncatecholaminergic fibers provide essential support for the maintenance of catecholamines in the forebrain. Lesions in the medial forebrain bundle produce a drop of 90 %, or more, of these important neurochemicals throughout the entire forebrain, even though the fibers in the medial forebrain bundle do not directly terminate in many of the areas in which the depletion is found. This has suggested to Heller (1972) that the polysynaptic systems of the medial forebrain bundle govern the synthesis of at least some forms of neurotransmitters in the forebrain. Apparently they do not act only as a transport system for catecholamines from the brain stem. The maximal decline in norepinephrine found after lesions of the medial forebrain bundle may require as much as 12 days. In contrast, there is a rapid decrease in the amount of dopamine found in the caudate nucleus after lesions of the nigrostriatal pathways. Heller concludes that these pathways do act as a transport system for dopamine to the caudate nucleus but that the medial forebrain bundle acts in a different way: by controlling the synthesis of the neurochemicals in the forebrain itself.

From the information which has been presented, some idea of

the enormous complexities of the structures of the limbic system should now be apparent, as well as the system's ability to regulate neural and neurochemical activities throughout the brain. Each of the limbic system structures is made up of many different components with many pathways interconnecting one region with another, but all have a close relationship with the hypothalamus. Accordingly, the limbic system seems best defined in terms of its connections with the hypothalamus. In subsequent chapters, the various components of the limbic system will be discussed separately, in terms of their functional contributions to behavior.

Chapter 2
THE HYPOTHALAMUS

Neural systems of the hypothalamus influence many types of behavior, but the most frequently studied behaviors are those closely related to physiological functions, e.g., food and water ingestion and sex behavior. This is because many areas in the hypothalamus are involved in the regulation of the thermal, hormonal, osmotic, and nutritional balances of the body, and cells in this area are responsive to information arising in the internal and external environment. Beyond this, however, the hypothalamus is also involved in the regulation of somatic activities and the level of arousal in other forebrain regions of the brain.

However, the limbic system's influences on behavior extend far beyond those actions directed toward the maintenance of particular physiological conditions or balances. They involve many subtle aspects of learning, memory, motivation, and performance. They include effects which may be described in terms of cognitive acts, strategies, and hypotheses. Because of the intimate relationships of the septal area, amygdala, hippocampus, and cingulate cortex with the hypothalamus, it may serve us well to begin our study with this area, where all of the limbic structures' influences converge. This assumes that the hypothalamus may be the key to understanding the limbic system just as the dorsal thalamus may be the key to understanding the neocortex.

Because of my view that it is important to break with traditional ways of looking at the hypothalamus only as a regulator of physiological systems, I will begin with a landmark in research on brain functions which also helped change prominent theories of behavior: the discovery of pleasure centers in the brain.

Pleasurable Reactions

In 1953, Drs. James Olds and Peter Milner began a whole new approach to the analysis of brain activities as related to behavior with their discovery of rewarding effects produced by electrical stimulation of the brain. I have heard that at the time of their discovery Olds and Milner were attempting to determine the behavioral effects of electrical stimulation of "arousal systems." While testing their animals in a tabletop enclosure, they noticed that the animals seemed to be attracted to the corner of the enclosure in which they had received the stimulation. The animals seemed to "like" this area. This led Olds and Milner to give the animals an opportunity to make responses which would produce their own brain stimulation. Simply enough, they arranged a situation whereby the animals could depress a lever in an operant chamber. Pressing the lever activated control devices which sent small amounts of electrical current between the electrodes implanted deep in the animals' brain, exciting nearby tissues. The report of this experiment is now a milestone in the history of brain—behavior research (Olds and Milner, 1954).

This experiment was a turning point in the theoretical analysis of brain—behavior relationships. Until the time of the Olds and Milner experiment, the analysis of the brain's effects on behavior was dominated by "behavioristic" approaches. These included those developed and made popular in the world of experimental psychology by Clark Hull, Kenneth Spence, and B. F. Skinner, and their associates. These theories were based on the assumption that behavior could be explained by the development of rules describing the relationship between the stimuli affecting the organism, the responses made by the individual, and the conditions under which rewards were obtained. Behavior was to be explained on the basis of measurable events: stimuli, responses, and rewards. The theories were barren of any reference to the individual or his plans, experiences, or beliefs.

The discovery of brain regions which, when electrically stimulated, seemed to produce rewarding effects began an era of greater freedom in the scientific description of behavior. It did so because the behavior of the animals seemed most easily explained on the basis that the animals would perform responses of several different kinds to obtain electrical stimulation in certain brain regions. The goal of their efforts was most easily described in terms of obtaining a pleasurable experience. Thus the experiences of the organism had to become a factor in describing or explaining behavior. Pleasure and pain became accepted as legitimate terms, once again, for scientists trying to discover the neural bases of behavior. In short, the results of Olds and Milner helped break down the strong theoretical fortress of artificial concepts developed by learning theorists. Their results justified explanations of experimental data in hedonistic terms.

The debilitating effects of the behavioristic S-R theoretical structure on experimental studies of the brain and behavior can hardly be overestimated. In the 1930s, 1940s, and 1950s, the results of behavioral research were difficult if not impossible to publish if they failed to use the popular behavioristic techniques or failed to describe the results in terms of approved jargon. Words such as *cognition, reasoning, emotion*, and *hypotheses* were taboo. In my opinion, the report of Olds and Milner was the turning point in this historical trend, although others had recognized the intellectual poverty of such theories before.

At first, the report of Olds and Milner, as well as subsequent publications, dealing with self-stimulation phenomena was criticized as being "nonbehavioristic." Critics argued that better explanations of the behavior could be found within the S-R framework and that "feelings" of "affective experiences" need not be attributed to the animals whose brains were being stimulated. Nevertheless, as experiment mounted on experiment, it became evident that the most useful way to describe the behavioral effects of the brain stimulation was indeed in terms of the elicitation of positively rewarding, or pleasant, experiences. Reports from people whose brains had been stimulated in the reward regions have indicated that the experience obtained is, in fact, pleasant (Bishop et al., 1963).

The change of orientation of scientists in the brain—behavior area should not be interpreted as an overthrow of a strict scientific methodology for a looser and less demanding one. It was an overthrow of a theoretical structure which was too narrow and imposed too many constraints on the ideas which could be investigated. It is always important to be able to define precisely what is done in an experiment and to have theories in which the variables manipulated can be defined and understood by others. The fact is that as yet we do not have truly satisfactory theories of brain functions or of behavior, but progress toward better theories should not be inhibited by the dogmatic acceptance of inadequate ones.

The Location of Pleasure Regions

Olds and Milner first discovered rewarding or pleasant effects by stimulation of the septal area. But further investigations soon found sites in many areas of the brain which produced positively rewarding effects when electrically stimulated. These include some parts of all of the structures of the limbic system and some of the surrounding transitional cortical areas. Some of the regions which produce positively rewarding effects when stimulated are now well established. These include the lateral septal area, certain portions of the amygdala, some parts of the hippocampus, and the medial forebrain bundle and lateral hypothalamus.

In general summary, it can be said that the most "rewarding" regions of the brain are found along the base of the brain in the general region of the lateral hypothalamus and medial forebrain bundle (Olds and Olds, 1963). Perhaps the purest form of pleasurable effects is produced by electrical stimulation at posterior reaches of the hypothalamus, just ahead of the mammillary bodies. However, it is doubtful that the medial forebrain bundle is the only neural system involved, since lesions of the lateral hypothalamus do not disturb self-stimulation elicited from all forebrain electrode placements (e.g., Valenstein and Campbell, 1966). Boyd and Gardner (1967) have suggested that there are multiple hypothalamic pathways involved in the mediation of rewarding effects and that lesions in any one of them would produce a reduction in, but not a total abolition of, self-stimulation effects.

Early investigators of the effects of electrical brain stimulation concerned themselves with the regions stimulated, the electrical parameters of the stimulation, and the nature of the behavior which was elicited by the brain stimulation. Each of these represents an area of research unto itself. In regard to the electrical parameters of the stimulation, many types of pulses and pulse trains have been applied to the brain with rewarding effects. Some of the simplest systems for producing brain stimulation work quite well. For example, stimulating the brain with ordinary 60-cycle AC current with the appropriately reduced amperage to nondamaging levels often is more successful than the use of fancy biphasic square-wave stimulators. The significance is that self-stimulation behavior is easily obtained if the electrodes are correctly positioned in the brain and is not dependent on the use of specific parameters of stimulation.

Pain and Punishment

About the time that Olds and Milner were discovering that rewarding effects could be produced by electrical stimulation of the brain, Delgado et al., (1954) were finding behavioral effects produced by brain stimulation which indicated that an aversive or painful state had been produced. Hungry animals were shown to avoid food associated with stimulation, but, more important, the stimulation could serve to motivate the learning of an avoidance task. In this way, the stimulation was comparable to the effects of noxious electrical stimulation applied to the periphery of the body. It became reasonable, therefore, to consider these stimulation effects as aversive to the animal.

An interesting result stemming from brain stimulation studies is that animals will work both to turn on the electrical stimulation of the brain and to turn it off if it is left on long enough (Bower and

Miller, 1958; Roberts, 1958). This sort of result has been found in most of the brain regions which have been studied. The most positively reinforcing zones, namely the posterior aspects of the lateral hypothalamus, seem to be ones in which the animal will accept prolonged periods of stimulation without acting to turn it off. But for most other areas the animal seems to prefer limited amounts of electrical stimulation. These observations led to the notion that electrical stimulation of certain brain regions can activate both a postively rewarding "pleasure system" and a negatively rewarding "punishment" system. In those instances where an animal will act both to turn on brain stimulation and to turn it off, it might be assumed that the positively motivating system is activated first by the electrical stimulation but that when it continues the punishment system becomes activated. As this happens, the rewarding effects become antagonized by the activation of the punishment system. In fact, the balance must be changed in favor of the aversive system since the animal turns it off.

There are a host of assumptions which must be made in this type of explanation. These include assumptions pertinent to differential thresholds for cells (or fibers) activated by the electrical stimulation in the positively and negatively rewarding system, habituation of the positive system, or recruitment in the negative system. It does seem clear, however, that electrical stimulation often has a mixed character, having both positive and negative qualities. Furthermore, these opposite qualities can interact with each other, stimulation in a predominantly positive area reducing effects mediated by the negative systems and vice versa. Rewarding brain stimulation can mask the effects of peripheral pain in man (Heath and Mickle, 1960) and animals (Cox and Valenstein, 1965), as well as attentuate the effects of stimulation of aversive regions (Routtenberg and Olds, 1963). Stimulation of aversive regions can attenuate the behavioral effects produced by stimulation of reward areas (Olds and Olds, 1962).

It might well be asked if any brain stimulation which influences behavior has some positive or negative affective quality. At least for their work with tegmental sites, Olds and Peretz (1960) have suggested that there can be three types of systems of effects produced by electrical stimulation. Two of these are related to the affective reactions of the organism: the positively and negatively rewarding systems. The third system is one which produces changes in arousal. Certain portions of the tegmentum produce both behavioral and electrical signs of arousal when stimulated. This stimulation is without affective tone since the animals do not act to turn it on or off. Thus there may be systems which modulate the arousal of the animal without necessarily producing pleasure or pain. It is likely that stimulation of most regions of the brain produces some combinations of activity of the affective and the arousal systems.

The Location of Pain Regions

The midbrain central gray and periventricular regions, the region of the medial lemniscus in the midbrain, and the ventromedial nucleus of the hypothalamus all seem to produce the strong aversive reactions (Delgado et al., 1954).

The midbrain regions which produce aversive effects when stimulated can be rather clearly defined, but this definition is greatly reduced in the diencephalon. Some painlike effects have been produced by stimulation of nuclei of the thalamus but less frequently in the hypothalamus. Responses resembling those indicative of fear have been reported from the ventral aspects of the posterior nucleus and from the zona incerta (Roberts, 1962). Stimulation of the ventromedial nucleus has produced rage (Roberts, 1958) and has also produced escape reactions (Olds, 1960). However, the conclusion commonly reached is that stimulation of almost any region of the hypothalamus produces mixed, ambivalent effects (Olds and Olds, 1963).

Ball (1972) has found that self-stimulation can be produced by stimulation of the ventromedial nucleus if the animals are tested with high current levels over several days. After several days of testing at high current levels, the animals begin to show stable self-stimulation behavior at much lower current levels. At this time, the response rates of the animals become comparable to those of animals having electrodes implanted into lateral hypothalamic regions. These results make the association of the ventromedial nucleus with a forward extension of a punishment system subject to question.

Various nuclei of the medial thalamus have been implicated with the forebrain projections of aversive systems (Casey, 1966).

Recently, it has been found that electrical stimulation of the medial forebrain bundle in the lateral hypothalamus and of the midbrain reticular formation produce opposing effects on the discharge of single units in at least two medial thalamic nuclei (Keene, 1973; Keene and Casey, 1973). These nuclei are the dorsomedial and the paracentral. Since the medial forebrain bundle stimulation is generally considered to be rewarding and the reticular formation stimulation to be aversive, these opposing effects may be an important clue as to the brain regions which monitor the relative activity in opposing hedonic systems.

The relationship of the hypothalamus to aversive systems cannot be considered in terms of a simple dichotomy of affective mechanisms existing independently of other neural systems. Hoebel and Thompson (1969) have shown, for example, that escape reactions and self-stimulation rates produced by lateral hypothalamic stimulation are influenced by the animal's weight. If an animal is made overweight by forced feeding, its escape reactions to brain stimulation increase and its self-stimulation rates decrease. It is as if making an animal overweight reduces the rewarding aspects of lateral hypothalamic stimulation and enhances the negative aspects.

These observations point out that the effects of brain stimulation must be considered in terms of the internal environment of the animal. But the external environment and the animal's past experiences also play determining roles. For example, in one experiment cats with electrodes implanted into the diencephalon were trained to make a response which caused a door to open between two compartments. One compartment was "dangerous" since the animal received electrical footshocks in it. The other was "safe" since the animal was never punished in it. After the response which opened the door between the compartments and allowed the cats to gain access to the "safe" compartment was well established, they were given identical electrical brain stimulation in both compartments. Stimulation applied to the animal while it was in the dangerous location produced the learned response which opened the door leading to safety. The same stimulation applied in the safe compartment made the animal relax and go to sleep. This is the "dual effect" of brain stimulation described by Grastyán (see Grastyán, 1968).

Elicited Behaviors

Electrical brain stimulation can produce very specific behavioral acts which occur at the time the brain is being stimulated. When a behavior is reliably elicited by electrical brain stimulation it is called "stimulus bound" or "elicited."

Elicited behaviors are typically measured in open situations where the animals can roam freely. What happens when the brain of an animal is stimulated at a rewarding site in this open situation in which many kinds of responses can be made? One of the most common elicited behaviors is simply a general increase in exploration and orienting movements. Frequently, however, elicited behaviors are more specific. They could be licking from a water bottle, eating a food pellet, gnawing on a block of wood, drinking water from a dish, or a sexual or aggressive act. Often these behaviors will be produced by electrical stimulation at intensities too low to obtain positively rewarding effects.[*] Elicited behaviors are not the consequences of an activation of a motivational system. To be sure, eating and drinking can be reliably produced by electrical stimulation in hypothalamic areas. Nevertheless, these behavioral acts are not actions directed toward the alleviation of induced motives for food or water. They seem to be patterns of behavior which are elicited without regard to the satisfaction of particular motives.

Important behavioral sequences which frequently occur must be organized at the midbrain, brain stem, or spinal cord levels, since no known lesion of any nucleus or tract rostral to these regions alters these acts to any appreciable degree. The contribution of the hypothalamus, and other forebrain areas, is to modify and regulate the expression of these organized behavioral sequences. The term "command area" can be used to describe brain stem and spinal cord systems responsible for organized acts such as eating, gnawing, licking, lapping, sexual acts, aggression, and many other types of unlearned behaviors.

---

[*] The entire volume 2, issue number 4 (1969) of *Brain, Behavior and Evolution* is recommended to the reader. It contains theoretical reviews by Valenstein, Cox, and Valenstein, by Roberts, and by Caggiula.

These command areas are fully organized neural systems which are capable of coordinating the many subcomponents of behavioral acts, taking into consideration the sensory feedback arising from each of the subcomponents. The subcomponents are woven into the fabric of a complete behavior sequence. The job of understanding behavior must include the question of the neural mechanisms of the forebrain selectively facilitating or inhibiting the many different command areas at different times.

In this light, stimulation of the hypothalamus can be considered to activate selectively a command area governing the expression of one behavioral sequence when an elicited behavior is produced. Influences from other forebrain regions are funneled into the midbrain and brain stem through fibers of the medial forebrain bundle. As a result, it would be expected that, from time to time, electrodes in the hypothalamus would be in the immediate vicinity of nuclei or fiber tracts which exert a special influence on one or another "command area." With this perspective, the phenomena of electrically elicited behaviors are not surprising. Probably it is more surprising that electrical stimulation of the hypothalamus or the medial forebrain bundle sometimes fails to elicit some behavioral act.

Changes in Elicited Behaviors

If an electrode is placed into a hypothalamic region which, when stimulated, reliably produces a particular behavior, it might be thought that electrical stimulation of this region would continue to produce this response for evermore. However, this is not the case. For example, if the elicited response is licking water from a drinking tube, the question can be asked, "What would happen if the electrical stimulation were applied when a drinking tube was no longer in the animal's environment?" A theory based on the facilitation of a command center for licking might predict that a licking response would be made to any object available. A motivational theory which considers the elicited behavior to indicate the induction of thirst would predict that the animal would engage in some other form of behavior directed toward the incorporation of fluids. In fact, however, the removal of the drinking tube eliminates the licking response during periods of electrical stimulation but fails to elicit other forms of water-oriented behavior, such as lapping water from a dish. Therefore, the behavior produced by the electrical stimulation of the brain is dependent on the available objects in the environment but cannot be explained by the induction of particular physiological motives.

If an animal has been stimulated in an environment containing many types of objects, and has demonstrated a particular elicited behavior, then the removal of the object supporting this behavior causes a disruption of the elicited behavior. The behavior is specifically tied to a specific environmental support object. Even though no other behavior immediately becomes prominent when the environmental support object is removed, the animal can develop a new behavior correlated with the electrical stimulation and directed toward a different support object. This new elicited behavior is often quite different from the one made formerly. The change in elicited behaviors can be produced by stimulating the animal over a prolonged period of time while it is in the presence of other objects. For many animals, at least, a new behavior will emerge which cannot be predicted from the original elicited behavior. This means that an animal originally drinking from a drinking tube when electrically stimulated might start gnawing wood or eating food just as readily as lapping from a water dish after a prolonged bout of stimulation without the drinking tube available. If the original environmental support object is replaced in the animal's environment, the animal does not give up the new behavior sequence it has developed in place of the initial elicited behavior. The electrical stimulation of the brain without the preferred support object has changed the animal. It has a new and relatively permanent behavior associated with the brain stimulation.

These results overthrow one possible explanation which would have provided a relatively simple account of the change in elicited behaviors. It might have been that the electrode was in a region which facilitated one command zone (drinking from the tube) more than it facilitated another behavior command system (gnawing on a block of wood). The total amount of facilitation of a behavior command zone would be the summation of (1) the effect produced by the hypothalamic stimulation and (2) the facilitation derived from the presence of appropriate environmental support objects. In this type of explanation, the absence of the environmental support object for the initial behavioral sequence (licking drinking tube) reduced the total amount of facilitation of its command zone below a threshold amount. Prolonged electrical stimulation might have increased facilitation for the second (gnawing on wood) system to a position of dominance. Accordingly, the replacement of the environmental support object for the first elicited behavior should have immediately reinstated the primary behavior. But this does not happen. This indicates that a more or less permanent reorganization has occurred in the central nervous system which is reflected in the maintenance of the new elicited behavior.

Valenstein now believes that these behavioral phenomena might be based on the activation of the "reward system" in conjunction with a specific behavioral act. This could produce a "stamping in" of the behavior occurring at the time of the electrical brain stimulation. The changing from one elicited behavior to another would reflect a modification in the neural apparatus of the brain such that a new behavioral disposition related to available environmental support objects has become maximally facilitated by the electrical brain stimulation. The behavioral disposition has been called the "prepotent" behavioral tendency of the animal (Valenstein, 1969).

The hypothesis that the behavior elicited by hypothalamic stimulation is a result of a "prepotent" or dominant behavioral tendency is attractive, yet presents certain difficulties. According to this theory, if each of two pairs of electrodes were placed into a behavior-facilitating system, the same "dominant behavior" should be elicited through both pairs of electrodes. Valenstein et al. (1969) have found that electrical stimulation of the lateral hypothalamus through different pairs of electrodes does not always elicit the same response. For example, a specific elicited behavior is often produced at one electrode site while general exploratory activities are elicited at the other (Cox and Valenstein, 1969). In some cases, it is possible to change the behavior elicited from one site so that it is similar to that produced at the other location. Gallistel (1969) found that when a posterior hypothalamic electrode elicited sexual behavior and a lateral hypothalamic electrode elicited eating, later retesting indicated that both behaviors could be elicited from each placement.

It is not possible to establish a stimulus-bound behavior simply by pairing electrical stimulation of the brain with the spontaneous occurrence of a behavioral response or by stimulating the animal while it is under the influence of a particular biological motive. Valenstein and Cox (1970) found that stimulating the hypothalamus while the animal was eating did not establish elicited feeding. Repeated pairings of a behavior and the electrical stimulation are of help only when the electrical stimulation *was* able to elicit the response in the first place.

It must be remembered that electrical stimulation of the hypothalamus does more than elicit specific behaviors. It also changes an animal's reactions to sensory stimulation. For example, Flynn (1967) has carefully noted changes in a cat's responsiveness to stimulation applied around its face when the hypothalamus is stimulated. He considers the stimulation to both potentiate the sensory reactions and increase the effectiveness of the stimulation in initiating responses related to eating and aggression. The potentiation of responses can be quite specific. Certain points in the hypothalamus of a cat will elicit attacks on the experimenter but not on a rat. Stimulation at other hypothalamic points will lead to attacks on a rat but not on the experimenter. Nevertheless, these different responses could be caused by effects produced in the animal which are not as specific as might at first appear. The extent to which the animal is afraid might help determine whether or not attack would be directed toward a large (experimenter) or a small (rat) stimulus. In addition, it is difficult to determine the relative contribution of response and sensory contributions to an observed behavioral act. Does the exaggerated tendency to respond to a stimulus applied to the cat's muzzle indicate a facilitation of the sensory input, the effectiveness of the input in directing behavior, or the response mechanisms involved? These questions are difficult to unravel experimentally.

Self-Stimulation, Arousal, and Elicited Behaviors

Since animals will press levers or perform other acts to obtain electrical stimulation of the hypothalamus, they can be said to be "motivated" by the brain stimulation. Since brain stimulation can be used as a reward for learning or performance in many types of situations, it must also have reinforcing properties. Therefore, electrical stimulation of the hypothalamus has both reinforcing and motivating qualities. The question arises as to whether or not these components can be separated anatomically or physiological-ly. The distinction between the motivational and rewarding prop-erties of brain stimulation has been emphasized by several authors (e.g., Deutsch and Howarth, 1963; Gallistel, 1964).

Huston (1971) has reported studies in which he measured the amounts of electrical stimulation needed to affect three types of "motivation-sensitive" behaviors: (1) the production of stimulus-bound eating, drinking, or copulating, (2) the facil-itation of operant response rate on a fixed-ratio schedule, and (3) the "release" of a previous extinguished response. Then he compared the current levels required to obtain these behaviors with the current required to support self-stimulation at the same electrode sites. The thresholds for all three types of "motivation-sensitive" behaviors were well below the threshold for self-stimulation. This could be interpreted to mean that self-stimulation effects depend on the activation of a high-threshold reward system which is independent of the lower-threshold motivation-sensitive systems.

Rolls (1971) has pointed out that two fairly clear patterns of behavior are observed associated with self-stimulation in different brain regions. The behavioral syndrome produced by medial forebrain bundle—lateral hypothalamic stimulation includes hyper-activity, a high rate of responding in an operant situation, a lack of habituation to the stimulation, and sometimes the production of elicited behaviors. This pattern is similar to that described by Huston for his "motivation-sensitive" effects. Self-stimulation induced in other brain regions, including some limbic locations, is associated with reduced activity, low rates of operant response, rapid habituation of response rate, and sometimes poststimulus "rebound behaviors" (see Milgram, 1969). These results suggest the possibility of two (or more) reward systems in the brain.

In a further extension of this line of thinking, Rolls studied the effects of rewarding brain stimulation on activities of single neurons in the brain stem. For his rewarding effects, he used electrodes in the medial forebrain bundle and in the nucleus accumbens septi. Stimulation at both locations produced good self-stimulation behavior but affected brain stem units quite differently. The nucleus accumbens septi stimulation affected only a few cells in the brain stem, while stimulation of the medial forebrain bundle affected a large number. Stimulation at the two sites could also be differentiated on the basis of the changes produced in the electrical activities of the neocortex. Stimulation of the medial forebrain bundle produced an arousal response in the cortex, while stimulation of the nucleus accumbens did not. The electrical effects produced in the neocortex by the stimulation of the medial forebrain bundle lasted beyond the actual period of stimulation. Some behavioral effects do, also. For example, the act of running in a linear runway to obtain electrical brain stimulation must be "primed" by stimulation given in the start box before every trial (Gallistel, 1969), but priming of a behavior rewarded by electrical brain stimulation does not require the use of the electrical stimulation of the *brain*. Peripheral electrical stimulation of the animal's feet will also work (MacDougall and Bevan, 1968). This suggests that stimulation of the medial forebrain bundle could produce rewarding effects by facilitation of one neural system and produce increased behavioral activation by facilitation of a different system. In fact, Rolls and Kelly (1972) suggest that the hypothalamic stimulation could antidromically excite cells in the brain stem whose collaterals reach other cells in the same area. The brain stem cells affected in this secondary fashion could be responsible for the activation and arousal produced by the hypothalamic stimulation. On the other hand, Keene and Casey (1970) have shown that electrical stimulation of the lateral hypothalamus produces orthodromic excitatory effects on neurons in the brain stem reticular formation which are also influenced by noxious peripheral stimulation.

From these studies, it is clear that stimulation of the lateral hypothalamus produces at least three quite distinctive effects: (1) specific behavioral acts, (2) the activation of behavior, reflected in several ways, including increases in the rates of responding and the release of previously extinguished behaviors, and (3) rewarding effects. A dissociation between general arousal and rewarding effects is emphasized by the fact that self-stimulation can be obtained by stimulation in regions which, when stimulated, produce few, if any, signs of behavioral or electrographic arousal. Changes in performance occurring as a consequence of limbic or hypothalamic stimulation or lesions could be due to effects produced on either the arousal or the reward systems but must always be considered in the context of the animal's internal and external environment.

Relations with the Autonomic Nervous System

For many years, the anterior hypothalamic regions have been associated with parasympathetic activities in the autonomic nervous system and the posterior regions associated with sympathetic activities. This generalization comes from observations by many investigators of the effects produced by stimulation of hypothalamic sites. Like many generalizations, however, it is inaccurate in several ways. The simple dichotomous breakdown into anterior and posterior regions is misleading, since these regions are well organized into different nuclear groups. The dichotomy tends to neglect the importance of finer anatomical divisions. Hess (1949) has pointed out another difficulty. This is that stimulation of the hypothalamus always elicits both autonomic and somatic changes. Therefore, he proposed the terms "trophotropic" and "ergotropic" to describe the effects of stimulation of the anterior and posterior hypothalamus, respectively. "Trophotropic" effects would include parasympathetic activities but in addition the correlated activities of the somatic musculature associated with the conservation of bodily energies and with activities of the internal organs related to digestion and elimination. The term "ergotropic" was used to include reactions of both smooth and striate muscles directed toward the mobilization and expenditure of the body's resources.

The terms "trophotropic" and "ergotropic" extend our horizons. They emphasize that the effects produced by hypothalamic stimulation extend beyond the autonomic nervous system and even beyond the somatic nervous system. Trophotrophic reactions include changes in the electrical activity found in the neocortex which indicate decreased arousal. Ergotropic reactions include the desynchronization of the electrical activity of the cortex. Speculations about the role of the ergotropic and trophotropic systems in behavior have been advanced before by Gellhorn (e.g., Gellhorn, 1970).

   The ergotropic reactions mediated by the hypothalamus may play an important role in activating and maintaining behavioral sequences. Such a role would be comparable to the "motivational effects" produced by hypothalamic stimulation described above. It seems likely that some "critical amount" of activation of hypothalamic arousal systems is essential both to the "initiation" and the "maintenance" of all behavioral acts. Furthermore, it might be hypothesized that the stronger the ergotropic system activity, the more energetic and quicker will be the response. I have suggested that an ergotropic balance activity may be essential to the continuation of behavioral episodes and that the hippocampus provides one means of adjusting this balance (Isaacson, 1972a). I think now that the term "ergotropic" is not quite the best term since it has been so closely associated with posterior regions of the hypothalamus. The energizing systems could well be associated with the medial forebrain bundle, which extends well beyond the posterior hypothalamus.

   Usually the ergotropic and trophotropic systems cooperate to maintain a balance between the two systems appropriate to the environmental circumstances. Normally, the greater the activity in one, the less activity there will be in the other, since the two stand in a mutually inhibitory relationship. However, this balance can be upset so that great amounts of activity can occur in both systems at the same time. This simultaneous activation of the two systems is found during convulsions.

   While the terms "ergotropic" and "trophotropic" suggest unitary anatomical or functional systems, this need not be the case. It may well be that each "system" is really a collection of specific neural subsystems which share the potential of increasing or decreasing arousal. These separate neural systems could be those involved with the regulation of specific behaviors related to aggressive, sexual, feeding, drinking, or other goal-oriented behaviors. Each of these systems could act to provide degrees of somatic and automonic activation appropriate to its own actions.

Lesions of the Lateral Hypothalamus

   Lesions of the lateral hypothalamus produce aphagia and adipsia (Teitelbaum and Epstein, 1962). Animals with such lesions will die unless they are tube-fed after the operation. If this is done, however, the animals can, over time, come to begin to eat food and ultimately to drink water. The animals begin to eat food usually before they begin to drink water spontaneously. Teitelbaum and Epstein described four stages in the recovery of animals with lesions of the lateral hypothalamus. These recovery stages can be described as follows: In stage 1, the animals will eat some wet and palatable food. In stage 2, the animals will spontaneously regulate their food intake and body weight on the wet and palatable foods. (In stage 1, the animals will not eat enough to provide themselves with their necessary metabolic requirements.) In stage 3, the animal will eat dry food provided that they have an appropriate water balance. The animals have to be hydrated artificially by stomach tubes in order to eat dry foods and maintain themselves in a reasonable nutritional state. In stage 4, the animals will drink water spontaneously and will survive on a dry food diet. Teitelbaum et al. (1969) have suggested that the recovery process which occurs after lateral hypothalamic lesions represents a behavioral recapitulation of the mechanisms responsible for the development of regulated food intake after birth.

Recovery is never really complete. For example, even in stage 4 the animals drink water only after eating. The animals seem to be wetting their mouths in order to eat the dry food. In addition, these animals are always finicky about their food. They reject food which has already been adulterated with an unpleasant substance more readily than normal animals do. Animals which have recovered from the lateral hypothalamic damage do not reach the same body weights as normal animals despite normal levels of food intake.

Powley and Keesey (1970) have pointed out that the aphasic and adipsic condition following lateral hypothalamic lesions can be greatly reduced if the subjects are starved before the lesions are made. In some cases, prelesion starvation can even prevent the usual aphagia and adipsia. Some animals actually overeat after the lesion. Powley and Keesey suggest that the effect of the lateral hypothalamic lesion is to reset bodily mechanisms for a new ideal "target weight" (probably reflected in the amount of fat in the adipose tissues) which is less than that of normal animals. The effect of a ventromedial hypothalamic lesion could be to establish a new target weight which is higher than that of normal animals.

Therefore, the aphagia or hyperphagia which follows hypothalamic destruction could be explained as attempts of the animals to reach their new target weights. Animals made overweight before ventromedial lesions show only slight overeating afterward (Hoebel and Teitelbaum, 1966).

When animals are fed intragastrically after the lateral hypothalamic lesions are made, they are usually maintained at something approximating their preoperative weight levels. According to the Powley and Keesey position, keeping the body weights elevated by artificial means just postpones the inevitable. It is worth noting that their theorized "recovery" does not occur after the hypothalamic lesions. After the lesions, the animals merely start to eat, or do not eat, to attain their "ideal" weights. Furthermore, if lesions of the lateral hypothalamus result in the setting of a lower target weight and lesions of the ventromedial hypothalamus result in the setting of a higher target weight, then it might be possible for lesions in each to offset each other, at least to some extent. Preliminary data from Keesey's laboratory tend to support this possibility (Keesey, personal communication).

The feeding systems of the brain have been associated with neural systems using adrenergic transmitters (see Grossman, 1960; Slangen and Miller, 1969; Leibowitz, 1970). It is perhaps not too surprising, therefore, that the injection of norepinephrine into the ventricles can restore the drinking of milk in aphagic and adipsic animals with lateral hypothalamic damage (Berger et al., 1971). At least this occurred if the animals had progressed beyond recovery stage 1. These data suggest (a) that the effects of the lesions are related to alterations in noradrenergic systems and (b) that the mechanisms underlying feeding still exist after lateral hypothalamic damage, although they are inactive unless stimulated by the norepinephrine. If "recovery" does occur, it is not a restoration of neural connections essential for normal feeding but rather a restoration of facilitatory influences on intact neural systems.

Furthermore, there is evidence suggesting that abnormal catecholaminergic reactions occurring near the site of the lesion play an important role in the development of the lateral hypothalamic syndrome. When an inhibitor of catecholamine synthesis, α-methyl-p-tyrosine, was given to animals near the time at which the lateral hypothalamic lesion was made, the animals failed to exhibit the syndrome (Glick *et al.*, 1972). The same kinds of effects have been found in the study of paralysis resulting from compression of the cat spinal cord. Suppression of the localized release of norepinephrine by treatment with the same drug produced much greater recovery of motor activities than would otherwise have occurred (Osterholm and Mathews, 1972). From the study of the cat spinal cord, it is clear that the extent of the motor impairment is associated with the release of norepinephrine in the region of the compression.

The level of norepinephrine in the brain is reduced by undernourishment in infant rats (Sereni *et al.*, 1966; Shoemaker and Wurtman, 1971). If starvation in the adult rat produces a similar reduction in brain norepinephrine, it might be possible that the starvation-produced elimination of the lateral hypothalamic syndrome need not be explained on the basis of "target weights" but rather on a decrease in catecholamine supplies. This possibility should be investigated in the future.

A Modification of the Lateral Hypothalamic Syndrome

Ellison (1968) has devised a technique which produces a lesion circumscribing the hypothalamus. The technique isolates the hypothalamus and prevents its communicating with the rest of the brain. The technique has been used in both cats and rats (Ellison and Flynn, 1968; Ellison *et al.*, 1970). If the lesion extends to include the far lateral reaches of the hypothalamus, the animals become permanently aphagic and will starve to death. Recovery does not occur even when the animals have been maintained by forced feeding for over 100 days. Oddly enough, the animals are not finicky about their food. They will swallow food if it is placed in their mouths. Thus they do not actively reject food as do animals with the lateral hypothalamic syndrome. The animals seem to have lost the appetitive drive to seek food, but they do not find the taste of food aversive. The aversion to the taste of food may arise from a hyperactivity of medial hypothalamic systems still available to the animals after lateral hypothalamic lesions.

If the lesions do not extend quite so far laterally, the animals will accept, but not seek, food almost immediately after the lesion. Nibbling of food returns in a few days and spontaneous eating in a little over a week. Eating sufficient to maintain weight returns in about 2 weeks. This smaller lesion leaves some parts of the lateral hypothalamus intact and in communication with the rest of the brain. This smaller circumscription of the hypothalamus apparently removes aversive components of the syndrome from being exhibited, presumably because of the isolation of the medial hypothalamus. This, in combination with some intact lateral tissue, allows the animals to enter into "recovery" stage 4 soon after the lesion. Ellison suggests that the normal lateral hypothalamic syndrome represents effects produced by the elimination, or reduction, of lateral hypothalamic influences and by the disinhibition of the medial satiety (aversive) system.

Although the data discussed in the preceding paragraphs are related to food consumption, certain more general principles may be inferred. These include the fact that the usual lateral hypothalamic lesions which affect food and water intake probably do not destroy any neural systems essential to the behavior. Rather, they seem to reduce facilitatory influences which, at least, are adrenergically mediated in the case of eating. Lesions of the lateral hypothalamus must, to a greater or smaller extent, interrupt the catecholaminergic and serotonergic pathways to the forebrain. Therefore, the effects of the lesion must include those produced by the reduction in these transmitters in the brain rostral to the lesion. Restoration of the affected behaviors can follow appropriate pharmacological treatments either at the time of the lesion or much afterward. Furthermore, lesions of the lateral hypothalamic areas are likely to change activity in the medial regions, and vice versa, so that the consequences of a lesion in one location could be due to the reduction of activity in that location and abnormally high activity in the other.

Escape Behavior

M. E. Olds and Frey (1971) have reported that lesions in either the medial or the lateral hypothalamic areas eliminate escape responses elicited by electrical stimulation of the aversive systems of the midbrain. These results are somewhat surprising if one considers the lateral hypothalamus to be a part of a positive reinforcing system which normally acts in opposition to a pain or punishment system. A disruption of the positive reward system might be expected to produce exaggerated escape behaviors, and in fact there have been reports of increased reactions to painful stimuli after lateral hypothalamic lesions, as will be mentioned below.

A lesion-produced disruption of the aversive system of the medial hypothalamus could reduce the effectiveness of pain in regulating behavior, but how can the effects of lateral hypothalamic lesions be explained? If the medial forebrain bundle— lateral hypothalamus system is considered to be a region which mediates the activation of dominant behavioral sequences, then the results make sense. The lesions would have eliminated or diminished the neural mechanisms which are responsible for the initiation and maintenance of the behavior. Indeed, Olds and Frey suggest this possibility:

> The basis for the dificits produced by lateral hypothalamic lesions lies in the damage inflicted in the positively reinforcing system or in the excitatory forces initiating and maintaining behaviors. (p. 17)

Lesions in the medial forebrain bundle can produce an enhanced reflexive reaction to painful stimulation. However, this has been shown to be a consequence of the lesion producing a reduction in the serotonin content of the forebrain, presumably by the interruption of fibers originating from the raphe nuclei and ascending through this fiber bundle, and not due to the disruption of a "reward system." Treatment of the animals with the immediate precursor of serotonin (DL-5-hydroxytryptophan) restores normal reactivity to pain (Yunger and Harvey, 1973). These results point out that it is difficult to ascribe the behavioral effects of hypothalamic lesions or stimulation directly to anatomical systems without taking the status of neurochemical systems into account. Furthermore, the results of Yunger and Harvey make the first possible explanation offered by Olds and Frey most unlikely and leave the second as the viable alternative. In addition, this second proposal explains why stimulation of the lateral hypothalamus enhances escape responding rather than diminishing it (Olds and Olds, 1962). The hypothalamic stimulation is eliciting and energizing the dominant response of the situation.

Sensory Neglect

Electrical stimulation of the lateral hypothalamus facilitates the elicitation of various aggressive responses in the cat by sensory stimulation (Flynn, 1967; MacDonnell and Flynn, 1966; Bandler and Flynn, 1972). Recently, the opposite effect has been reported to follow lateral hypothalamic damage in the rat (Marshall et al., 1971). The lateral hypothalamic lesions greatly reduced the ability of the rat to orient to stimuli contralateral to the side of the lesion.* There was recovery from this sensory neglect which proceeded in a rostral–caudal direction. Sensitivity on the face and snout recovered first, followed later by areas of the midsection and the flank. Sensory neglect was found for many types of stimuli. Food was less frequently approached and eaten when presented on the side contralateral to the lesion than on the ipsilateral side. The elicitation of mousekilling was nonexistent when the mouse was on the contralateral side, even in established mouse killers. The animals did not use information arriving from the side opposite to that of the lesion to accept food or initiate attack behaviors. Marshall et al. interpreted their results in terms of the ability of the rat to integrate the sensory information with effective behavior patterns which are of biological significance to the animal. In a subsequent study, Turner (1973) found a similar, transient contralateral neglect to arise from unilateral lesions of the amygdala and argued that there is presumptive evidence for these effects to be mediated by amygdalohypothalamic fibers coursing through the ventrofugal fiber system. It is tempting to think of these results as due to effects produced by damage to systems mediating reward or behavior activation in the hypothalamus. But this need not be the case. The lesions of the hypothalamus interrupt ascending fibers which are responsible for the maintenance of normal serotonin and norepinephrine levels in the forebrain (Heller, 1972). The sensory neglect could be a consequence of the depletion of these neurotransmitters rostral to the lesion and not of a disruption of the hypothalamus per se.

---

* It is of interest that these animals also showed an impaired motor ability on the contralateral side, especially in the use of the limbs to right themselves and to resist gravity.

Ventromedial Hypothalamic Lesions

The most prominent effect reported to follow lesions of the ventromedial nucleus of the hypothalamus is a permanent hyperphagia and obesity (e.g., Heatherington and Ranson, 1942). Reports of obesity (and other symptoms) have been made in the human where there is suspected damage of medial hypothalamic regions (e.g., Killeffer and Stern, 1970). While the general effects of ventromedial lesions are often described in terms of a reduction in the effectiveness of a satiety mechanism (Epstein, 1960; Teitelbaum and Campbell, 1958), there are a number of surprising behavioral and physiological changes found in animals following such lesions. Not all of them fit in with any simple explanation of the lesion effects. One such change is that while animals with such lesions overeat and gain weight they are finicky about the taste of their food (Teitelbaum, 1955). They will turn away from food adulterated with quinine or other distasteful substance at levels that will not deter normal animals.

Although there have been reports that animals with ventromedial lesions will not "work" to obtain the additional food requirements (e.g., Miller *et al.*, 1950; Teitelbaum, 1957), more recent evidence suggests that they do behave as if they were hungrier than nonlesioned control animals. Kent and Peters (1973) tested their subjects postoperatively on a variable-interval schedule of reinforcement in an operant task under various food deprivation levels. The lesions did not enhance responding when the animals were tested at 80% of their preoperative weights. As food deprivation was lessened, however, the control animals reduced their response rates while the rates of lesioned animals remained high. Under low to moderate food deprivation, the lesioned animals started to run a straight alley for food rewards more quickly than did control animals, and their rate of food ingestion in their home cages was higher under all conditions of deprivation. Kent and Peters suggest that other authors may have inadvertently confused a heightened emotionality of the animals which was exaggerated by the training conditions with a diminished interest in working to obtain food.

Animals with ventromedial lesions tend to accumulate fats,

sometimes at the expense of other body tissues (Han, 1967). Their behavior is strongly regulated by taste factors, so much so that if the taste of food is removed by intragastric feeding, the animals will fail to depress the lever in an operant task to feed themselves (McGinty *et al.*, 1965). There are, unfortunately, a number of issues which remain unresolved concerning the effects of these lesions on obesity. These involve the issues of the interaction between the lesion itself and various hormonal changes (see Hoebel, 1971, for a discussion of these and other related issues).

Selective Lesions in the Hypothalamus

Obesity can be produced by a 1-mm cut through the area just along the anterolateral edge of the ventromedial nucleus (Gold, 1970), but, as mentioned above, the isolation of the ventromedial nucleus along with some portions of the lateral hypothalamus does not produce obesity. Instead, it produces a modified form of the lateral hypothalamic syndrome (Ellison, 1968).

Several attempts to trace degeneration from the lateral hypothalamus to the ventromedial nucleus have been without success. However, such projections recently have been described using an ammoniacal silver degeneration technique (Eager *et al.*, 1971). Knife cuts which separated the medial and lateral hypothalamic areas, more or less, produced finicky food behaviors and a mild hyperphagia if the animals were given their preferred foods. This "hyperphagia" developed after a period of aphagia and adipsia which lasted 2–3 weeks. Cuts made at the outer border of the lateral hypothalamus produced a long-term aphagia and adipsia. Cuts made at the far lateral aspects of the hypothalamus produced only transient adipsia and aphagia (Grossman and Grossman, 1971).

In a subsequent experiment, Grossman (1971) found that transverse cuts made anterior or posterior to the ventromedial nuclei of the hypothalamus produced hyperphagia and hyperdypsia. These effects were noticeable immediately after surgery and were not preceded by a period of aphagia and adipsia as found when connections between the medial and lateral hypothalamic regions were severed. Taken together, these studies from Grossman's laboratory indicate that neural fibers concerned with eating behaviors project rostrally, laterally, and caudally from the ventromedial area and even to regions lateral to the border of the hypothalamus itself. The more pronounced effects obtained by Grossman from transverse cuts made posterior to the ventromedial nuclei suggest the greater significance of caudally directed fibers. In 1946, Brobeck had suggested that fibers extending from the ventromedial nuclei to the mammillary complex and beyond were important for feeding behaviors. This suggestion was given further support by the work of Gold *et al.* (1972), in which hyperphagia was found after asymmetrical lesions involving a knife cut rostral to the ventromedial nucleus on one side of the brain and destruction of the mammillary body on the other side of the brain. This indicates that such lesions disrupt different aspects of a common system that goes through or near the mammillary complex and the ventromedial nuclei. There is some evidence that lateral hypothalamic systems related to feeding can be traced below the hypothalamus into the midbrain (Gold, 1967). This approach should be extended to include the hyperphagia response associated with the medial systems.

Transverse sections made just behind the ventromedial nucleus interrupting the descending fibers from a large portion of the hypothalamus have been reported to interfere with the acquisition of a two-way active avoidance task. If the transverse cut is made just ahead of the ventromedial nucleus, there is no effect on the acquisition of the avoidance response (Grossman and Grossman, 1970).

However, there seem to be substantial, indeed even con- tradictory, effects produced by making the transverse cut behind the ventromedial nucleus and its destruction by electrolytic techniques. Lesions of the ventromedial nucleus produce a facilitation in acquisition of a conditioned avoidance response, not an impairment (Grossman, 1966, 1972). Maybe this discrepancy is due to the fact that the transverse sections made by Grossman and Grossman (1970) interrupted the periventricular system as well as the medial hypothalamic efferent fibers. Even so, the animals with the transverse sections did acquire the two-way active avoidance problem. Their impairment consisted primarily of an increase in the number of trials required for the animals to begin making avoidance responses consistently. This deficit is not unlike that found in animals with damage to the amygdala. Parasagittal cuts in the hypothalamus also affect avoidance behaviors. Sections which separate the medial from the lateral hypothalamus produce a severe deficit in the two-way avoidance, while cuts made at the lateral border of the hypothalamus produce a facilitatory effect (Grossman, 1970).

Lesions of the ventromedial nuclei of the hypothalamus have also been reported to produce an impairment in passive avoidance behaviors (Kaada *et al.*, 1962; McNew and Thompson, 1966; Sclafani and Grossman, 1971). Recently, Gold and Proulx (1972) found that these lesions also produced an impaired ability to avoid a saccharin solution which was associated with sickness produced by injections of apomorphine. Lesions which interrupt descending influences from the medial areas of the hypothalamus have also been shown to enhance components of the copulatory response in male rats, reducing the postejaculatory interval and allowing ejaculations to occur after only a few intromissions (Heimer and Larsson, 1964). The effect seems to be due to disruption of the medial aspects of hypothalamus and not the medial forebrain bundle (Heimer and Larsson, 1966–1967).

If hyperphagia is the most prominent behavioral characteristic found after destruction of the ventromedial nuclei, savageness and aggression must rank a close second. Both effects can occur together. Indeed, one of my own most striking memories is of huge, fat, and extremely hostile cats with ventromedial hypothalamic lesions which I observed many years ago at the University of Iowa. When they observed laboratory visitors through the bars, thankfully strong bars, of their cages, they appeared to have a singular interest in attack. They gave every sign of dedication to the goal of destroying the visitor. Their great size made the threat something not to be taken lightly.* Reports of such fierce attack behavior after ventromedial hypothalamic lesions have been reported in rat, cat, and monkey (Eclancher and Karli, 1971). However, rage and attack are not always found after lesions of the ventromedial

---

* The only comparable ferocity I have ever observed in the rat is that produced by olfactory bulb lesions. Not every animal with such a lesion is hostile, but if ferocity occurs the animals can show well-directed, permanent, and intense attack behaviors.

nucleus, and sometimes only a relatively minor increase of aggression is found. There is a possibility that hyperphagia and aggression are correlated consequences of lesions in the ventromedial nucleus, but different mechanisms may be involved.

A dissociation of the mechanisms responsible for active avoidance learning and intraspecies aggression was reported by Grossman and Grossman (1970). Transverse cuts through the anterior hypothalamus reduced aggressive acts but did not affect avoidance performance. Aggressive behaviors were not affected by the posterior sections which did influence avoidance behaviors despite the massive amount of fiber destruction involved. The measurement of changes in aggressive behaviors is undoubtedly a complex matter, and the evaluation of the anatomical systems involved will be no less difficult. In the cat, Chi and Flynn (1971) have described separate anatomical pathways descending into the midbrain related to quiet biting attacks and to the more full-scale aggressive reactions. The time would seem ripe to combine the lesion and mapping studies, now only used by different workers with different species, to understand the various systems involved more completely.

Neurochemical Systems

In recent years, considerable attention has been directed toward understanding the neurotransmitter substances related to hypothalamic and limbic activities. As one example, Stein (1969) has proposed that the neural systems of the basal forebrain which subserve the pleasure system are noradrenergic. Systems involved with aversive reactions and the suppression of behavior are thought to be cholinergic. In a recent statement of this theory, Stein et al. (1972) suggest that rewards tend to release behaviors from inhibitory influences of the periventricular system. The signal of a rewarding event or the experience of pleasure activates the norepinephrine-producing cells in the brain stem whose axons project into the forebrain via the medial forebrain bundle. Some of these axons reach to the periventricular system and inhibit the activity in it. They may do this directly and also indirectly by inhibition of cells in the limbic system which normally facilitate cells in the periventricular system. These intermediary cells of the limbic system are thought to be the ones using acetylcholine as their transmitter. Signals of punishment are thought to enhance the periventricular system activity either directly or indirectly by the activation of serotonergic cells in the dorsal raphe and other brain stem regions. Axons from these cells may facilitate the periventricular cells directly or exert their influences by stimulating the limbic system cholinergic cells. A diagram of this arrangement is given in Figure 11.

This adrenergic-reward theory is based on a number of different types of experimental observations, including the facts that stimulation of the reward regions of the lateral hypothalamus produces a release of labeled norepinephrine in regions anterior to the stimulated region (Stein and Wise, 1969) and that drugs which enhance adrenergic activity facilitate self-stimulation while those that deplete the available adrenergic supplies also decrease self-stimulation (see Stein, 1969). Even so, caution in unqualified acceptance of the identification of the reward system with an adrenergic system should be exercised for both chemical and behavioral reasons. For example, self-stimulation behavior

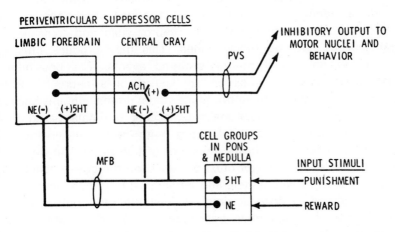

Figure 11. Diagrammatic representation of possible relationships between reward and punishment systems. Reward system acts to release behaviors from suppression by periventricular system. Abbreviations: NE, norepinephrine; MFB, medial forebrain bundle; 5HT, serotonin; PVS, periventricular system; ACh, acetylcholine. From Stein *et al.* (1972).

can be maintained despite lesions of the anterior medial forebrain bundle which substantially decrease the amount of norepinephrine available in the forebrain.

Several authors (e.g., Stein, 1969; Stein et al., 1972; Carlton, 1969) have proposed that the most medial systems of the hypothalamus, especially those of the periventricular system, are involved with the suppression of behavior. The ventromedial nuclei of the hypothalamus are considered to be a component of inhibitory system, and investigations have been made to determine if the inhibitory mechanisms of this nucleus are cholinergic. Cholinergic blockade of the ventromedial nucleus produces a disinhibition of bar pressing for milk (Margules and Stein, 1969), and responding is enhanced in other types of tasks as well (Rożkowska and Fonberg, 1971). This same cholinergic blockade does not affect the consummatory act of eating.

The administration of amphetamine which potentiates the release of norepinephrine from synaptic vesicles produces opposite effects on feeding and on self-stimulation. Amphetamine raises the threshold for feeding behaviors but lowers the threshold for self-stimulation behavior when both are elicited from the same lateral hypothalamic electrode (Miller, 1960; Stark and Totty, 1967; Hoebel, 1969).* It should be remembered that the injection of drugs directly into the brain may produce conditions so a-physiological, so unnatural, that receptor sites and transmitter mechanisms may be overwhelmed. This may produce effects which do not reveal normal synaptic events. The possibility also exists that too small an application of a neurochemical produces effects which are not found under normal circumstances in the brain. This should make us accept the data based on intracranial administration of drugs with certain reservations. Confirmation of hypotheses concerning transmitter substances and their roles in behavior must be based on the convergence of many lines of research, including intracranial drug administration, but also including systemic drug administration and iontophoretic application of presumptive transmitters onto single cells; each individual method has its own inherent limitations.

---

* A possible explanation of this observation could be based on differential effectiveness of amphetamine according to the level of activation in the feeding system.

Investigations of the central nervous system neurochemistry of food and water intake have revealed a part of the great complexities related to the interaction of α- and β-adrenergic subsystems. Since a large portion of this literature is specific to food-oriented behaviors, it will be presented below in a condensed format.

The Neurochemistry of Eating

In studies where the limbic system has been stimulated chemically, adrenergic stimulation has elicited feeding responses and cholinergic stimulation has elicited drinking (Grossman, 1969; Fisher, 1969). One subsequent direction of research has been the attempt to refine the understanding of the regulation of feeding behaviors. Some investigators have postulated that there is an antagonism between the α- and β-adrenergic systems in the hypothalamus (Leibowitz, 1970). The α-adrenergic system is thought to be involved with the initiation of eating, while the β-adrenergic system is considered to be involved in the suppression of eating and this involvement with the termination of feeding leads to a possible association with the medial hypothalamic satiety mechanisms. Evidence for such a view comes from the fact that the intrahypothalamic injection of α-adrenergic agonists produces eating while β-adrenergic agonists injected into the same area inhibits eating, even in food-deprived animals. The injection of an α-adrenergic antagonist blocks eating, while the injection of a β-antagonist seems to reduce "satiety." Leibowitz believes that α-adrenergic terminals inhibit medial satiety neurons, thus releasing feeding centers in the brain stem from the normal suppression after eating. The β-adrenergic terminals are inhibitory on lateral hypothalamic feeding neurons.

Actually, the picture drawn by Leibowitz is rather more complicated when the anatomical locations are taken into considerations. She has found that there are important regional differences in the reactions of animals to the localized injection of the adrenergic compounds. Alpha-, but not beta-, adrenergic substances are effective when injected into the ventromedial nucleus of the hypothalamus. Beta-, but not alpha-, adrenergic substances are effective when introduced into the lateral hypo-thalamus.* This indicates that the cells of the ventromedial nucleus are α-sensitive and those of the lateral hypothalamus are β-sensitive. The cells of the ventromedial nucleus are assumed to be α-adrenergic sensitive but to exert their inhibitory effect on lateral hypothalamic systems by means of a β-adrenergic transmitter. In short, they are thought to receive α-coded messages and send β-coded messages.

A similar, but not identical, system is thought to hold for the lateral hypothalamic neurons. This area is thought to contain β-sensitive cells and to project their influences to cells in the brain stem by an unknown transmitter system. The adrenergic brain stem cells affected by the lateral hypothalamic neurons then send axons to the ventromedial hypothalamic area and release their α-adrenergic substances there. Thus the effect of the ventromedial nucleus on the lateral hypothalamic cells is direct, while the effect of the lateral hypothalamus on the medial is indirect and includes a relay in the brain stem. Despite this difference in the two systems, lateral and medial, they are postulated to stand in a mutually inhibitory relation to each other.†

This theory must assume that norepinephrine is synthesized in the hypothalamus, and this is a debatable point. It is in opposition to the view that only cells in the brain stem synthesize this putative transmitter. The belief that norepinephrine synthesis is restricted to the brain stem is based on the fluorescence technique developed by Dahlström and Fuxe (1964). There is suggestive, albeit indirect, evidence that some norepinephrine is synthesized in the forebrain (Heller, 1972). Therefore, while theories like that of Leibowitz which rest on the synthesis of norepinephrine at nonbrain stem sites must be treated with skepticism, they should not be rejected out of hand.

Margules (1970a, b) has presented a different theory of feeding which is also related to α-adrenergic and β-adrenergic ac-

---

* The perifornical area of the hypothalamus was found by Leibowitz (1970) to be the only area in which both α and β-adrenergic substances produced effects. The significance of this area for the regulation of eating is unknown at the present time.
† It should be pointed out, however, that many of the effects of electrical stimulation of the ventromedial nucleus are excitatory and not inhibitory on cells of the lateral hypothalamus (Van Atta and Sutin, 1971).

tivities. In his theory, the β-adrenergic system is thought to mediate inhibition of eating on the basis of taste factors. The α-adrenergic system is also considered to be an inhibitory system. It inhibits eating on the basis of physiological satiety, and regulates eating on the basis of caloric requirements rather than on the taste of the food. Heightened activity in either system can inhibit eating behavior.

Since the theories of Margules and Leibowitz are so different, it might be anticipated that a resolution between them could be easily achieved by empirical test. Unfortunately, this is not the case because of the possible effects of different amounts of adrenergic compounds when applied to brain tissue. As an example, one problem with the Leibowitz theory is that it does not deal specifically with the finicky behavior of animals with ventromedial hypothalamic damage. In one experiment, Margules tested rats after the hypothalamic injection of an α-adrenergic blocker. Leibowitz had reported that this procedure suppressed eating of food pellets. Margules found no suppression of the drinking of sweet milk. In fact, the animals overdrank this food substance. On the other hand, if the milk was made somewhat distasteful with quinine, the animals stopped drinking. If dry food pellets and quinine-adulterated milk are considered to produce an unpleasant taste, then the effect of the administration of the α-blocking drug would be expected. According to the Margules theory, the animals should be responding primarily on the basis of the taste system after the injection of the α-adrenergic blocking drug since the suppression mechanisms arising from the satisfaction of caloric demands was eliminated. According to Margules, the administration of a β-adrenergic blocking drug should release the animal from aversive taste controls. The animals should accept more unpalatable food than normal animals (Margules, 1970b).

The results of several other types of experiments can be explained by the Margules theory if the results of deprivation are to make the animals more sensitive to taste factors. The greater the deprivation, the greater would be the preference for sweet, highly palatable foods (see Jacobs and Sharma, 1969). This suggests that when deprivation is severe, food intake would be regulated more by the β-adrenergic system than the α-adrenergic system. Under conditions of minimal deprivation, food intake would be regulated more by the α-adrenergic than the β-adrenergic system. Thus the effects of agonists or antagonists of the two adrenergic subsystems should be different under different degrees of deprivation.

Theories of the neurochemistry of feeding should be able to explain the effects of amphetamine. Margules suggests that amphetamine releases norepinephrine from synaptic terminals and thus excites α-adrenergic receptors which signal satiety. This should suppress eating, at least in the mildly deprived subject, and produce the anorexic effects normally reported for the drug. On the other hand, Leibowitz (1970) suggests amphetamine has two types of effects: (1) an α-adrenergic effect which stimulates eating and (2) a β-adrenergic effect which inhibits it. It effects on the β-adrenergic system are considered to be predominant. This has the effect of stimulating the satiety mechanism in her model. She tested this idea by giving amphetamine to animals along with a β-adrenergic blocking drug. The anorexic effect of the amphetamine was lost. The administration of an α-adrenergic blocking drug along with amphetamine enhanced the anorexic effects of the drug. Further support for this idea comes from the report that the intracranial injection of norepinephrine will counteract the anorexic effects of amphetamine (Berger et al., 1971).

There are other conditions during which amphetamine can lead to an increase in eating as opposed to the usual anorexic effects. These are conditions of extreme deprivation coupled with the offering of highly palatable foods (described in Berger et al., 1971), or when eating is initiated by high-intensity stimulation of the lateral hypothalamus (Thode and Carlisle, 1968).

Why does norepinephrine injected into the hypothalamus initiate eating in terms of the Margules model? Increased stimulation in either the α- or the β-adrenergic system should suppress eating behaviors. Margules suggests that it does because small amounts of norepinephrine only activate a membrane pump at the synapse which stimulates the uptake of this drug. Accordingly, small amounts of norepinephrine *reduce* the effective amount of this transmitter at the synapse. Greater amounts would, at some point, overcome the increased activity of the membrane pump and be effective as an agonist to adrenergic activities. According to the Margules theory, this amount would lead to the suppression of eating rather than to initiation.

The Neurochemistry of Behavioral Suppression

The application of some forms of norepinephrine into limbic structures can release behaviors which have been suppressed by punishment. Margules (1968) demonstrated this with injections into the amygdala in rats. The damage caused by the introduction of the cannulae into the amygdala produced passive avoidance deficits, but these deficits were enhanced by the application of norepinephrine through the cannulae. Margules interprets these results to mean that the amygdala is under the inhibitory control of adrenergic fibers with origin in the brain stem and which pass through the medial forebrain bundle system. The function of the norepinephrine is to inhibit ongoing activities of the amygdala and thus indirectly to release behaviors being suppressed by the amygdala. Stein (1969) has suggested that all of the noradrenergic fibers going to limbic areas are inhibitory. According to his view, the unlearned tendencies to approach stimuli in the environment are suppressed by the limbic system. When the limbic system is inhibited through activation of the medial forebrain bundle, this is accomplished through the noradrenergic components of the system.

This theory, and others like it, consider the limbic system to be all of a piece—to exert inhibitory or facilitatory influences on another system in a homogeneous way. This is probably too broad a generalization. Furthermore, limbic system damage, at least in some regions, has the effect of potentiating the animals' reactivity to low doses of amphetamine. It is not clear that this could be adequately explained only as a reduction of facilitation supplied to the periventricular system as proposed in Stein's model.

In the 1972 version of their theory, Stein, Wise, and Berger consider the possible significance of the fact that the ascending noradrenergic system has two major branches. The dorsal branch originates in the locus coeruleus and reaches to the neocortex and hippocampus. The ventral branch takes origin in the brain stem reticular formation and projects mainly to the hypothalamus and ventral forebrain regions (Fuxe *et al.*, 1970). Both of these adrenergic pathways are thought to be involved in the mediation of rewarding effects. The ventral pathway is thought to be concerned with the motor acts of the individual: activating and supporting them to completion. The dorsal pathway is considered to be associated with facilitating *thought* (italics mine). The reader can not help but be struck with the realization of how openly respected neuroscientists, like Stein and his colleagues, talk about "thought," using it as an accepted psychological term in experimental and biological contexts. This is an excellent example of how far the biobehavioral sciences have turned away from a hidebound stimulus–response behaviorism and toward terms found in common language and in theories with a cognitive or humanistic basis.

Carlton (1969) has emphasized the role of the cholinergic system in the suppression of responses. One example of response suppression is the decline in the magnitude of responses over repeated trials referred to as "habituation." Carlton argues that the cholinergic system is responsible for habituation. Habituation can be related to the difference between rewards and reinforcements. If the effects of rewards are resistant to habituation while those of reinforcements are not, then reinforcements could be transmuted into rewards by decreasing the effective cholinergic supplies.

The role of response suppression in the learning of new responses is of major importance. For example, in the original learning of a problem, an anticholinergic drug should enhance acquisition. The response to be learned would be less likely to be suppressed by moment-to-moment changes of the animal relative to the environment. This effect should be most prominent at the beginning of training. But once a response had been acquired there should be a disruption of performance, since animals given anticholinergic drugs should not be able to achieve as high a stable level of performance as animals not given the drug.

No neurochemical system operates in isolation. Activity in one system will influence the behavioral effects produced by changes in another, and several systems must act synergistically to affect behavior. For example, there is also evidence that the degree of catecholaminergic activation is related to behavioral suppression. Anticholinergics tend to release suppressed behaviors, whereas drugs which enhance catecholaminergic activity tend to increase the suppression. Furthermore, the situation becomes even more complicated when it is recognized that the experiences and actions of the animal affect the chemistry and physiology of the animal. Therefore, the effects of an anticholinergic drug on behavior can be complex and depend in part on the nature of the training circumstances, the level of training, and whether or not older, established responses need to be inhibited for the new task to be learned successfully.

The Mammillary Bodies, the Mammillothalamic Tract, and the Cingulate Cortex

The mammillary bodies are a special collection of nuclei at the posterior boundary of the hypothalamus. Most of the studies directed toward understanding their contribution to behavior have investigated the effects of sectioning *one* of the pathways arising from them, the mammillothalamic tract. Since this tract is the initial component of a system reaching the anterior thalamic nuclei and progressing, after synaptic "relay," to the cingulate cortex, these structures will be considered together. However, it should be noted that the behavioral studies which involve sections of the mammillothalamic tract are disrupting only one pathway from the mammillary nuclei. The other major efferent pathway, leading to the tegmentum, usually is unaffected by the lesion.

Lesions of the Mammillothalamic Tract

In his dissertation at the University of Illinois, Krieckhaus (1962, 1964) studied the effect of mammillothalamic tract (MTT) lesions in cats, extending observations made earlier by two of his mentors, Thomas and Fry. He found, as they had before, that either complete or partial destruction of the MTT (produced by ultrasound) adversely affected the retention of a two-way active avoidance task. A much less striking deficit was found after MTT lesion in a one-way active avoidance task. At that time, Krieckhaus interpreted his results in terms of an enhanced tendency of the lesioned animals to "freeze," i.e., crouch and become immobile under the stress of his testing situation.

Subsequently, Thomas *et al.* (1963) found that ultrasonic lesions of the MTT failed to affect the retention of a visual discrimination learned for a positive reward. They also trained lesioned animals in the two-way active avoidance task. This was a study of the postoperative acquisition of the avoidance problem as opposed to previous studies in which the retention of the problem was examined. They found rather mixed results. Seven of the 11 animals studied acquired the problem within the number of trials usually required by intact animals, but four animals failed to learn the task at all. This study indicated that disruption in "memory," as a global concept, could not account for the behavioral changes produced by the MTT lesions, although the question of the effects of the lesions on the postoperative acquisition of the avoidance problem was not answered in a definitive fashion.

In 1965, Krieckhaus found that the behavioral changes produced by MTT lesions in the rat mimicked those found previously in the cat. The lesions reduced the retention of the two-way active avoidance task. He also found that the performance of the lesioned animals could be greatly improved by administration of amphetamine before testing. It had been shown before that amphetamine improves the active avoidance performance of normal animals as well as those with hypothalamic lesions (Cardo, 1960). The drug also enhances exploratory behavior and reduces "freezing." Therefore, Krieckhaus believed that the beneficial effect of the amphetamine was primarily to reduce the enhanced freezing response of the lesioned animals which, in turn, produced a beneficial effect on the avoidance behavior.

Later, Krieckhaus and Chi (1966) began to question the explanation of the avoidance task deficits based on an enhancement of the freezing response. They reported data which showed that the retention deficit could be found in animals which did not have any exaggerated signs of fear or freezing. They also found that when the cats with MTT lesions were subjected to training conditions which should have increased fear, their performance actually improved. Later, Krieckhaus (1966) reported that conditioned emotional responses were not enhanced by the MTT lesions. He concluded that the increased occurrence of freezing found in previous studies had been a consequence rather than the cause of the retention deficits.

Krieckhaus and Lorenz (1968) found that cats were much differently affected by MTT lesions when trained in a lever-press task to avoid shock than when they were trained to press a lever to acquire milk. This suggested that the deficits were not due to an inability to perform the required response but were linked to the motivational systems required to avoid the punishing electrical shocks. Krieckhaus et al. (1968) also found that the deficit produced by the MTT lesions was unrelated to the difficulty of the task. The retention deficits seemed to be related to the willingness of the animals to undertake the required response, since once the animal was induced to begin a behavioral sequence in a T-maze, it made the correct choice in a successive brightness discrimination problem. This reluctance to undertake a behavioral response was also found in a study by Krieckhaus and Randall (1968). These authors found that MTT animals were not impaired in learning a spatial discrimination for a water reward using a T-maze, either in terms of trials required for learning or in terms of errors. They were, however, slower in leaving the start box at the beginning of a trial.

Thompson (1964) and Thompson et al. (1964) have reported that lesions of the MTT or the mammillary bodies per se resulted in an impairment of the ability to perform a spatial discrimination in a T-maze in order to avoid electrical footshocks. The results of Krieckhaus and Randall, discussed above, point out that animals with the MTT lesions are not generally impaired in such tasks, since they can perform them when working to obtain water when thirsty. However, the behavior of animals with MTT lesions can be altered in tasks other than those based on avoidance of shock. Krieckhaus and Randall (1968) found data supporting earlier results obtained by Thompson in that the MTT lesions improved performance on a reversal task even when the water reward was used.

At the present time, it appears that lesions of the MTT lead to disturbances of certain types of behaviors learned on the basis of punishment and that the impairment cannot be described as a general loss of memory, since some tasks learned for positive rewards are unaltered by the lesions. *The most significant obser-*

*vation is that animals with MTT lesions are slow or reluctant
to begin new behavioral acts.* This observation must be considered
in the context of related changes in behavior caused by lesions
of the limbic system which affect the animals' willingness to
initiate or continue behavioral sequences.

The Cingulate Cortex: Avoidance Tasks

Most of the early observations made of animals with lesions
of the cingulate cortex failed to find any behavioral consequences.
Such disturbances as were found were described as "transient,
apparently minimal, and difficult to appraise" (Pribram and
Fulton, 1954, p. 39). The lesions made in the Pribram and Fulton
study were restricted to the anterior cingulate regions. Performance
was measured in a delayed response task and in a visual discrimination problem, and no effects were found. A reduction in the
duration of retreat and withdrawal behaviors was noted when the
expected reward was omitted after a correct response, but a similar
reduction in this emotional reaction was found after other types
of prefrontal lobe lesions, too. Pribram and Weiskrantz (1957)
found more rapid extinction of a two-way active avoidance
task after anterior cingulate lesions when the lesioned animals
were tested after a 1-week recovery interval. Reconditioning of the
active avoidance task was also impaired. Shortly afterward, other
types of behavioral deficits resulting from cingulate lesions
came to be reported in the literature. For example, Brutkowski and
Mempel (1961) found that dogs with anterior (but not posterior)
cingulate lesions seemed unable to restrain their responding
to a nonrewarded stimulus. The ability to respond correctly to
the positive stimulus was retained. These authors interpreted their
results in terms of a loss of the "inhibition" required by the
animals to refrain from responding on negative trials, i.e., those
trials on which a response did not lead to a reward.

Lubar (1964) reported that anterior cingulate lesions did not
affect the learning of a one-way avoidance task and actually
potentiated the learning of a passive avoidance response, at least
as measured by how many trials were required to extinguish
the avoidance response. Furthermore, these effects of cingulate
destruction were antagonistic to the effects of septal area de-

struction which diminished an animal's ability to form a passive avoidance response. Combined cingulate–septal area lesions produce an animal with essentially unchanged passive avoidance behavior. Lubar proposed a direct antagonism between the influences mediated by the cingulate cortex and the septal area.

If there is such an antagonism, it should be reflected in the learning of a two-way active avoidance task. King (1958) was the first to report a facilitation in the acquisition of this task after septal lesions, and now there are reports of impairments in the task produced by cingulate destruction (Peretz, 1960; Thomas and Slotnick, 1962; McCleary, 1961). Lubar and Perachio (1965) found an impairment in two-way active avoidance conditioning in cats after cingulate lesions. They noticed enhanced freezing responses in the animals with cingulate lesions and advanced the hypothesis of an enhanced fear response to account for their observations, as Krieckhaus had done to account for effects of damage to the MTT. However, once again, this hypothesis has not been confirmed in subsequent studies. Kimble and Gostnell (1968), for example, failed to find any evidence for an enhancement of fear after cingulate lesions, using two different behavioral measures, although a substantial impairment in active avoidance conditioning was found.

In a subsequent paper, Lubar et al. (1966) suggested that the impairment found after cingulate cortex lesions was due to damage of the visual neocortical areas of the cat brain incidentally produced when these areas were undercut as the cingulate lesions were made. However, the actual observations made by Lubar et al. were that damage to the lateral or posterolateral gyri could produce deficits in two-way active avoidance conditioning. A direct experimental test of their hypothesis was not undertaken in this study.

The explanation offered by Lubar et al. (1966) for the impairment of avoidance conditioning (i.e., damage to visual cortex) may have merit for the cat but does not seem appropriate for studies in which the rat cingulate cortex is destroyed. In some studies using the rat, cortical control lesions were made which were more likely to interrupt the visual system than were the cingulate lesions. These control lesions were ineffective in altering two-way active avoidance behavior (e.g., Kimble, 1968).

In addition, Trafton *et al.* (1969) found that lesions of several different regions of the anterior cingulate areas, far removed from the visual system, were effective in impairing the active avoidance conditioning. Therefore, while the "visual cortex" of the cat may participate in the regulation of some of the behavioral mechanisms underlying avoidance behavior, the anterior cingulate regions make their own contributions.

The avoidance impairment produced by cingulate lesions is not absolute. For example, if animals are trained in an avoidance task under conditions of food deprivation, the usual deficit may be substantially reduced (Thomas and Slotnick, 1963). This effect could well be mediated by an alteration in the motivational or the arousal level of the organism such that the heightened arousal produced by the lesions actually "offsets" the effect of the lesion.

Other Behavioral Contributions of the Cingulate Cortex

Lesions made in the cingulate cortex lead to the disruption of the orderly sequencing of behaviors. For example, Stamm (1955) has shown that the sequential organization of the behavioral acts used by rats to produce an appropriate nest and to retrieve their young pups was disturbed if the rat "mothers" had cingulate damage. Both anterior and posterior cingulate lesions were reported to disrupt the sequential behaviors of an ethologically significant nature. On the other hand, Wilsoncroft (1963) found that the greatest behavioral effect was produced by lesions of the anterior cingulate region.

The most extensive analysis of the effects of cingulate damage on maternal behaviors has been made by Slotnick (1967). In general, the lesioned animals appear to be confused. They go out to retrieve pups, to gather nesting materials, or to engage in other nest-building operations, but fail to complete the behavioral sequence in a normal fashion. The animals may drop a pup half way back to the nest or bring the pup back to the nest and then remove it again.

The disruption of the sequences of these ethologically significant behaviors produced by the cingulate lesions led to further studies of the effect of the lesions on other types of behaviors in which the temporal order of responding was critical.

Barker and Thomas (1965, 1966) studied the acquisition of a single runway problem in which rewards were provided only on alternate trials. The animals with lesions in the anterior cingulate areas were greatly impaired in the mastery of the problem. Animals with posterior cingulate lesions were not. For animals with the anterior cingulate lesions, the degree of retrograde destruction in the anteromedial thalamic nuclei was correlated with the behavioral impairment. Subsequently, Barker (1967) found an impairment in the performance of the alternation of bar-press responses in an operant situation.

An appealing suggestion related to one aspect of the behavioral deficit produced by cingulate damage comes from a study by Glass et al. (1969). They propose that the lesioned animals are unable to anticipate the emotional consequences of their behaviors both for rewards and for punishments. Another possibility relates to the fact that the behavior of the lesioned animals could also be described on the basis of an *increased* tolerance to frustration. The results of Gurowitz et al. (1970) support such an interpretation. These investigators found that cingulectomized animals had greatly diminished inhibitory re- actions normally found when the magnitude of rewards is reduced (i.e., the Crespi effect).

Both of these interpretations are related to the forecasting of future, stressful events and could be related to the mobilization of the body's resources in preparation for them. Several years ago, I was associated with the beginnings of research aimed at testing this possibility more directly. Using a paradigm for evalu- ating the reduction of circulating eosinophils as a measure of stress (Gollender et al., 1960), Gollender (1967) was able to show that cingulate destruction eliminated or reduced the conditioned stress response but did not change the unconditioned response. Pursuing this general idea in a different way, Liebeskind (1962) found that animals with neocortical damage could become adapted to the stress of being tumbled in a Noble–Collip drum. Destruction of the cingulate areas, however, impaired the ability of the animals to profit from prior stress experiences.

In man, surgical disruption of the cingulate system has been attempted for the relief of pain (Foltz and White, 1962). Apparently, this procedure is of value to some patients but it is not uniformly successful. In tests of cognitive function after cingulectomy, the greatest changes observed were in nonverbal tasks which required temporal ordering or sequencing (Faillace *et al.*, 1971). This result would be expected on the basis of the results obtained from animals. Earlier reports that destruction of the cingulum bundle was without effects on cognition were based on verbal testing procedures alone, and it may be that the destruction of the cingulum influences only certain nonverbal processes. Supporting this lack of effect of cingulum destruction on verbal behavior is the report of Fedio and Ommaya (1970) that bilateral lesions of the bundle did not affect tests of intelligence or memory even though electrical stimulation of the left (but not the right) cingulum did so before the coagulation which produced the ultimate destruction. These authors suggest that the stimulation-produced memory effects are a result of indirect stimulation of structures at a distance from the site of stimulation via interconnecting fiber systems.

Earlier, Foltz and White (1957) and Foltz (1959) in monkeys and Foltz and White (1966) in man reported that lesions of the cingulum bundle decreased withdrawal reactions to morphine. In a study with rats, Trafton and Marques (1971) found that rats with anterior cingulate lesions failed to show behaviors which were indications of addictive behavior. The behavior of the lesioned animals was less opiate oriented than that of rats with control lesions (some of which included the septal area) both during the period when the addiction was being formed and after total drug withdrawal. However, not all subsequent reports have shown beneficial effects of cingulum lesions on drug dependence. For example, Wikler *et al.* (1972) found that cingulum lesions did not alter the signs of specific morphine withdrawal in the rat. These signs include "wet dog" shaking and a decrease in temperature measured in the colon. Therefore, the effects obtained in these several studies could reflect the attenuation of the anticipation of future pleasures or punishments while leaving unaltered the fundamental physiological alterations induced by the morphine.

Lesions of the mammillothalamic tract seem to be related to the initiation of behaviors, and once the animal starts performing a task it can learn, remember, and perform it. The deficit in initiating behaviors seems to be specific to the motives used to induce the behavior. An impaired ability to utilize spatial aspects of the environment may also be found in animals with damage to the tracts. Neither type of deficit should be considered to be uniquely associated with the mammillothalamic tract, since similar effects can be found after damage to other parts of the limbic system.

The effects of lesions of the cingulate cortex depend on the subregions affected. Anterior cingulate lesions are more related to impairments in withholding or suppressing responses than those of the posterior region. As noted in the preceding chapter, the anterior and posterior subregions of the cingulate cortex receive different projections from the anterior nuclear group of the thalamus. An interaction with treatments that affect the arousal of the animals is also implied on the basis of the behavioral changes induced in the lesioned animals by amphetamine administration and by changes in the motivation circumstances under which the animals are tested.

Studies of the effects of cingulate lesions in the rat have involved the production of midline cortical damage. Unfortunately, as reported in the previous chapter, the midline cortex of the rat is probably not comparable to the midline cortex of other animals as defined on the basis of the fibers it receives from the thalamus. Of special importance are the projections from the dorsomedial nucleus. Lesions of the midline cortex, whether in the rat or other species, are likely to interfere with fibers of neural systems in or near it. These include the cingulum bundle and the supracallosal fibers of the fornix. Therefore, it becomes difficult to evaluate separately the effects of destruction of the cingulate cortex, the cingulum bundle, or the superior fornix, either behaviorally or anatomically.

Reflections and Summary

It was with the discovery of "rewarding areas" in the brain that psychology and the related fields of neurobiology finally were able to overthrow overly strict behavioristic traditions. These traditions had inhibited the development of theories concerning man and his behavior by excluding the use of cognitive and affective terms in the explanation of behavior. "Pleasure centers" in the brain provided a physiological basis for introspective reality.

The reward systems of the brain seem to be coextensive with the pathways of the medial forebrain bundle in the lateral hypothalamus and with components of it which reach into some limbic system structures. There are also systems in the brain which mediate aversive effects and others which can alter behavior without changing affective tone. None of them is simple or unitary. For example, the aversive systems are complicated in that animals will learn to avoid brain stimulation applied to some sites but not others, despite the fact that animals will learn to escape stimulation in both. This result may be due to the intimate relationship of some affective sites with behaviors related to ethologically significant events. For example, if electrical stimulation were to mediate both aversive experiences *and* a behavioral tendency to freeze in order to escape from a predator, it would be difficult to train an animal to make an active avoidance response on the basis of this stimulation. In general, the significance of ethologically important factors in determining the responses to brain stimulation has been too often ignored. Mendelson (1972) has shown that the preferred duration of rewarding brain stimulation can be increased or decreased by the objects available in the animal's environment.

The elicitation of specific behaviors by means of hypothalamic stimulation is well established and seems to be best explained on the basis that the stimulation facilitates "command centers" at midbrain or brain stem levels for unlearned and learned response patterns. From the fact that the elicited behaviors can be changed by changes in the environment, it can be assumed that the electrodes do not stimulate the behavioral "command centers" directly. Apparently, the brain stimulation can facilitate behavioral sequences which are likely to occur given the animal's genetic endowment, the general and specific stimuli of the environment, and the animal's prior experiences.

Rewarding and behaviorally energizing effects must be distinguished in hypothalamic stimulation experiments. Elicited behaviors, the release of extinguished responses, and increased rates of responding in operant tasks can be produced at intensities below that required to support self-stimulation behavior. The release of previously suppressed behaviors can also be obtained by cholinergic blockade of the ventromedial nucleus of the hypothalamus or by adrenergic stimulation with the limbic system. Rewarding effects can be elicited at sites which do not facilitate behavior generally.

Electrical stimulation of the hypothalamus can lead to opposite behavioral effects depending on the behavioral tendencies made dominant by the environment. This is most easily seen in the case where the same electrical stimulation can lead to an active escape response or to drowsiness and sleep, dependent on the compartment in which the animal is located. The stimulation seems to potentiate any type of response sequence which is dominant at the moment of stimulation

Under some conditions, lesions of the hypothalamus produce drastic changes in eating and drinking, as well as in other behaviors (e.g., sensory neglect), which seem to be recovered over time. It is of interest to me that those behaviors in which postoperative recovery is found are also those in which the immediate effects of the lesions can be mitigated by changes in body weight or by chemical therapies at the time of surgery. Probably the control of body weight is governed by neural systems located in far lateral parts of the diencephalon and perhaps involving some portions or tracts of the basal ganglia (see Morgane, 1961).

In many ways, the ventromedial nucleus of the hypothalamus, and perhaps the medial aspects of the posterior hypothalamus more generally, seems to be antagonistic to the functions of the lateral hypothalamus and the medial forebrain bundle. Interconnections exist between these regions, and it seems reasonable to conclude that these fibers mediate a reciprocal inhibition, yet there is opposing evidence to the effect that the medial and lateral hypothalamus often facilitate each other. This complication is but one of the several difficult matters which must be explained before full understanding of the hypothalamus is achieved. While the lateral regions undoubtedly are rich in adrenergic fibers and the medial hypothalamus is correspondingly rich in cholinergic fibers, there is extensive controversy as to the roles played by these and other neurochemical systems in behavior.

The distinction between the energizing (motivational) and

rewarding effects mediated by the lateral hypothalamus is not easy to keep in mind. This distinction is of considerable importance for understanding the neurochemistry of hypothalamic activities, even though there is still some uncertainty as to whether reward effects occur when the hypothalamus is being stimulated or when the stimulation is over and a poststimulus rebound occurs (Molnár and Grastyán, 1972). The distinction can be made more apparent by an example. If an animal makes a response which produces a rewarding effect, this response will come to be dominant in that situation. In the future when the medial forebrain bundle is stimulated, the dominant response for that particular situation will be facilitated. When electrical stimulation is used to provide the reward response rates should be extremely high. But electrical stimulation of the medial forebrain bundle at intensities below that required to elicit rewarding effects also will amplify response rates. Perhaps the role of reward is to make a particular response dominant in a situation, and whatever response is dominant will be expressed when the medial forebrain is activated. Theoretically, it should be possible to determine if the neurochemistry of the reward effect is the same as that of the energizing effect. The evaluation of the effect of drugs on the response rate emitted by the animal for electrical brain stimulation is probably not adequate to determine such a difference—if it exists.

The energizing and rewarding effects mediated by systems of the lateral hypothalamus are opposed by two regions: (1) the anterior hypothalamus and (2) the medial hypothalamus. The trophotropic reactions which are mediated by the anterior regions seem related in some fashion to the satiety systems of the ventromedial nuclei. As yet, however, the relationship between the two regions has been little investigated. Because both areas seem to be greatly involved in effecting changes in neural activity and behavior in response to changes in the internal environment and because of their possible antagonism to the lateral hypothalamus and medial forebrain bundle, such investigations would be most profitable.

Chapter 3

THE AMYGDALA

As with other regions of the limbic system, the amygdala has close ties with the hypothalamus, although it differs from other limbic structures in also having a close relationship to the basal ganglia. Thus the amygdala has a special place among the subcortical nuclear masses in being intimately involved in both limbic and striatal activities. This dual association suggests that there would be a corresponding division within amygdalar nuclei. As mentioned in the first chapter, there is a basic differentiation among the nuclei of the amygdala into corticomedial and baso-lateral groups, with the corticomedial group thought to be more closely linked to the basal ganglia (Crosby et al., 1962). In this connection, however, it is surprising that the lateral and basal nuclei of the amygdala are extremely rich in cholinesterase in the rat (Girgis, 1972). High acetycholine and cholinesterase activities have been associated with the basal ganglia to a greater extent than with the limbic system. On this basis, the corticomedial division might have been anticipated to be the one with the greatest cholinergic activity. However, as will be discussed later, it is doubtful that the diverse functions of the amygdala can be definitely related to any known anatomical groupings. In any case, as with other limbic structures, the amygdala is not homogeneous with regard to either structure or function.

In this chapter, I will present some of the behavioral contributions made by the amygdalar complex. General changes in behavior produced by the stimulation or destruction of the amygdala will be considered first, followed by a discussion of more specific changes.

General Effects Produced
by Amygdala Stimulation or Lesions

In the context of this chapter, and certain subsequent ones, I will distinguish "general" from "specific" effects produced by lesion or stimulation techniques. By these terms, I do not mean to imply more than that some of these effects, the "general" effects, can be observed in a wider range of situations than others, the "specific" effects. For example, stimulation of the amygdala might produce heart rate changes in many situations. If it did, then it would be considered a general effect. But if the heart rate effect were found only in a particular type of situation, say when the animal was tightly restrained, it would be considered under a specialized heading. It will be admitted that all behavioral effects produced by lesions or by stimulation are probably neither general to all situations nor entirely specific to one situation, but it is helpful to organize the available literature on this basis.

Autonomic Effects

Electrical stimulation of the amygdala does produce effects on autonomic activity, including heart rate and respiration. Both bradycardia and tachycardia have been produced by stimulation of the amygdala (e.g., Koikegami et al., 1957). The slowing of the heart rate produced by amygdala stimulation can be abolished by atropine or vagotomy, whereas the tachycardia effects are not influenced by section of the vagal nerves. The increase in heart rate response is presumed to be of sympathetic origin, whereas the bradycardial reaction is thought to be secondary to interruption of normal reflex functions induced by the stimulation (Reis and McHugh, 1968). The location of the electrodes in the amygdala is important in determining the direction of the heart rate changes, as is the anesthetic used in the experiment (Mogenson and Calaresu, 1973). Presence of afterdischarges induced by the stimulation can influence the intensity of the reaction, but not the type of effect which occurs. For example, if the electrode is in a region of the amygdala which produces a bradycardial response, this will be greatest if an afterdischarge is elicited. Changing the frequency of stimulation or reducing its intensity so as not to produce afterdischarges will only change the magnitude of the heart rate slowing (Reis and Oliphant, 1964). In paralyzed animals, Bonvallet and Bobo (1972) found that decreases in respiration were obtained from stimulation of the lateral parts of the central nucleus, the lateral nucleus, and the small cell division of the basal nucleus. A decrease in heart rate often accompanied a corresponding respiratory change. Respiratory increases, frequently associated with cardiac acceleration, could be produced by stimulation of the amygdala; however, there seemed to be no clear pattern of localization of these effects. Stimulation of the magnocellular portions of the amygdala produced an initial decrease in respiration followed by a "rebound" increase. The heart rate changes were closely associated with the changes in respiration.

Changes in the galvanic skin response (GSR) have also been found to result from stimulation of the amygdala and the subsequent afterdischarges (Lang et al., 1964). The "middle regions" of the amygdala have been found to be the most effective for production of the GSR effects. A close correspondence with basolateral or corticomedial divisions was not found. These observations on the galvanic skin response were substantiated by observations in which the GSR was decreased or abolished by lesions of the amygdala (Bagshaw et al., 1965). Lesions of the amygdala tend to eliminate the autonomic, but not the somatic, components of the orienting reflex in monkeys. In addition to a reduction of the GSR, heart rate and respiratory reactions were not found even though the lesioned animals still could exhibit orienting reflexes. Somatic reactions and activation of the cortical EEG associated with the orienting reaction remained after the lesions (Bagshaw and Benzies, 1968). The association of the amygdala with the orienting response, or portions of it, is related to the observation that stimulation of the amygdala can produce orienting reactions (Ursin et al., 1967, 1969).

Orienting and Habituation

The orienting reflex or reaction is, of course, of great significance to all animals. The complete orienting reaction includes the suppression of ongoing behaviors, the orienting of the body and receptor toward the new stimulus, changes in the peripheral autonomic nervous system, and, perhaps less obvious, preparations for associating the new stimulus with memories from the past and expectancies of the future.

In a recent study using a camera to record eye fixations on visual targets, Bagshaw *et al.* (1972) were able to demonstrate that when responses to particular visual stimuli were not rewarded, monkeys with destruction of the amygdala made fewer observing responses than normal monkeys. Visual orientation toward unfamiliar stimuli was greatly reduced by amygdala damage. These results suggest that the lesions produce animals which pay less attention to their visual environment and which react less to changes in the visual world around them. On the other hand, when the animals with amygdala lesions are rewarded for attending to visual stimuli, as in visual discrimination problems, they can learn them as readily as normal animals (Schwartzbaum and Pribram, 1960), despite their apparent inattentiveness. Lesions of the inferotemporal cortex, on the other hand, produce animals which have great difficulty in learning visual discriminations but which exhibit more visual orienting responses than intact animals in nonrewarded conditions. The monkeys with inferotemporal lesions also react toward novel conditions in a visual display in the same fashion as do normal subjects. It may be that amygdala lesions alter the animals' willingness to respond toward novel events unless there is a substantial "payoff" (reward) for doing so. This idea is supported by previous studies in which the behavior of the animals with amygdala lesions could be explained on the basis that the lesion altered the willingness of the animal to undertake new responses (Pribram *et al.*, 1969). In essence, the lesioned animals can orient toward new stimuli but are reluctant to do so unless adequate justification is provided.

Destruction of the amygdala alters the rate of habituation of locomotor activity, while not influencing its peak levels. Furthermore, the locomotor activity of animals with amygdala damage is not overly enhanced by external stimulation, as is sometimes found after damage to the frontal lobes. Monkeys with amygdala lesions do not exhibit the incessant pacing often found in animals with frontal lobe damage. The failure of locomotor activity to habituate is confined to tests made when the amygdala-lesioned animals are placed in unfamiliar circumstances. The animals are not overactive in their home cages (Schwartzbaum *et al.*, 1961).

Emotional Changes

Fonberg and Delgado (1961) studied the reactions of cats both to short periods of amygdala stimulation and to chronic stimulation of the structure lasting over 24 hr. They found that the brief periods of stimulation could interrupt certain kinds of behaviors. These included eating, as well as the responses learned to obtain food. The interruption of behaviors produced by amygdala stimulation was specific to food-oriented behaviors. This is related to studies which have found that lesions of the amygdala can produce overeating and even voracious attacks on food in some animals, including man (Pribram and Bagshaw, 1953; see Pribram, 1971). If the stimulation applied to the amygdala by Fonberg and Delgado did not produce afterdischarges or obvious motor effects, it would not disrupt playing behaviors or alert the animal if it was resting. Chronic stimulation of the basolateral nucleus which lasted for periods of 24 hr produced decreased activity and food intake. In general, the animals seemed to be relaxed and purred a great deal. They were not impaired on previously learned avoidance behaviors unless afterdischarges or obvious motor effects were produced by the electrical stimulation.* The animals adapted to this type of stimulation and came to eat as well as to bar-press for food over the course of the 24-hr period.

On the basis of studies of animals with lesions in different regions of the amygdala, Fonberg (1973) now believes that there are two antagonistic divisions relative to eating and emotional

---

* In contrast, prolonged stimulation of the cingulate cortex produced increased activity, signs of anxiety, and hyperirritability.

reactions: (1) a dorsal—medial region which, when lesioned, results in aphagia and a loss of emotional tone and (2) a lateral division which, when lesioned, produces hyperphagia and an enhancement of pleasure. The net effect of a lesion in the amygdalar complex is determined by the extent to which the *balance* of impulses over the two systems is affected. If a lesion were to affect the two amygdala areas equally, the balance of activities would be unaltered and no change in food behavior observed.

Emotional changes were also observed as a function of lesions in the two systems. After lesions of the dorsal—medial region, dogs ceased to be friendly and became fearful, sad, and sometimes aggressive. After a second lesion of the lateral area, the dogs became happy, played, showed affection, and enjoyed eating again. The balance between the two amygdala systems had been restored, according to the Fonberg interpretation.

In another type of study, stimulation of the amygdala was found to suppress aggressive activities of the animals, including aggression induced by hypothalamic stimulation (Egger and Flynn, 1962). However, regional differences within the amygdala again must be considered. Whether or not attack and aggressive behaviors will be facilitated or inhibited by stimulation of the amygdala is related to the region in which the electrode is located.

Ursin and Kaada (1960) stimulated the amygdalar complex with chronically implanted electrodes. They found a dissociation of fear (flight) and aggressive behaviors. Flight and fear responses could be obtained from the rostral regions of the amygdala, including the lateral nucleus, the periamygdaloid area, and the central nucleus. Defense or aggressive reactions could be obtained from the medial and the caudal aspects of the amygdala. These regions in the cat, as mapped out by Ursin, are shown in Figure 12. As can be seen, the flight and defensive regions do not correspond to the established nuclear division of the amygdala. It may be of importance that the stria terminalis is thought to have a preponderance of fibers from the caudal portions of the amygdalar complex (Nauta, 1961) and that it projects predominantly to medial hypothalamic structures, especially in and around the ventromedial nucleus. F. A. King (personal communication) was able to show that the attack behavior elicited by

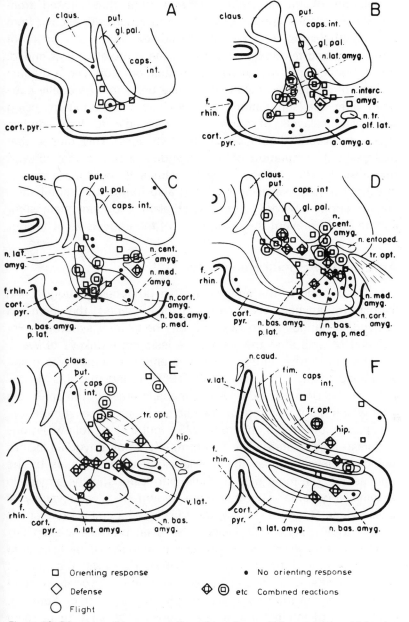

Figure 12. Diagrammatic representation of locations within amygdala which when electrically stimulated produce orienting, defensive reactions, flight, or combined reactions. Symbols are explained in figure. Courtesy Dr. Holger Ursin.

stimulation of the amygdala differed from that elicited from stimulation of the hypothalamus. The attack behavior elicited from the hypothalamus was begun immediately with the onset of stimulation and terminated as soon as the stimulation was ended. On the other hand, the amygdala stimulation produced a gradual buildup of aggressive behaviors. These behaviors gradually subsided after the stimulation was terminated. In addition, using subthreshold levels of current, he was able to find additive effects between stimulation at the two sites. This means that subthreshold stimulation of the amygdala would summate with subthreshold stimulation of hypothalamus to produce a suprathreshold aggressive response. King also found that septal stimulation applied before either hypothalamus or amygdala stimulation could prevent the occurrence of the aggressive behaviors.

Arousal and Social Reactivity

Destruction of the amygdala often produces a sluggish and hypoactive animal. Weiskrantz (1956) coined the term an "amygdala hangover" to describe this behavioral syndrome. For a period of time after the lesion, the lesioned monkeys of Weiskrantz were droopy and paid little attention to what was going on around them. In the cat, Ursin (1965) found that this "hangover" results primarily from lesions made in areas of the amygdala from which flight reaction can be elicited by electrical stimulation, whereas in the dog Fonberg (1973) found it to follow lesions in dorsal—medial areas. The longterm effects of amygdala lesions include a depression in the normal aggressive activities of the animals. For the most part, animals with lesions in the amygdala become very tame. This has been shown in a wide variety of species (see Goddard, 1964a, for a listing of some 43 references on this topic). Amygdala lesions can even produce a calm demeanor in animals made rageful and hyperreactive by lesions in the septal area (King and Meyer, 1958). However, the general behavioral effects produced by lesions of the amygdala depend on the regions of the amygdalar complex damaged (e.g., Fonberg, 1973). It is of interest that in the opposum, at least, there seem to be opposite effects produced by lesions of the amygdala and the pyriform cortex, the former leading to the expected placidity and the latter producing an increase in aggression (Hara and Myers, 1973).

Along with the enhanced placidity and tameness found after near complete amygdala lesions, there is a reduction in the interactions found between the lesioned animals and other animals of their own species. This is reflected in the reduction in social rank found after the lesions (Rosvold et al., 1954; Fuller et al., 1957). Bunnell (1966) has attributed the social effects produced by amygdala lesions in terms of a raised threshold for reactions produced by social stimuli. Animals suffering from amygdala lesions can exhibit normal aggression and fighting if the conditions and the stimuli are strong enough. In particular, amygdalecto-mized animals produce as much shock-induced fighting and aggression as normal animals (Finch et al., 1968). Shock-induced aggression is certainly a condition in which the environmental circumstances are most impelling. Thus the ability to exhibit aggressive behaviors has not been impaired. The animals are merely reluctant to do so.

The effects of amygdala lesions can be contrasted with those produced by the septal area. Jonason and Enloe (1971) found that amygdala lesions produced a reduction in social contacts made by the lesioned animals while septal lesions produced an enhancement of social contacts. They explained this on the basis of an enhancement or facilitation of prepotent responses produced by the septal lesions. This normal tendency for social contacts was facilitated by the septal lesions and reduced by amygdala lesions.

The effects of amygdala lesions cannot be explained simply as a reduction in all types of behavior. Galef (1970) studied the effects of amygdala lesions in wild Norway rats. He found these animals to be more aggressive toward humans, mice, and other rats than the domesticated laboratory animals. As would be expected, the wild rats were tamer after the lesions and exhibited fewer aggressive acts. However, the wild rats were also more timid in novel feeding situations than the domesticated laboratory animals. This means that they did not begin eating in an unfamiliar situation as quickly as did the tamer, laboratory animals. After the amygdala lesions, however, these animals began to eat in unfamiliar circumstances more readily. As measured by the time required to begin eating in unfamiliar circumstances, they were less timid after the amygdala lesions.

In studies of free-roaming monkeys in the jungle habitat, A. Kling (personal communication) found that animals with amygdala lesions quickly became social isolates. They did not interact with others in the monkey tribe and soon wandered off, probably to die. They did not respond to the social signals given out by the other monkeys and they did not initiate social interactions. These effects are not a unique consequence of amygdala destruction. Myers and Swett (1970) observed monkeys with anterior temporal lobe damage which were allowed to roam freely over an island near Puerto Rico. These lesions, which did not invade the amygdala, also made the animals into lonely, asocial creatures without affinity for their group. Their survival times in the jungle were only a few weeks, on the average.

Stimulation of the amygdala can produce arousal reactions of many different kinds. These arousal effects are widespread and involve many neural systems, both autonomic and somatic. In some ways, they are reminiscent of the effects found from stimulation of the midbrain reticular formation (e.g., Feindel and Gloor, 1954) There is ample evidence of differentiation within the amygdala for this behavioral dimension, too. Kreindler and Steriade (1963) have reported that stimulation of the dorsal amygdala produced effects which were quite different from those found after stimulation of its ventral regions. High-frequency stimulation of the dorsal regions produced desynchronization of neocortical rhythms, whereas the same stimulation of ventral regions induced synchronized rhythms and sleep patterns in the neocortex. In addition, stimulation of the ventral regions could produce seizure discharges during the time of stimulation, whereas stimulation of dorsal amygdala produced seizure discharges only after the stimulation had ended. The arousal systems of the amygdala seem to be independent of the midbrain reticular formation since the arousal effects produced by amygdala stimulation can be found after lesions of the midbrain reticular formation. The cortical arousal effects initiated from the dorsal amygdala stimulation can suppress epileptiform discharges produced by the application of penicillin to the neocortex (Kreindler and Steriade, 1964). In addition, the activation of the neocortex by amygdala stimulation can also occlude evoked potentials in the neocortex (King *et al.*, 1953).

Studies of Learning and Memory

The tameness found in animals after amygdalectomy seems to reflect a decrease in emotionality, at least in response to many conditions and signals from the environment. This reduction in emotional responsiveness may be related to the changes in behavior found in formal tasks used to study learning and memory.

Aversive Conditioning

The effects of amygdala lesions have been studied in many types of learning situations, but probably the most intensive study has been made on animals performing in avoidance tasks. The learning of an avoidance task is related to the intensity of the electrical shock used as punishment or, more accurately, to how the animals experience the shock. The amygdala lesion could alter the pain sensitivity or alter reactions to pain. In the monkey, lesions of the amygdala seem to change the threshold for reactions to punishing electrical shocks (Bagshaw and Pribram, 1968). In the rat, Kemble and Beckman (1969) tested the escape reactions of animals with amygdala damage to the sequential administration of 0.5-, 0.1-, and 1.0-mA footshocks. They found the lesioned animals to react more quickly than control animals at the low intensity levels but more slowly at the high intensity level. This effect might be related to the fact that the animals were first tested with the lower shock levels. In a second experiment, Kemble and Beckman found escape latencies lower than those of control animals under the 1.0-mA condition when this shock intensity was the only one given to the animals. Animals with amygdala lesions had very similar escape latencies to the first experience of electrical shock at all intensities. In other words, the animals responded with the same speed regardless of the intensity of shock employed, while the speed of the control animals' reactions was influenced by the shock levels. Since impairments of avoidance learning produced by lesions are evaluated relative to the performance of control animals, the level of shock employed could be of great significance for the results obtained.

In one of the earlier studies of avoidance conditioning, Horvath (1963) found some impairment in two-way active avoidance (shuttlebox) learning after amygdala lesions, but the effects were not large. In this study, cats with lesions of the basolateral complex were the most impaired, and indeed there was some suggestion that damage to the corticomedial group could attenuate the effect of the basolateral damage. Horvath also found that the retention of the two-way active avoidance response was reduced after the basolateral lesion. No lesion effect was observed on a passive avoidance task or in one-way active avoidance problems. The effect of the amygdala lesion on the retention of the shuttlebox task found by Horvath is somewhat surprising since Fonberg et al. (1962) failed to find a retention deficit on a well-established preoperative avoidance response in dogs after damage to the amygdala.

King (1958) failed to find any debilitation in the two-way active avoidance task in terms of the number of responses made, although there was an effect on the speed with which the responses were made. The animals with the amygdala lesions were much slower in making the avoidance response, barely accomplishing it in the interval between the onset of the CS and the onset of the shock. This is an important point, since there is evidence to suggest that one of the major difficulties of the animals with amygdala lesions is their reluctance to initiate behavioral acts.

Deficiencies in the two-way active avoidance task as a consequence of amygdala lesions in the cat have been observed by Kling et al. (1960). Their deficit was in terms of the number of trials required to begin making avoidance responses. Once the animals had begun to make avoidance responses, learning seemed to progress naturally and at the same rate as found in the intact animals. Suggestion of a similar deficit was found in the rat after lesions of the stria terminalis by Fred Pond and me (unpublished observations). Animals with lesions involving the stria terminalis were found to require more trials to begin avoidance responding, but once avoidance responding had been initiated, learning progressed as in normal animals.

In general, amygdala lesions do not change behavior in passive avoidance tasks (e.g., McNew and Thompson, 1966). One exception is a study by Ursin (1965) in which lesions of the medial nucleus of the amygdala produced an impairment in passive avoidance behaviors. Specific details of training are important. A deficit in one-way active avoidance behavior was found by McNew and Thompson, as well as by Ursin, using a task in which the animals were not picked up between trials. The influence of handling between trials is important and probably adds to the emotionality of the animal in the training task. Tasks without handling between trials probably allow the animals to be evaluated at lower arousal or emotionality levels than when they are handled between trials. Handling between trials may also produce some disorientation of the animals or distract the animals from the specific requirements of the task. In any case, task parameters are of great significance in the evaluation of avoidance deficits after amygdala lesions. Such deficits are not a necessary consequence of amygdala damage. For example, no decrement in avoidance behavior was found in a bar-press avoidance task for either a tone or a visual signal following amygdala lesions (DiCara, 1966).

One important observation made by Ursin in his study of the one-way active avoidance problem was that the animals failed to initiate their responses despite "fullblown" emotional reactions in response to the CS. The lesions were in the flight zone (fear zone) of the amygdala. This suggests more evidence for a dissociation between the expression of behavior and emotional reactions.

While animals with amygdala lesions are somewhat loath to begin responses under certain conditions, they are quick to give them up. Rapid extinction of two-way active avoidance tasks and panel-pressing avoidance reactions have been observed in monkeys (Pribram and Weiskrantz, 1957; Weiskrantz, 1956; Weiskrantz and Wilson, 1955, 1958). Moreover, animals with amygdala lesions will often simply refuse to respond to two-choice maze problems. This has been found when training the animals in reversal procedures. The lesioned animals seem to have an enhanced tendency to stop all responding when confronted by disrupting events and nonreinforcement, despite the fact that they exhibit more "vicarious trial and error" movements at the choice point of the maze (Kemble and Beckman, 1970).

Lesions of the amygdala also disrupt the formation of conditioned emotional responses. In this task, the emotional reaction is measured by the extent to which operant responding is suppressed during the presentation of a tone or visual stimulus which was associated in the past with some form of noxious stimulation, usually electrical footshock. The degree of suppression of the response during the presentation of the tone is a measure of the degree to which an association has been made between the signal and the painful stimulation. Usually, it is thought that the animals become "afraid" of the signal and that this fear produces responses incompatible with bar pressing. These incompatible responses lower the rate of bar pressing for food or water. However, in brain-damaged animals when a conditioned emotional response cannot be established or is less than in control animals, this does not mean that the lesioned animals are less fearful of the stimulus. It could be that the brain-damaged animals are just as afraid of the stimulus as their normal counterparts but have lost an ability to suppress ongoing behaviors. A seeming dissociation between emotional responses and the expression of the emotions in behavior was noted by Ursin after amygdala damage (mentioned above). Furthermore, explanations of the conditioned emotional response based entirely on the failure of animals to consolidate or incubate a fear response are inadequate. Using a bar-press avoidance, Campenot (1969) found that animals with amygdala lesions performed poorly on the task the first day of training but on the second day showed anticipatory responses to the signals in a normal fashion. On the second day, they did learn the task, but as training continued on the second day, the animals' behavior began to deteriorate once again. The interpretation of this behavior cannot be based on the failure of the animals to consolidate the fear response on the first day of training, since it was expressed quite well in behavior on the second day. Campenot suggests that the more adequate explanation must be based on an alteration in the animals' ability to suppress previously learned behavior sequences. The interruption of conditioned emotional response formation reported by Thompson and Schwartzbaum (1964) to follow amygdala lesions could represent a change in emotional reactivity or response inhibition or both. A debilitation in the suppression of responses not based on the conditioning of a fear response has also been reported by Schwartzbaum *et al.* (1964).

Goddard (1964*b*) studied the effects of continuous stimulation of the amygdala on several types of behavioral problems.* He found that stimulation of the amygdala impaired two-way active avoidance behavior but failed to have any influence on the learning of a Lashley III maze for a food reward. Normal acquisition of a one-way active avoidance response was observed, although this response extinguished more rapidly than it did in normal animals. There was also a disruption of the formation of conditioned emotional responses. To further investigate the effect of amygdala stimulation on the formation of conditioned emotional responses, in one group of subjects Goddard applied the stimulation only during the period during which the CS was presented and in another group for 5 min after the painful shock which was paired with a tone. He found that the pairing of the tone with the amygdala stimulation did not affect the formation of the conditioned emotional response, whereas stimulation of the amygdala after the painful shock did. At that time, he proposed that stimulation of the amygdala produced a disruption in the "consolidation" or the "incubation" of the fear response. †

In 1969, Goddard modified his previous hypothesis on the basis of new information. In this more recent study, he stimulated the amygdala with injections of carbachol and found a disruption in conditioned emotional responses and a passive avoidance task but found no effects on behavior in the one-way active avoidance response. The disruption of the passive avoidance behavior occurred only when the training had been distributed over several days and not when massed training was given to the animals.

---

* The stimulation used by Goddard was a 60 cycle/sec stimulus ranging in current level from 3 to 13 μA. The stimulation was applied the entire time the animal was in the training situation. The stimulation was adjusted so that it was below threshold for any observable motor effects.

† Pellegrino (1965) reported that noncontingent continuous stimulation of the amygdala interfered with the learning of a passive avoidance response. Lidsky *et al.* (1970) challenged the results of Pellegrino on the basis of probable artifactual interactions between the grid-shock and the brain stimulation circuit. The issue of such interactions was discussed by Schwartzbaum and Donovick (1968) and Schwartzbaum and Gustafson (1970).

Goddard noted that retention was impaired only when the animals were required to suppress previously learned behaviors. The ability to withhold responses on the basis of associations with noxious events seemed to be lost. The carbachol injection into the amygdala seemed to eliminate the ability of the animals to inhibit responses based on fear motivation.

The results and conclusions of Goddard (1964*b*, 1969) have been challenged by Lidsky *et al.* (1970). These investigators failed to find any amnesic effects as measured by conditioned suppression of an operant response on a licking response produced by subseizure stimulation of the amygdala. If the current used in stimulating the amygdala was raised enough to support self-stimulation, it still was without effect. Only when the intensity of the stimulation was raised even further, to the point that seizures were observed, did any behavioral deficit in retention occur. The fact that seizures initiated in the amygdala spread widely throughout the brain makes the association of the amnesic effect with any particular structure tenuous. In addition, Lidsky *et al.* suggest that "state-dependent" effects result from the amygdala seizures.

McIntyre (1970) has made observations which may help to clarify the discrepancy between the Goddard and Lidsky *et al.* experiments. He found that stimulation of the amygdala was effective in disrupting the development of a conditioned emotional response if the stimulation was given after the amygdala had been previously stimulated sufficiently to produce what is called "kindling." Stimulation of the amygdala after the CS–shock pairing in the absence of kindled reactions to stimulation failed to disrupt the formation of the conditioned emotional response.

The term "kindling" refers to the effects produced by brief periods of electrical stimulation applied at regular intervals but separated by hours to days (Goddard *et al.*, 1969). Slowly, with repeated stimulation, the brief stimuli come to have greater and greater effects. Afterdischarges begin to occur after the stimulation and then are found bilaterally after unilateral stimulation. Later, the afterdischarges spread to brain regions beyond the amygdala and finally come to produce fullblown motor seizures. Thus the same stimulation repeatedly applied to a particular brain area comes to produce more and more intense reactions as it is applied time and again. Yet to produce the kindling effect the periods of stimulation must be spaced with at least several hours between them. Massing the periods of stimulation together prevents the kindling effect. The kindling effect is more or less specific to the brain region being stimulated, and it does not reflect a general change in the reactivity of the brain (Racine, 1972), although there is some interfacilitation between kindling effects produced in the amygdala and the septal area.

As mentioned above, McIntyre was able to show an amnesic effect from stimulation of the amygdala after it had been "kindled" but not otherwise. The stimulation did produce convulsions in the kindled animals, and therefore the question of whether the amygdala itself was critical to the behavioral impairment must be considered. McIntyre found that seizures produced by stimulation of the "anterior limbic field" after it had been kindled failed to produce the same amnesic effects as stimulation of the amygdala.* He also suggested that the amnesic effect may be due to the postictal depression which results from the amygdala stimulation in the kindled animals. Animals given the CS–shock pairing while in the postictal period failed to demonstrate conditioned suppression to the CS in later testing.

In general, then, McIntyre reaffirmed the importance of the amygdala in the formation of a conditioned emotional response but at the same time he failed to support Goddard's 1964 results. In the 1964 study of Goddard, the brain stimulation had been applied for prolonged periods of time, however, and it is possible that some unusual electrical seizure activity had developed and been propagated to areas which were important for the later demonstration of the conditioned emotional response. If the propagation of abnormal activity to a particular region or system of the brain is critical, the amygdala apparently has greater access to it than the anterior limbic field.

In a recent study, Bresnahan and Routtenberg (1972) studied the effects of unilateral stimulation of the amygdala during the learning of a stepdown passive avoidance task measured 24 hr after the animals had been trained. Stimulation of the amygdala

---

* The anterior limbic field designates an area of neocortex in the rat which lies along the dorsal, anterior surface just lateral to the cingulate cortex (Goddard et al., 1969; Hudspeth and Wilsoncroft, 1969).

occurred only during acquisition. Their results indicated poorer performance when the medial nucleus was stimulated but not if other areas of the amygdala were stimulated. Their electrographic records indicated that stimulation-induced seizures could not account for their results. On the other hand, since the stimulation was given during acquisition and not during retention, a pure memory effect cannot be assumed. It is possible that the stimulation produced a different "state" of the organism during acquisition than occurred during testing and the dissimilarity of the states accounted for the performance differences.

Response Suppression in Appetitive Tasks

The ability of animals with destruction of the amygdala to inhibit responses has been studied in many types of tasks in which the animals work to obtain positive rewards. These studies should be considered in the context of the changes related to food and water regulation which may follow amygdala lesions. Unfortunately, the data available in the literature are not consistent. There are about as many reports of decreased food intake as of increased food intake after amygdala lesions (see Goddard, 1964a). In some cases, a decrease in food intake is found immediately after the lesion which is replaced by an increase later on. In addition, lesions of the amygdala can also lead to indiscriminate incorporation of inedible objects such as in animals with the Klüver—Bucy syndrome (Klüver and Bucy, 1939), which results from extensive damage to the temporal lobes (Rosvold et al, 1951).

Even though animals with amygdala lesions may become hyperphagic, they do not become overly motivated to obtain food. Rather, there is some evidence that cats and monkeys are less motivated to obtain food after amygdala lesions (Masserman et al., 1958) and are relatively insensitive to conditions of food deprivation and rewards (Schwartzbaum, 1960, 1961). Kemble and Beckman (1970) found that animals with amygdala lesions seemed to be less sensitive to the amounts of the incentives provided than were control animals but suggested that this was due to a perseveration of the speed of response first acquired with the initial incentive conditions.

This apparent perseverative quality of behavior after amygdala lesions could affect the outcome of experiments evaluating changes in food motivation, or not, depending on the design of the experiment. The necessity of examining any experiment to determine if the perseveration of first-learned responses could influence later testing is obvious.

A comparison of the ability to inhibit responses following amygdala or hippocampus lesions was undertaken by Schwartz-baum *et al.* (1964*b*). These investigators found that animals with amygdala lesions increased the number of responses made during conditions when reinforcements were not being obtained. These results tend to indicate an inability of the animal with amygdala damage to withhold responses under conditions of nonreinforce-ment. This effect was not found after small lesions of the hippo-campus (a reasonable control lesion) which indicates that the effect did not follow all limbic lesions, although this does not mean that such changes would not occur after more radical destruction of the hippocampus.

Schwartzbaum and Poulos (1965) found that amygdala lesions impaired the acquisition of successive reversals and learn-ing sets in monkeys. In their experiment, the monkeys were unable to withhold responses to irrelevant aspects of the stimuli and had trouble suppressing responses learned in the past but which no longer led to rewards. Reactions to the new "situations" presented by the reversal and learning set conditions lasted longer than in control animals. These results are not unlike those found after orbital frontal lesions in monkeys (Butter *et al.*, 1963). These similarities in lesion-produced effects could be expected on the basis of the strong interconnections between the amygdala and nearby temporal lobe areas and the orbital frontal regions of the monkey neocortex. A learning set impairment has also been found by Barrett (1969). Eleftheriou *et al.* (1972) found impaired learning of successive reversals in the deermouse following lesions in the cortical or basolateral amygdala but not after lesions of the medial nuclear group.

In a subsequent study, Elias *et al.* (1973) found that lesions of a particular area of the amygdala do not always produce the same kinds of behavioral effects in different strains of mice. Mice of the C57Bl/6J strain with damage to the lateral nucleus evidenced an impairment in learning the second reversal after damage to the medial nucleus, while mice of the BALB/cJ strain were impaired in learning the first reversal. This indicates that an appropriate analysis of lesion effects on behavior must include consideration of the animal strain used and the exact anatomical structures destroyed, as well as the behavioral requirements of the task. Henke *et al.* (1972) trained animals on two different reinforcement schedules in the same operant situation. The animals responded on two "signaled" variable-interval (VI) schedules each day. After behavior had become stable on the two concurrent schedules, one of the signaled VI schedules was changed to extinction. Normal animals showed greatly enhanced response rates in the periods during which they could obtain reinforcements on the remaining VI schedule and stopped responding in the nonrewarded periods. The animals with amygdala lesions did not show an increased rate of response during periods of reward on the remaining VI schedule but did stop responding in the nonrewarded periods. Hencke *et al.* believe that the increase in responding found in the normal animals reflects a heightened emotionality or arousal resulting from the frustration induced by the change of one of the VI schedules to extinction. The amygdala-lesioned animals respond less because their emotional reactivity is decreased by the lesion. However, the failure to increase responding on the still active VI schedule could also be interpreted as a perseveration of the previously acquired rate of responding. The emotional reactions of the animals with amygdala lesions could be as great as those of normal animals but their behavior need not reflect them. The same issue arises in connection with experiments in which an incentive is made less attractive. White (1971) has shown that animals with lesions of the amygdala perseverate in drinking a water solution adulterated with quinine to a greater extent than normal animals. This could be interpreted as an example of perseveration of behavior in the face of an unpleasant consequence of the response, although an explanation in terms of the raising of a threshold for unpleasant tastes could also explain these data. However, this threshold explanation cannot be applied satisfactorily to all types of situations in which perseverative behaviors are found after amygdala lesions. For example, Bagshaw and Pribram (1968) found that amygdala-lesioned monkeys had a *lower* threshold for responses to electrical stimulation of the skin as measured by the galvanic skin response. Despite this lower threshold, however, lesions of the amygdala eliminated the galvanic skin response component of the orienting reflex and prevented the galvanic skin response from being conditioned to neutral stimuli. Some discrepancies are to be found in the literature, however, since Pellegrino (1968) failed to find impairments in reversal learning following amygdala lesions in the rat. Pellegrino's results once again stress the importance of regional differences in the amygdala system. Using rats, he found that lesions of the basolateral nuclear amygdala, but not the corticomedial group, produced deficits in performance on problems in which a suppression of the response was necessary for success. The problems studied included a passive avoidance task, the DRL operant task (in which responses must be delayed for a given interval to obtain reinforcement), and a spatial alternation task. Performance on these tasks was possible for the lesioned animals only if external cues were provided.

Using the DADTA apparatus developed in Pribram's laboratory (Pribram *et al.*, 1962), which allows stimuli of various kinds to be displayed on any or all of 16 panels, Barrett (1969) studied the behavior of monkeys with amygdala damage as they learned to make responses to two stimuli in a specified order. In one condition, the monkeys had to respond in an experimenter-determined order; i.e., on the first opportunity they had to respond to the panel having an "H" displayed on it and on the second opportunity to respond to the panel with an "M" displayed on it. On both opportunities to respond, panels with both letters were displayed. The amygdalectomized animals learned this response faster than did intact monkeys. In Barrett's other condition, the numbers "4" and "8" were displayed on each of two opportunities to respond. To obtain a reward, the animals had to select on the second occasion the number they had not selected on the first occasion. In this task, the animals with amygdala destruction were substantially impaired. Barrett interpreted this impairment as a consequence of the animal's inability to use "internally ordered" sequences. However, there are several differences in the tasks other than whether the experimenter or the animal determined the order of responding to the two cues. For example, in the experimenter-selected order of response condition, the stimuli could appear in any of the 16 locations of the DADTA apparatus, while in the subject-determined order condition only four locations were used. Therefore, I do not believe that it is possible to conclude with absolute assurance that the significant difference between the two conditions is the method of selection of the order of responses to the stimuli. What is most interesting about Barrett's results is the superior performance of the amygdalectomized animals when they learned to respond to the "H" and "M" in order, despite the fact that the stimuli occurred randomly over the 16 panel locations. This entailed a visual search for the "H" and "M" and then the learning of the "H—M" sequence.

Transfer and Transposition

In a series of experiments, the ability of monkeys with lesions of the amygdala to transfer what has been learned in one task to a somewhat modified training condition has been studied. Some of these studies involve the use of a "transposition paradigm." For example, monkeys have been trained to respond to the lighter of two gray panels for a food reward. After acquisition of this problem, they were tested with the previously rewarded light gray panel paired with an even lighter gray panel. The normal monkeys responded to this altered condition by pressing the lighter of the two gray panels. They behaved as if they had learned to respond to the relative brightness of the two gray panels. However, the animals with lesions of the amygdala distributed their responses equally between the two gray panels when tested with the new lighter gray panel. This type of behavior would be expected if the lesioned monkeys perceived the changed test conditions as an entirely new circumstance, one unrelated to the former conditions of training (Schwartzbaum and Pribram, 1960). A similar observation was made by Bagshaw and Pribram (1965). They found that while normal monkeys trained to respond to the larger of two squares selected the larger of two new circles, amygdalectomized monkeys responded equally to the two new stimuli. Of special interest is the fact that animals with lesions of the amygdala generalized their responses in a normal fashion when tested for stimulus generalization.

Douglas (1966) has raised some serious issues about the conclusions drawn from the transposition experiments mentioned above. He points out that the study by Bagshaw and Pribram was actually an investigation of postoperative retention, with all of the training being given before surgery. The transposition tests were made after the removal of the amygdala. Douglas also points out that the transposition deficit found by Schwartzbaum and Pribram occurred only in one of two experiments reported in their article. The results of the second experiment with the same animals could be interpreted as indicating an exaggerated degree of transposition. The animals in the second experiment were given half of the trials with a medium gray matched against a light gray and on the other half of the trials they were given the medium gray with a dark gray. Responses to the medium gray were always reinforced. Normal monkeys quickly learned to respond to the medium gray, whereas the amygdalectomized animals made many more mistakes when the light gray and the medium gray were paired and few with the medium gray—dark gray pair. It was this pair that had been used in original training of the discrimination. Douglas argues that an enhanced degree of transposition would have led to the larger number of errors during testing with the two light shades of gray. In the first Schwartzbaum and Pribram procedure, only a few (12) test trials for transposition were given. To further study the problem, Douglas tested animals with amygdala lesions and with hippo-campus lesions and control animals in a transposition test where acquisition training was given postoperatively and more test trials were given. He found no evidence for a transpositional deficit in either group of lesioned subjects. For various reasons, Douglas believes that the seeming impairment in transpositional response found previously was due to the altered reactions to novel stimulus conditions found in the amygdalectomized animals. Errors produced by the enhanced novelty reactions were mistaken for the absence of transpositional abilities. In a subsequent paper, Douglas and Pribram (1969) found that lesions of the amygdala produced an exaggerated distractibility to novel stimulus conditions on the first occasion that a distracting stimulus was presented but that this overreaction soon habituated to levels of the control animals. Changes in the position or the nature of the distracting stimulus produced renewed distractibility of the lesioned animals which again declined rapidly in the monkeys with amygdala lesions.

If stimuli of the environment are to be used by the animal in guiding its behavior, they must be detected and evaluated. After lesions of the amygdala, or at least some portions of it, the animals give fewer signs of orienting toward unexpected stimuli (Bagshaw *et al.*, 1972) but can use the visual information if sufficient justification is provided. They can use these stimuli to form new behavior patterns and to pause in their reactions when the unexpected occurs (Douglas and Pribram, 1969). Under certain conditions they overreact to novel stimuli, and this can interfere with the efficient performance of an ongoing behavioral act.

But what is a novel stimulus? By experimental definition it is a stimulus which is unexpected, something added to the environment of the animal as it is engaged in a behavioral act. The performance of any behavioral act suggests that the animal has developed a set of hypotheses about its environment and the payoff of certain behavioral reactions in that environment. The animal has expectations about relevant and irrelevant aspects of the environment. The introduction of a new stimulus can be useful in obtaining rewards or relief from environmental oppressions or it can be irrelevant to them. Therefore, reactions to unexpected or to the expected stimuli can be useful or not, depending on the relationship of the stimulus to the payoff to be found in the environment.

A novel stimulus is one for which the animal is unprepared. It has not been evaluated for possible relevancy. It has not been tested for its potential contributions to behavior. The animal with destruction of the amygdala is reluctant to undertake the evaluation of novel stimuli unless it has good justification for so doing. This justification is based on the creation of a sufficient motivational state and the induction of a belief that there is a course of action open to the animal which will lead to attenuation of the motivational conditions. Thus if the animal is led to believe that differential responding to visual cues can improve its conditions, it can learn to do so. If it finds that running will lead to escape or avoidance of an electrical shock, it will do so. It is as if the animal with amygdala damage is reluctant to take the "first step," to begin a new form of behavior. Once it does begin, it can and will learn readily to do what is consistent with the reward structure of the environment. The reluctance to begin new acts includes those related to observing and investigation as well as to new forms of learned reactions.

Reflections and Summary

Based on anatomical, physiological, and behavioral considerations, the amygdala is clearly a heterogeneous structure. For some purposes it may be considered as a bipartite structure, but its functional divisions do not always correspond to the common nuclear divisions of a corticomedial and a basolateral subgroup. When stimulated, the more dorsal portions of the amygdala facilitate arousal reactions while the more ventral aspects produce a decrease in arousal and sleep. The association of the amygdala with food intake seems to be clearly demonstrable, but the actual effect, i.e., an increase or decrease, depends on the regions stimulated and on whether or not afterdischarges are produced.

The amygdala is associated with the expression of emotional behaviors, but once again whether or not the influence is facilitatory or inhibtory depends on the regions stimulated or destroyed. Stimulation arriving over the stria terminalis is likely to be inhibitory on the medial hypothalamus, and if the medial and lateral hypothalamic areas are reciprocally inhibitory this could produce an enhancement of many activities including those related to aggressive behaviors. The facilitation of fear and flight behaviors from stimulation of the anterior amygdala could represent a facilitatory effect on anterior regions of the hypothalamus, whether it be direct or mediated via inhibitory influences from the lateral systems.

On balance, the amygdala's contributions seem to be on the excitatory side. Lesions of the amygdala produce a tame and placid animal, one which apparently exhibits a trophotropic balance. The change may be in the amount of stimulation required to release aggressive behaviors, since the ability to demonstrate them is not lost.

Overall, animals with amygdala destruction seem to be characterized by a syndrome which includes an apparent insensitivity to certain types of environmental changes, greater tameness and placidity, and less interest in the social signals sent by other of their species. They seem to be content with their particular lot and relatively unconcerned about changes in the rewards given them or the conditions which motivate them to action. They seem loath to initiate new behaviors in many situations and are willing to give up established behavior patterns readily.

Chapter 4

THE SEPTAL AREA

As in the previous chapter, I am going to examine some of the behavioral effects produced by stimulation and lesions of the septal area, beginning with those of a general nature and proceeding to ones of greater specificity. The purpose is to understand the nature and diversity of these changes and hopefully to place them in a more general context based on the relationship of the septal area to the hypothalamus and other limbic system structures.

General Changes Following Septal Lesions

Emotionality

Rats and mice with lesions made in the septal area often exhibit increased rage reactions and hyperemotionality immediately after surgery. These characteristics are sometimes called the "septal syndrome" (Brady and Nauta, 1955). They disappear over time, usually lasting between 2 and 4 weeks. For some reason, these changes are not usually found in animals of other species. In particular, the hamster (Sodetz et al., 1967) and the monkey (Buddington et al., 1967) do not seem to exhibit a septal syndrome after lesions, although some hyperemotionality has been described in cats (Moore, 1964). The fact that the hyperemotionality dissipates rapidly over time after septal lesions in rodents stands in contrast to the long-lasting hyperemotionality found after lesions of the ventromedial nucleus of the hypothalamus (Singh, 1969) or after lesions of the olfactory bulb.*

While the septal syndrome becomes diminished after surgery, time alone is not the only essential factor. The more the animals are handled, the faster the hyperemotionality abates. In a recent report, Gotsick and Marshall (1972) found that with daily handling normal emotionality could be acheived as early as 6 days after surgery. If the animals were not handled for 6 days postsurgically, they were hyperemotional for the first day of handling (the seventh postoperative day) but not afterward. Some animals were handled 12 times on the first postoperative day, and within this day no decline in hyperemotionality was detected. This suggests that the reduction on hyperemotionality is due to a combination of handling and the simple passing of time. It is of special interest that when the animals had returned to "normal levels" of emotionality, they were actually easier to pick up and remove from their cages than normal animals.

The age of the animals at the time of lesion also affects the hyperemotional reactions of the animals. Lesions made shortly after weaning in Wistar rats produce only a transient period of hyperemotionality, whereas lesions made at 55—65 days of age produced more persistent effects (Phillips and Lieblich, 1972). Castration of the animals early in life prevented the enhanced emotionality from occurring after the septal lesions. However, for castration to be effective it must be accomplished before the thirtieth day of life.

In recent years, there have been several attempts to define the relationship of particular regions in and around the septal area to the "septal syndrome." Clody and Carlton (1969) have found an absence of the rage response and even a decrease in emotionality after lesions restricted to the medial septal nucleus. Turner (1970) has suggested that nuclei presumably associated

---

* Lesions of the olfactory bulb do not always produce a hyperemotional animal. Why these lesions sometimes do and sometimes do not produce hyperemotionality is unknown.

with the basal ganglia (nucleus accumbens septi) and in particular the long fiber tract from the amygdala to the hypothalamus, the stria terminalis, are more involved in the production of the septal syndrome than are the septal nuclei themselves. These results are in contrast to the work of Harrison and Lyon (1957), who found no structural or functional differentiation within the septal area insofar as the rage response was concerned. My own observations, although limited, indicate that the septal syndrome can be produced by lesions limited to the septal complex although there is no doubt that there are regional differences in the septal area in terms of the frequency with which the syndrome is produced by lesions.

As with lesions made in other limbic areas, the functional contributions made by particular subregions may not be entirely consistent from one animal to another even within the same species or strain. Nevertheless, if the septal area is lesioned in rats and mice, the transient periods of hyperemotionality and aggression are found quite frequently. It is difficult to evaluate the significance of this syndrome, however, since it is found only, or primarily, in rodents. It must be considered to be an important phenomenon, even if poorly understood, not because of what it tells us about the behavioral significance of the septal area, but because it offers a way in which transitory changes in the brain resulting from damage may be investigated.

After the initial hyperemotionality abates, rats with septal lesions still do not react in a normal fashion to stimulation. For example, animals with septal damage have been reported to be more sensitive to footshock than normal animals (Lints and Harvey, 1969). Lubar et al. (1970) found no difference in the footshock threshold of animals with septal lesions but did find that their reactions to the footshock were greatly enhanced, and I think this is probably the appropriate interpretation. It is not so much that the painful shocks are detected at lower levels of stimulation by the lesioned animals but rather that their reactions to the stimulation are greater.

In other experiments, septal lesions have been found to produce an increased sensitivity to light. Lesioned animals exhibit an exaggerated photophobic reaction (Donovick, 1968;

Green and Schwartzbaum, 1968). Flashes of light presented to the animals with septal lesions produce enhanced levels of locomotor activity relatively resistant to habituation. Since habituation occurs less with more intense stimulation, it suggests that the reactivity must be studied at various intensities of stimulation. It is also of interest that while the lesioned animals exhibit exaggerated motoric reactions to the light flashes, they exhibited progressively reduced visual evoked potentials, and on this basis the animals would be described as having greater habituation (Schwartzbaum et al., 1972a, b). This indicates that the effects of septal lesions on behavior and on electrical potentials may be quite different. Looking at either measure of "reactivity" alone would be misleading, revealing only one aspect of the effects produced by the septal lesions.

Exaggerated motor responses to various types of stimulation may characterize the animal with septal area destruction, as suggested by the increased reactivity to footshock described above, but this general overreactivity does not imply that the animals will be more ready to interact with their environment. Carey (1969) showed that lesions of the posterior septal area produced animals which seemed to be *less* motivated in operant tasks, based on responses produced to obtain a water reward, despite their well-established increase in *ad libitum* water consumption (see below). This suggests that while septal area lesions may change the animals' reactivity to external stimulation, they may not change the animals' readiness to engage in actions aimed at relieving or alleviating the stimulating conditions.

Water Consumption

An increase in the amount of water consumed by animals with septal lesions has been frequently observed (e.g., Harvey and Hunt, 1965; Donovick and Burright, 1968). It may be related to changes in the taste of various substances produced by the lesions. Beatty and Schwartzbaum (1968a) found that septal lesions enhanced the animals' licking of a sucrose solution at various concentrations, and in addition these authors showed that the increased sucrose intake could not be explained on the basis of either increased hunger or increased thirst. They suggested, as did Donovick *et al.* (1969), that the lesions alter the animals' reactivity to tastes by enhancing approach reactions to pleasant tastes and increasing aversive responses to unpleasant tastes. Such an observation was made by Carey (1971). In his study, animals with septal lesions took in less quinine-adulterated water while drinking more water with saccharin in it. Carey's results could not be explained on the basis of a change in taste threshold; rather, the animals had changed reactions to the tastes. In a recent study, Kemble *et al.* (1972) found that these accentuated taste aversions and preferences habituate rapidly and the differences between the lesioned animals and controls disappear with continued exposure to the test solutions.

The increase in water consumption found after septal lesions could be interpreted as an attempt to make normal laboratory food taste better through adulteration with water. Thus the increased water consumption would be secondary to changes relative to reactions to good and bad tastes. Nevertheless, hyperdipsia occurs when no food is available, as found by Harvey and Hunt. As a consequence, other supplementary explanations must be sought which go beyond those based on changes in taste alone.

The increase in water consumption found after septal lesions has been related to a deficiency in the secretion of antidiuretic hormone by Lubar *et al.* (1968, 1969). This suggests that the increase in water intake is secondary to an excessive excretion of water. Antidiuretic hormone (ADH) is responsible for the recirculation of water through the kidneys and affects the water volume lost through urination. A deficiency in ADH results in the secretion of a more dilute urine and a greater loss of water. However, Blass and Hanson (1970) have argued that the increase in water intake found in septal-lesioned animals is a primary effect on systems which control water intake. They showed that the amounts of water drunk by animals with septal damage were not directly related to the amount of water lost through urination as would be expected on the basis of a deficiency in ADH secretion. In addition, they found that the drinking patterns of animals with septal lesions did not correspond to those of animals with reduced amounts of saliva, i.e., dry throats, which should occur if water volume had been depleted. Further, they found no differences in blood levels of sodium and potassium between the septal-lesioned animals and controls. This means that the increase in drinking could not be due to a hyponatremia (sodium deficiency). On the positive side, they found that septal-damaged animals did overdrink after subcutaneous injections of polyethylene glycol. This compound reduces the total amount of an animal's plasma volume. On the basis of all these observations, they suggest, therefore, that the increased water consumption of the animals with septal lesions is due to a disruption of a neural system which normally initiates, maintains, and terminates drinking in response to a decrease in the total fluid volume of the body.

Social Behavior

Animals of different species do not respond in the same way to septal lesions. Rats with septal lesions tend to be hyper-emotional and gregarious in open-field situations, but this has not been observed in hamsters (Johnson et al., 1972). Poplawsky and Johnson (1972) have shown that the increase in sociability, as measured in increased contact time among animals and greater submissiveness, arises from medial but not lateral septal lesions. A complicating factor in interpreting these results has been introduced by MacDougall et al. (1973). These authors report that while septal area lesions enhance the social contacts made by one subspecies of the deer mouse (gracillis), the lesions actually reduce the social contacts made by a subspecies which is less social (bairdi). This suggests that the effects produced by the lesions cannot be considered independently of the genetic endowments and characteristic behavior patterns of the animals. Indeed, the lesion effects may be best interpreted as potentiating the predominant behavioral tendencies of the animals, including those which are provided by their genetic endowments, but possibly those which have been acquired, also.

Animals with septal lesions tend to interact well with other members of their species and make a decreased number of aggressive responses to stimuli which normally induce such responses. Slotnick and McMullen (1972) found that mice with septal lesions were poor fighters. They were always defeated by normal animals. Their response to aggression exhibited by other animals was to run away, even when they had had experience in winning fighting bouts before the lesions were made. However, the septal lesion does not produce an inability to fight but rather a reluctance to do so. For example, enhanced fighting, induced by electrical shocks, was found in rats with septal damage when they were tested 85 days postoperatively (Wetzel et al., 1967). No increase in emotionality ratings was found in these animals at that time. As with the septal syndrome, the intensity of shock-induced fighting becomes less and less after surgery. The decline in the intensity of shock-induced fighting in septal-lesioned animals depends on the housing of the animals, among other things. If the animals are caged with other animals during the postoperative period, the enhanced tendency for shock-induced fighting disappears within 17 days. On the other hand, if the animals are housed by themselves, the animals show this exaggerated reaction up to 45 days postoperatively (Ahmad and Harvey, 1968).

Eichelman (1971) also found that septal lesions enhance shock-induced aggressive behaviors and in addition has reported a decrease in such behaviors after destruction of the amygdala.

The stimuli responsible for intraspecies aggressive acts are quite different from those leading to shock-induced fighting. Perhaps the discrepancy found between the two measures is related to changes in the threshold of the stimulation required to elicit aggression. In studying the effects of septal lesions in hamsters, Sodetz and Bunnell (1970) found increases in the aggressiveness of their submissive subjects. The animals were still submissive after the lesions but engaged in fighting behaviors more frequently than they had before. Apparently, the lesions had not made the animals incapable of exhibiting aggression but had made most animals less likely to do so under certain conditions.

Activity

Gotsick (1969) has studied the open-field behavior of animals with septal lesions and made comparisons with the behavior of animals with hippocampal lesions. He reports that animals with septal lesions did not exhibit the overall increase in activity exhibited by animals with hippocampal lesions. However, the animals with septal lesions had a high initial level of activity when first placed in an unfamiliar testing situation. The activity habituated rapidly and soon reached a level below that of the normal animals. The animals with hippocampal lesions did not have as high an initial value but habituated much less. Thus, as has been reported before (Douglas and Isaacson, 1966), the heightened exploration of animals with hippocampal destruction arises mainly from a failure in the habituation of exploration activity. At least this is true for animals with hippocampal lesions when activity is measured 2 or 3 weeks after surgery. Animals with septal lesions and hippocampal lesions also differed in their reactivity to the introduction of unfamiliar stimuli and the initiation of food or water deprivation. Both of these procedures increased the activity of animals with septal lesions but not the activity of animals with hippocampal lesions. The fact that the septal-lesioned animals show a rapid habituation of open-field activity to levels below that of normal animal fits with other observations that open-field activity is reduced after such lesions (Schwartzbaum and Gay, 1966; Corman et al., 1967).

Animals with septal lesions tend to become immobile, i. e., to exhibit gross bodily freezing responses, less frequently than control animals (Blanchard and Fial, 1968; Duncan, 1971; Trafton and Marques, 1971). The same reduction in freezing has been found after hippocampal lesions (Lovely et al., 1971). This reduction in bodily immobility under conditions of stimulation or stress may be related to the observation that animals with septal damage do not keep a bar in an operant chamber depressed for as long periods of time as normal animals. In effect, this allows them to make more responses per unit of time than animals which make a response and hold the bar down longer. Depending on the requirements of the task presented to the animal, this could be advantageous or not.

Changes in Performance on Learning Tasks After Septal Lesions—Avoidance Behaviors

Damage to the septal area produces many types of changes in the behavior of animals as they are trained in specific problems designed to test learning and memory. These are best considered in terms of the types of tasks with which the animals are confronted and the circumstances used to motivate the animals. First to be considered will be performance on tasks in which the animals attempt to avoid noxious stimulation. It is on these tasks that the behavioral effects of septal lesions have been most extensively studied.

Research on the effects of septal lesions on avoidance tasks gained significance and impetus from the work of McCleary. His hypothesis was that such lesions would impair mechanisms responsible for the suppression of behavioral acts (McCleary, 1961; 1966), although related work had begun several years earlier (e.g., King, 1958). McCleary undertook to extend the ideas of Kaada (1951), who found facilitation or inhibition of autonomic activities after stimulation of many limbic system regions. McCleary had the idea that these same areas might facilitate or inhibit somatic responses and even well-defined behavior directed toward specific environmental goals.

Accordingly, he made selective lesions in various limbic system areas, among them the tissue underneath the genu of the corpus callosum, including the septal area. It was in this region that Kaada had found inhibitory effects on autonomic activities resulting from electrical stimulation. McCleary found that animals with lesions in this region were inferior to other animals in their ability to suppress behavior in certain tasks, including those in which the animals had to stop responding to avoid punishment. On the other hand, the lesioned animals were not impaired in the learning of an active avoidance task.

Lesions in the cingulate cortex produced just the opposite effect. This was of interest since the cingulate area was one in which electrical stimulation facilitated autonomic activities. Thus the combination of the results obtained by McCleary and by Kaada produced a remarkable correlation between the effects of lesions and electrical stimulation in limbic structures. Behaviorally, some lesions impaired passive, but not active, avoidance learning, while other lesions did just the opposite. The lesioned areas which caused an impairment in the passive avoidance task were those which when stimulated inhibited autonomic activities. Some of these were in the septal area.

An impairment in the acquisition of passive avoidance tasks after septal lesions has been found by many authors (e.g., Kaada *et al.,* 1962; McCleary, 1961; Lubar, 1964). In addition, an impairment in withholding or suppressing responses (i.e., the passive avoidance deficit) is not restricted to training conditions in which electrical shock is used as the deterrent. When their drinking water is adulterated with quinine (0.025 M quinine hydrochloride), animals with septal lesions continue to drink more than do normal animals (Brown *et al.,* 1971). It should be mentioned that the evidence is not entirely uniform. For example, Gittelson *et al.* (1969) found greater response suppression in rats with septal lesions when quinine was used instead of electrical shock in a passive avoidance task. The apparent discrepancies in the literature probably are related to the conditions of testing the animals, and the results obtained in any particular experiment probably represent an exaggerated responsiveness to both absolute and relative tastes (e.g., Flaherty and Hamilton, 1971). They also may arise from an impaired ability to terminate established response sequences. In addition, Flaherty *et al.* (1973) have also shown that the time between the exposure to a particular taste and subsequent testing with a different taste plays an important role in determining the reactions of the animals with septal damage. These authors rewarded animals with a 32% sucrose solution and then tested them after vacations of various lengths from the training procedure with a 4% sucrose solution. The 32% solution is greatly preferred to the 4% solution. If a 4-day interval was imposed between the last day of 32% reward and testing with the 4% solution, normal animals still responded poorly to the new reward while the animals with septal lesions did not. Flaherty *et al.* believe this indicates that the animals with septal lesions forget their experiences with the favored solution more readily than normal animals and consequently fail to show the usual depressive effect when tested with the less preferred solution after even a few days' intermission between tests.

Septal lesions produce an enhanced acquisition of two-way active avoidance problems. This observation was first reported by King (1958). This effect has been demonstrated in several strains of rats (Deagle and Lubar, 1971), guinea pigs

(Lown et al., 1969), mice (Carlson, 1970), and squirrel monkeys (Buddington et al., 1967). In a few studies, this facilitation has not been observed. For example, LaVaque (1966) found no difference between animals with septal lesions and normal animals in the acquisition of the two-way active avoidance problem, and Dalby (1970) also failed to find the facilitation. In the Dalby experiment, however, a high hurdle was used to differentiate the two types of compartments. Some motor actions may be difficult for animals with limbic damage, and the motor demands presented by the hurdle could interfere with the expression of what is being learned. In addition, the cues differentiating the two compartments of the shuttlebox are of importance. F. A. King (personal communication) found that the greater the differentiation of the compartments, the *less* facilitation will be shown by animals after septal damage. When the compartments are poorly differentiated, the septal animals will show enhanced performance relative to that of the normal subjects. The same thing has been shown in animals with hippocampal lesions, which are also facilitated in the two-way active avoidance problem (Isaacson, unpublished observations). The effect of the cues provided to differentiate the two compartments is to make the problem more or less difficult for the normal animals. Normal animals learn least well when the two compartments are the same color and best when they are different colors. A barrier can also help to differentiate the compartments provided it is not so high as to impede crossing between the two sides of the apparatus. Animals with septal or hippocampal lesions seem to learn the task as quickly under well-differentiated conditions and poorly differentiated conditions. Therefore, the best conditions for demonstrating the superiority of the animals with septal or hippocampal damage are those which make the problem most difficult for the normal animals, since it is against their performance that the enhanced responding of the lesioned animals will be shown.

While the septal lesions seem to produce animals which acquire the two-way active avoidance response more readily than normal animals, there are also reports that these lesions interfere with the acquisition of a one-way active avoidance problem (Kenyon and Krieckhaus, 1965; Liss, 1964, cited by Deagle and Lubar, 1971; Vanderwolf, 1964). All of these studies were done with hooded animals, and Deagle and Lubar suggest that an impairment of one-way active avoidance conditioning is not found after septal lesions in the albino rat. This hypothesis, however, has not been supported. For example, Hamilton (1972) was able to find a substantial deficit in one-way active avoidance using albino rats. Of special interest is the fact that the deficit was in terms of when the first avoidance response was made. After making the initial avoidance response, the animals with septal lesions quickly acquired the problem. This type of deficit is like that found in the learning of active avoidance tasks by animals with damage to the amygdala. In addition, Hamilton was able to show that animals with the septal lesions were insensitive to manipulation of the cues provided in the training environment. This imperviousness to irrelevant environmental cues in a training situation is also found after destruction of the hippocampus.

By and large, animals with septal lesions trained in avoidance tasks seem similar to animals with hippocampal destruction. Both types of animals show an enhanced rate of acquisition in the two-way avoidance task and an impairment in the acquisition of the one-way avoidance task. It should be emphasized that the changes in learning these tasks found in animals after septal area or hippocampal destruction are always relative to the performance of normal animals.

The facilitation of performance in avoidance tasks is not restricted to the two-way problem. Duncan and Duncan (1971) found improved acquisition of operant avoidance tasks, using both signaled and unsignaled footshocks, in animals with septal lesions. Similar results have been reported by Morgan and Mitchell (1969). Sodetz (1970) found that rats with septal lesions acquired an operant avoidance task more readily than controls and that this facilitation of performance could not be accounted for on the basis of a greater number of responses made by the lesioned animals. Schwartzbaum et al. (1967) showed the enhanced performance of septal-lesioned animals in the two-way active avoidance problem to be independent of shock level, the strength of the conditioned stimulus, the ambient level of illumination, and the gross hyperactivity of the animals. This contribution was especially important because it showed that the improvement in active avoidance conditioning shown by such animals was not secondary to heightened locomotor activity levels in these animals. This result was supported by the results of the study of Buddington *et al.* (1967) with the squirrel monkey.

Destruction of the neocortex can produce an impairment in the two-way active avoidance problem. However, if a septal lesion is made in animals which also have neocortical destruction, a facilitation in performance is obtained (Meyer *et al.,* 1970). A similar result has been found in studies of the effect of hippocampal lesions (Olton and Isaacson, 1968). It is tempting to think that the limbic lesion somehow overrides the changes induced by the neocortical lesion. However, it is also possible that the neocortical and the limbic lesions affect quite different aspects of behavior and that those produced by the neocortical damage are less influential in affecting avoidance behaviors than those resulting from septal area or hippocampal damage. This difference in interpretation could be most important. If the septal damage acted to "cure" the animal suffering from neocortical destruction, this would indicate a convergence of the effects of the two types of brain damage on the same output systems. If the two lesions act independently on behavior, then they probably act on different output systems. One approach to the matter would be to try to establish specific changes in behavioral tactics or strategies produced by the neocortical lesions and then to determine if these remain despite other behavioral changes produced by the subcortical lesions.

Response Inhibition in Appetitive Tasks

Another experimental approach to the response inhibition hypothesis presented by McCleary uses tests in which the animals are required to suppress established responses to obtain rewards when environmental contingencies change. Impairments following septal lesions have been found by several groups of researchers when training animals to perform on DRL operant schedules where animals must wait a predetermined number of seconds between responses (Burkett and Bunnell, 1966; Ellen *et al.,* 1964; Mac-

Dougall *et al.,* 1969). This impairment takes the form of an inappropriately high rate of responding and a decrease in the number of reinforcements obtained under DRL schedules. If the DRL paradigm is modified to make it into a discrete trial procedure, the abilities of the lesioned animals are not improved (Van Hoesen *et al.,* 1971). However, the impairment cannot be attributed to a failure of response inhibition, since Kelsey and Grossman (1971) used a shuttlebox DRL-30 task in which the septal-lesioned animals made more errors of "anticipation" than of "perseveration." In this task, the animals were trained to shuttle between two compartments, alternating presses on pairs of levers placed in each of the two compartments. To make a correct response, the animals had to wait 30 sec between the time a reinforcement had been produced and the time the next response was made. An anticipatory error was made by moving into the other compartment and responding on a lever in it before 30 sec had elapsed. This suggests that the DRL impairment is not due to a simple failure to inhibit responses. It is as if the animals could not restrain themselves from activating a learned strategy of behavior which involved several, alternating motor responses.

Animals with septal lesions show altered patterns of responding in fixed-interval and fixed-ratio schedules (Ellen and Powell, 1962*a, b;* Lorens and Kondo, 1969; Schwartzbaum and Gay, 1966). Higher than normal rates of responses were found in these schedules. The behavior change is especially prominent in the higher ratios of responses to rewards (Hothershall *et al.,* 1970). Johnson and Thatcher (1972) found that animals with septal destruction showed higher response rates on fixed-ratio schedules only when they were under strenuous food deprivation. The dependency of the excessively high response rate in fixed-ratio schedules on the nature of the motivational circumstances was also supported by Harvey and Hunt (1965). These authors found that a reduction in the deprivation of the lesioned animals allowed them to exhibit more adequate performance levels on schedules where reinforcements were given intermittently.

The ability of an animal to reverse a learned habit can be considered to be an indicator of the ability to suppress previously acquired responses. An impaired reversal of position habits was found by Zucker and McCleary (1964) and Schwartzbaum and Donovick (1968). Gittelson and Donovick (1968) also found a deficit in the reversal of a discrimination learned on kinesthetic cues. Once again, however, there is evidence that the septal lesion effects cannot be entirely explained on the basis of the failure to suppress specific responses. Animals with septal lesions can learn to switch from responding on a lever to which responses are no longer rewarded to one on which they are reinforced as quickly as control animals, despite their higher than normal response rates (Schnelle et al., 1971).

A number of studies using different behavioral paradigms have shown that animals with septal lesions are slower to extinguish responses than control animals in appetitive tasks (Butters and Rosvold, 1968; Pubols, 1966; Schwartzbaum et al., 1964a) and in the two-way active avoidance task (LaVaque, 1966). Perhaps the most interesting report is that the degree of resistance to extinction in animals with septal lesions depends on both the motivational circumstances of the animal and its past training history (Fallon and Donovick, 1970). Furthermore, there is evidence that animals with septal lesions can, under certain circumstances, extinguish their responses as fast as, or faster than, normal animals. For example, Brown and Remley (1971) found responses made to escape from footshock to be extinguished at the same rate by animals with septal lesions as by normal animals. In addition, Fallon and Donovick (1970) found faster extinction relative to control animals when the animals with septal lesions were tested under changed motivational circumstances.

A comparison can be made between the behavioral effects of septal and caudate lesions. Septal lesions impair the reversal of a spatial discrimination problem. Caudate lesions produce just the opposite effect: an impaired brightness discrimination reversal but not a spatial discrimination reversal (Schwartzbaum and Donovick, 1968). This suggests that the septal-lesioned animals are more capable of attending to, and/or utilizing, information from the external world in the form of brightness cues than they are in some tasks in which spatial locations must be associated with rewards. Dalland (1970) has noted that animals with septal area damage tend to perseverate responses to the relative brightness of two arms of a T-maze when they are being tested for spontaneous (nonrewarded) alternation of responses to the two arms. In contrast, she found that animals with hippocampal destruction tend to perseverate responses to the positions of the two arms of the T-maze. The fact that the animals with septal area damage seem to be most responsive to prominent visual cues, namely those used by experimenters to indicate correct responses or to differentiate arms of a T-maze, and less responsive to the visual (and other) cues indicating spatial location may seem to be at odds with data obtained from active avoidance conditioning studies. In such experiments, the animals with septal lesions do best, relative to normal animals, when the compartments of the shuttlebox are poorly differentiated. I suspect, however, that the lesioned animals may simply learn *to run* or to change their locations in the two-way active avoidance task and that they learn this regardless of the interior cues of the apparatus. What they learn, i.e., movement, may be quite different from that learned by intact animals. The latter may associate spatial locations with foot-shock contingencies. If this interpretation is correct, the animals with septal damage could evidence high levels of performance in the active avoidance task despite an impaired ability to use information about spatial localization. Furthermore, their impairment in passive avoidance tasks could reflect a failure to have made an association between a particular location and the punishing event. The animals with septal damage may have learned "signal means run," whereas the intact animals learn "signal means go to place *X*." The point of greatest interest is the possibility that the animals with septal lesions could be learning a qualitatively different response than are the intact animals. When the animals with septal damage perseverate responses after punishment in the passive avoidance task, they may be harder to suppress than the association of a place with punishment. On the other hand, it is possible that the septal damage produces a relative tendency to perseverate any acquired response strategy in the face of non-reward or punishment.

Some additional problems for the notion that septal lesions produce an inability to inhibit specific responses come from a study by Carlson *et al.* (1972). These authors found that septal-lesioned mice easily acquired differential running speeds on alternate trials in a straight runway when rewards were given only on every other trial. The lesioned animals also showed differential running speeds when rewards were not given on alternate trials but rather on signaled trials presented on a random basis. However, a difference was observed in performance of the lesioned and nonlesioned mice. The septal-lesioned animals learned best when a signal was given before nonrewarded trials, whereas the normal animals learned best when the signal preceded rewarded trials. Other problems for the response suppression hypothesis come from experiments demonstrating enhanced two-bar lever-press alternation (Carlson and Cole, 1970) and enhanced go, no-go alternation in an operant task (Carlson and Norman, 1971).

The evidence seems clear that a failure to inhibit specific responses is not characteristic of the animals with septal area destruction. They can learn solutions to problems which require responses to be made on an alternating basis and to use signals appropriately. If they have difficulties which are usefully described in terms of perseverative tendencies or a failure of inhibition, these must be considered in terms of a perseveration of an approach or strategy used to attack the problem. More generally, however, the most prominent characteristic of animals with septal lesions is a heightened tendency to initiate responses and an intolerance of waiting. They learn tasks quickly and once they have learned them seem ready to perform quickly and effectively.

Electrical Stimulation of the Septal Area

Electrical stimulation of the septal area was found by Olds and Milner (1954) to produce what appear to be rewarding effects in rats, and similar results have been found in other species. The septal area contains many regions from which rewarding effects can be obtained when electrically stimulated. The question arises, however, as to the mechanisms whereby these rewarding effects are achieved and how the septal area interacts with other brain regions which are also related to rewarding events. To study these questions, Miller and Mogenson (1971a) implanted electrodes into both the septal area and the lateral hypothalamus. Animals were trained to depress a bar to obtain electrical stimulation of the lateral hypothalamus at both low and high current levels. As might be expected, the animals responded at higher rates for the high-intensity stimulation. The animals were then tested with electrical pulses delivered to the septal area just before each pulse was applied to the hypothalamus. This produced an increase in the self-stimulation rate when the hypothalamus was being stimulated with low-intensity currents but a decrease in response rate when the hypothalamus was being stimulated by high-intensity stimulation. A similar result has been found by the same authors in a study of the effects of septal stimulation on hypothalamic unit activity. Stimulation of the septal area augmented neuronal discharges when activity was low but decreased them when activity was high (Miller and Mogenson, 1971*b*). These investigators interpret their data in accord with a model in which the septal area and hypothalamus exert mutual modulating influences on each other. They suggest that different fiber systems which course between the two areas may have different functional roles. The dorsal fornix system arising from cells in the dorsal and midline septal area is thought to exert facilitatory influences on the hypothalamus and the stria terminalis system, which contains fibers arising from cells in the ventral septal region thought to be inhibitory on the hypothalamus. These authors also note that Kant (1969) has proposed that two fiber systems in the medial forebrain bundle modulate the septal area in an antagonistic fashion. Thus the effects of stimulation of a large region of the septal area could activate two systems which exert antagonistic influences on the hypothalamus and other brain regions.

Some brain stimulation seems to produce pleasurable or rewarding effects, while stimulation applied to other brain regions produces effects which can be described as painful or aversive. What are the interactions between these two opposite effects produced by brain stimulation? In a preliminary report in 1963, Routtenberg and Olds found that stimulation of the septal area at an intensity below that required for maintaining self-stimulation attenuated escape reactions elicited from electrical stimulation of the tegmentum. This suggested a direct antagonism between rewarding and punishing effects produced by brain stimulation, at least as these two brain regions are concerned and under conditions in which the escape responses are produced by brain stimulation as opposed to peripheral shock. Subsequent investigations have extended this line of work by studying the effects of rewarding and punishing states elicited by central stimulation on aversive reactions produced by either brain or peripheral stimulation. Gardner and Malmo (1969) located sites in the ventromedial region of the septal area which produced aversive reactions when electrically stimulated. The dorsal and lateral regions of the septal area produced the pleasurable or rewarding effects on stimulation. Using these positive and negative rewarding zones of the septal area, Gardner and Malmo then studied the effect of stimulation of these zones on the time required for animals to escape from aversive stimulation induced in one of two ways, i.e., by electrical shocks applied to the skin of the neck or by stimulation of the dorsal tegmentum. They found that septal stimulation in the positively reinforcing zone of the septal area slowed down latencies for escape from the tegmental stimulation, whereas septal stimulation of the negatively reinforcing zones of the septal area facilitated the escape latencies. On the other hand, stimulation in either septal region shortened escape latencies when peripheral shock was applied to the skin of the neck.

The difference between pain produced by peripheral noxious stimulation and by central noxious stimulation is, of course, of considerable interest. For example, painlike responses produced by stimulation of dorsal tegmental sites do not seem to habituate, e.g., decrease with repeated periods of stimulation. This type of stimulation tends to produce an "arrest reaction" or immobility. The animals seem to habituate to the painful electrical shocks delivered to the neck, and these shocks do not produce arrest or immobility. In addition, it must be remembered that electrical stimulation applied to the skin of the neck may produce quite different effects from those produced by footshock. Breglio *et al.* (1970) have found a decrease in responsiveness to electrical footshock as a result of septal stimulation.

It is unfortunate that the animals cannot simply tell us whether the septal area stimulation makes the aversive stimulation seem more or less intense. Such reports might make the interpretation of the interaction between rewarding and punishing effects more understandable. As it is, we must fall back on hypotheses and inferences about the animals' behavior, and there are several different ways in which the data from the experiments of Routtenberg and Olds, Gardner and Malmo, and Breglio *et al.* can be explained. One possibility is that stimulation of some septal regions activates those behavioral tendencies which are predominant at the time of stimulation. This could be accomplished over the dorsal pathway described by Miller and Mogenson, mentioned just above. This behavioral activation could occur whether or not rewarding effects are also produced by the stimulation. Thus stimulation of the dorsolateral "rewarding" sections of the septal area would potentiate the running induced by shocks applied to the neck or the freezing responses induced by stimulation of the dorsal tegmentum or by footshock. When the running response is facilitated, the escape latencies are reduced and the escape reaction is accomplished more swiftly. When the freezing response is facilitated, the time required to escape is increased. This could be considered as reflecting an antagonism between the septal stimulation and the effects of the punishing electrical shocks. This sort of explanation is similar to that reported earlier with regard to the similar effects of medial and lateral hypothalamic lesions on escape reaction (pp. 79–80).

Finally, the question of the effects of medial–ventral septal area stimulation should be considered. This stimulation has been reported to facilitate escape reactions to *both* central and peripheral stimulation of an aversive quality. Probably the simplest form of explanation is the assumption of the elicitation of a direct aversive effect which adds to the existing negative state. This greater total amount of discomfort or pain would make for a greater urgency in executing the escape response. While this is an economical explanation at the present time, it seems almost too simple.

Ultimately, I believe, the medial septal area will be best understood in terms of mechanisms influencing hypothalamic or brain stem mechanisms rather than altering the experience of pain. The terms "pain" and "pleasure" must themselves be explained in terms of neural mechanisms involved. One approach would be the assumption that the medial septal area acts to intensify the predominant behavioral tendencies of the organism. Therefore, this stimulation could potentiate either aversive or appetitive motivations depending on what systems have been induced by the environment and by the past history of the organism.

Electrical stimulation of the septal region given before the onset of the conditioned stimulus has been shown to facilitate both one-way and two-way active avoidance conditioning (Carder, 1971). Electrical stimulation of the septal area also has been shown to disrupt performance in spatial reversal problems (Donovick and Schwartzbaum, 1966) but not the two-bar alternation problem. In this task, animals were trained to run between two compartments. Each compartment had two levers in it. The animals had to press the bars in an alternating sequence in each compartment. In addition, as described above, the animals had to wait 30 sec between bar presses to obtain a reward. Electrical stimulation of the septal region did not affect performance in this task, whereas the performance was impaired by lesions of the septal area (Schwartzbaum and Donovick, 1968).

Autonomic Effects Produced by Septal Stimulation

Electrical stimulation of the septal area produces several types of effects, and to this point we have been primarily concerned with those related to behavior in learning situations or circumstances in which an animal depresses a bar or lever to produce stimulation of its own brain. These behavioral effects may be related to changes in the activity of the internal organs mediated by the autonomic nervous system. The effects of septal area stimulation on the autonomic nervous system were studied extensively by Kaada (1951). He found that septal area stimulation generally produced inhibitory effects on the autonomic nervous system in the anesthetized animal. These observations led to the general inhibitory theory of septal area function postulated by McCleary (1961), mentioned before.

One direction of more recent work has been that of Holdstock and his collaborators. In one study, he found that electrical stimulation of the septal area produced a cardiac deceleration without any effect on the galvanic skin response (Holdstock, 1967). This effect was reduced by the systemic administration of methyl atropine or atropine sulfate, and consequently it was thought to be mediated by cholinergic fibers of the vagus nerve (Chalmers and Holdstock, 1969). On the other hand, Sideroff *et al.* (1971) believe that the bradycardia resulting from septal area stimulation is a result of compensatory rebound from a brief period of sympathetic activation. These authors detected increases in blood pressure resulting from septal area stimulation and considered the delayed, more prominent, cardiac deceleration to be a parasympathetic rebound. These authors also found a difference in the effects produced by stimulation in the lateral and in the medial septal areas. Stimulation of the lateral septal area produced a decrease in heart rate, whereas stimulation of the medial septal area produced a brief increase followed by a long-lasting decrease. Previously, Malmo (1965) had reported a cardiac acceleration from stimulation in the medial septal region.

Holdstock (1970) found normal acquisition of differential heart rate responses to different stimuli following septal lesions. He also found a clear dissociation between the increases in motoric activity and increases in the activity of the autonomic nervous system, and felt that a good general description of his results would be that the animals had lost normal sympathetic reactivity under certain conditions.

Stimulation of the septal area can influence drinking elicited by hypothalamic stimulation. Sibole *et al.* (1971) found that concurrent stimulation of the medial septal area region and the hypothalamus facilitates drinking, whereas electrode locations in, or near, the bed nucleus of the stria terminalis produce a reduction in drinking. These results are related to presumed differences between the fibers of the fornix and stria terminalis systems mentioned above. Chronic stimulation of the septal area decreases spontaneous drinking, even the drinking of animals which have been deprived of water for 24 hr. Of special interest is the fact that the septal stimulation does not reduce the incidence of drinking but shortens the duration of the drinking bouts (Wishart and Mogenson, 1970*a*).

Neurochemical Considerations

Proper understanding of the relationship of the septal area to behavior depends on understanding the role of the septal area in the various neurochemical systems of the brain. Lesions in the septal area have been found to produce decreased levels of acetylcholine in the cortex and in the hippocampus, but not in the brain stem (Pepeu *et al.,* 1971). Sorensen and Harvey (1971) found that the decrease in acetylcholine in the cortex occurred only in rats which were also made hyperdipsic by the lesions. But acetylcholine is not the only presumed neurotransmitter which decreases in the forebrain after septal lesions. Lints and Harvey (1969) found that the lesions produced a decrease in cortical serotonin levels, as well. Stimulation of the septal area has been shown to increase the acetylcholine output of the neocortex (Szerb, 1967), and Pepeu *et al.* (1970) found that the acetylcholine output does not increase in the neocortex of animals with septal lesions following the administration of amphetamine as it does in intact animals. Acetylcholine release from the neocortex may not be a sensitive or specific indicator of limbic system activities, since the release of this presumed transmitter substance from the cortex probably reflects the general arousal level of the animal more than it does the activity of specific neural systems.

The cholinergic blocking agent atropine when injected into the septal area produces animals deficient in passive avoidance behavior but unimpaired on position reversal and on the learning of a one-way active avoidance response. This indicates that the cholinergic blockade of the septal area produced by the atropine reproduces some, but not all, of the effects produced by lesions (Hamilton *et al.,* 1968). It does not affect activity or photophobia (Kelsey and Grossman, 1969). Cholinergic blockade in the medial and ventral aspects of the septal area produces enhancement of acquisition in the two-way active avoidance task. This mimics the effects produced by septal lesions. Since hippocampal lesions also produce a facilitation of two-way active avoidance learning (see p. 171*ff*), this may indicate that the septal–hippocampal system which mediates these activities is cholinergic in nature. In fact, Warburton and Russell (1969) have suggested that there is a cholinergic path of reticular formation origin which courses through the medial septal area and reaches the hippocampus. Whether or not this pathway is excitatory or inhibitory relative to behavior is uncertain, since while cholinergic stimulation often affects performance in avoidance tasks this need not be a sign of a general inhibitory effect. Holloway (1972), for example, found that carbachol injections into the medial septal area reduced the number of avoidance responses made by cats while at the same time shortening the latency of the avoidance responses which were made. Greene (1968) has reported that carbachol injections into the medial septal area increased open-field locomotor activity. These observations suggest that there are effects generally considered to be excitatory in nature which result from cholinergic stimulation of the septal area. Most likely, the effects of chemical stimulation of the septal area can best be considered in terms of specific changes induced and not in terms of more global behavioral changes such as alterations in excitability.

Septal lesions influence a variety of neurochemical systems in the brain, and therefore it is not surprising that such lesions influence the behavior of animals to adrenergic stimulation. There is evidence that different behavioral consequences of septal area lesions are selectively affected by amphetamine (Novick and Pihl, 1969). Novick and Pihl found that the drug produced an enhancement of locomotor activity in animals with septal lesions. A dose of 3 mg/kg produced incessant exploration and pacing to a greater extent than produced in control animals. The 9 mg/kg dose used by Novick and Pihl produced the stereotyped head-moving responses associated with large doses of amphetamine (probably owing to increased activity in the dopaminergic systems) described by Randrup and Munkvad (1972) equally in both septal-lesioned and sham-operated animals. Amphetamine did not alter the improved two-way active avoidance performance or the impaired passive avoidance behavior of the animals with septal lesions. At high levels of amphetamine, the drug did impair control animals in the passive avoidance task, but it was at this drug level (9 mg/kg) that the animals had greatly reduced locomotor activity in the open-field situation. In normal animals, high levels of amphetamine decrease locomotor activity but increase reactivity to unexpected stimuli, e.g., noise, air puff, or being captured, to a level near that of the septal-lesioned animals without the drug.

In the study by Holloway mentioned above, the effects of norepinephrine introduced into the medial septal area were partially antagonistic to those produced by the carbachol. These injections increased the latency of avoidance responses. In a recent study in my laboratory, Baisden (1973) has found that the destruction of adrenergic terminals in the septal area by 6-hydroxydopamine does not mimic all of the effects of electrolytic destruction of the septal area, although it does modify the behavioral effects of hippocampal destruction.

Reflections and Summary

The septal area is of special interest since it occupies a a central position between the paired hemispheres of the brain. Because of its central position, it resembles a funnel for impulses going to other forebrain areas.

The phenomenon of septal rage, found primarily if not exclusively in rodents, remains a conceptual problem, and the possibility that it is a consequence of damage to other neural systems rather than to septal nuclei themselves must be considered. Furthermore, regional differences within the septal area must be considered since lesions restricted to the medial septal area produce a tame animal rather than one with heightened emotionality.

The septal area seems to be more concerned with the regulation of water than of food intake, although it may also have some important influences on the animal's reactions to the tastes of both.

Animals with septal lesions show exaggerated reactions to a number of changes in the environment. These include reactions to footshock and aversion to light. Despite this overreactiveness, there is little change in the animals' desire to do something about the conditions leading to the enhanced reactions.

Septal lesions result in animals with an enhanced tendency to flee from opponents and to run in an active avoidance task. The facilitation found in two-way active avoidance tasks after septal lesions is not tied to heightened emotionality levels or to other procedural variables. There is a distinct possibility that animals with septal lesions may learn a different response than normal animals in avoidance tasks.

Animals with septal area destruction show an enhanced acquisition in two-way active avoidance tasks but are impaired in learning to withhold responses in passive avoidance tasks. They also are impaired in withholding responses on DRL schedules, but this deficit is linked to the degree of food or water deprivation to which they have been subjected.

A review of available information indicates that it is unlikely that an inability to withhold responses is a suitable explanation for the behavioral effects produced by septal area damage. Perhaps the most viable description of the lesioned animals is one which emphasizes their eagerness to undertake responses, intolerance of delays, and their readiness to acquire new behavioral problems of several different kinds. There is a suggestion that the lesioned animals may be deficient in using the spatial localization of rewards as the determining characteristic for new learning or reversals, but this defect is by no means absolute.

In other situations, electrical stimulation of the septal region seems to facilitate many types of behaviors, and it may activate whatever behavioral tendencies are dominant in the animal at the time the stimulation is applied.

If the transient hyperemotionality and "rage" which mark the rodent after septal area damage are ignored, the general characterization of such animals indicates them to be ones which are easily handled and have a pleasant disposition. They are gregarious, sociable, submissive, and difficult to arouse in social combat. Even so, the lesioned animals show greater reactivity toward many forms of environmental changes of both a positive and a negative character. The animals show some of the characteristics of animals with medial hypothalamic damage; e.g., they are finicky over their food and drink and react as if at least certain of their behaviors were released from chronic regulatory control.

Even on the basis of the incomplete evidence available, important differences must exist within the septal complex. The failure of researchers to consider the significance of the anatomical and functional differences within the septal region probably has led to some unnecessary confusions in the results reported in the experimental literature. The differences between the dorsolateral and the ventromedial septal areas need to be stressed even though they are probably not the only regional differences of significance. Speculations concerning the dorsolateral and ventromedial differences can, of course, take many forms, but my disposition would be to consider the dorsolateral septal area to be associated with systems regulating ongoing behavioral sequences and the ventromedial regions to be associated with the motivational systems. Following this line of thinking, both divisions of the septal area would exert regulatory influences on the hypothalamus and midbrain mechanisms. The dorsolateral aspect of the septal area would have its influence directed toward the lateral hypothalamus and the ventromedial division would affect medial hypothalamic systems. Electrical or chemical stimulation which is effective in activating cells in these two regions should potentiate either the predominant behaviors or the predominant motivational circumstances of the animal. Possibly, stimulation effective over a wide enough region would activate both. Lesions in the septal region could disrupt behavioral or motivational aspects of performance, depending on the location of the damage.

It is tempting to put these differences into an evolutionary perspective. Perhaps the association of the medial septal area with the medial hypothalamus reflects an early evolutionary development. The lateral septal region may have developed hand-in-hand with the lateral hypothalamus. The relationship of the dorsolateral and ventromedial divisions of the septal area to the hippocampus (to be discussed later) also suggests the importance of this division for the understanding of limbic system activities.

While this differentiation between regions of the septal area is of importance, there is undeniable evidence that the effects of septal area stimulation or lesions depend on the genetic endowment of the animals, their past histories, and their ongoing activities when behavior is evaluated.

Chapter 5

THE HIPPOCAMPUS

In this chapter, I will attempt to describe some of the behavioral contributions made by another of the limbic system structures, the hippocampus. I will follow the approach of the two preceding chapters, discussing the general changes produced by hippocampal destruction or stimulation first.

General Changes Produced by Hippocampal Damage

Two prominent changes in the behavior of animals after hippocampal destruction are (1) a greater willingness to undertake new behavioral acts and (2) a decreased tendency to become inactive or immobile under conditions of fear or stress. In essence, they are active animals, eager to begin new behavioral sequences, although they often fail to persist in a particular goal-oriented action as long as intact animals. In many ways, these changes are similar to those found after damage to the septal area. The increased tendency to be active and the reduced tendency to become immobile can be found in situations of significance to the animals. For example, when confronted by a cat from which there is no escape, rats with hippocampal lesions tend to be more active and to exhibit fewer freezing responses than do control animals. When they can escape from the cat, rats with hippocampal damage do so more rapidly than normal animals (Blanchard and Blanchard, 1972). In normal animals, fear can lead to attempts at active escape or immobility (freezing), but the animals with hippocampal lesions are more likely to respond with an active response than by freezing. The reduction in the number of freezing responses exhibited by animals with hippocampal lesions could be related to a decrease in the intensity of fear elicited by the threatening stimulus. Kim *et al.* (1971*b*) found a reduction in aggressive acts following hippocampal lesions. These authors also reported the animals to be less fearful in general. This may be related to the observation that hippocampal lesions also tend to produce a reduction in shock-induced aggression, which is independent of changes in the threshold of the animals to the electrical footshock (Eichelman, 1971). But, if fear is reduced after hippocampal lesions and if this is related to the reduction of the immobility response, the relationship may be complicated, since (1) a reduction in fear could cause a reduction in freezing, (2) a reduction in freezing could produce lessened fear, (3) a reduction in freezing could cause fewer behavioral signs of fear but the animals could have internal fear responses of an intensity equal to those found in normal animals, or (4) both the decrease in the immobility response and the reduction in fear could be caused by alterations in independent neural mechanisms. Certainly alterations in fear responses cannot account for the changes found in active avoidance paradigms in which the animals with hippocampal lesions learn some problems (e.g., two-way active avoidance) more readily than intact animals.

Animals with hippocampal lesions tend to have normal circadian rhythms. However, during the daytime, when sleep is the predominant occupation of nocturnal animals, rats with hippocampal lesions tend to sleep less than control animals (Jarrard, 1968; Kim *et al.*, 1970). Even though the animals sleep less during the day, the occurrence of sleep episodes and of slow-wave sleep actually increases within the daylight period. Fast-wave sleep (REM sleep) is reduced, probably due to the reduction of the length of sleep episodes. Lesions restricted to the neocortex also produce a reduction in the occurrence of REM sleep. The results of Kim *et al.* (1971*a*) show that animals with hippocampal lesions show an increase in the frequency with which many behavior patterns, including sleep, are undertaken but the durations of the activities are so much less that the total time spent in them is also less than that of normal animals.

The greatest increase in activity of all varieties is found at night, when rats with hippocampal lesions seem greatly energized (Jarrard, 1968). In addition, rats and mice with hippocampal damage seem to be most aroused during conditions of dim illumination. This implies an interaction of conditions of ambient illumination and the effects produced by the lesion.

Some forms of activities show a consistent pattern of increases in the frequency with which they are undertaken without a change in the total time spent in them. In one report by Kim et al. (1970), these behaviors included visitations to the foodwell and grooming during the evening hours. Glickman et al. (1970) found that gerbils with hippocampal lesions tend to engage in many activities more frequently than their normal counterparts, even though the total time spent in the activities is unchanged or even reduced. All of these results indicate a heightened activity of the systems associated with the initiation of behavioral sequences.

Locomotor Activity

It is now well established that animals with hippocampal lesions exhibit enhanced locomotor activity in certain types of situations. A number of studies, reviewed by Douglas (1967) and Kimble (1968), have reported this hyperactivity in open field situations. The enhanced activity seems to result from a failure of the lesioned animals to reduce their locomotor activities within a testing session or between days. On the other hand, hyperactivity is not found when the animals are tested in small test chambers or in activity wheels. Therefore, it would be a mistake to consider the animals as hyperactive under all circumstances. They only are hyperactive in test situations where there is adequate space for extensive locomotor activity. DeFries and Hegmann (1970) have shown that in the mouse, at least, there are several independent genetic factors related to specific types of activity. Running in activity wheels and locomotion through open fields represent two genetically independent factors. The data from experiments with animals suffering hippocampal lesions also testify to the independence of these two factors, since the animals are slightly active in activity wheels but more active in open fields.

Recently, McClearn and Isaacson have studied the effect of hippocampal lesions on the activity of mice inbred to be high or low in locomotor activity. Lesions of either the hippocampus or the posterior neocortex produced increased activity in the low-activity strain but a decrease in the activity of the high-activity strain. The reduced locomotor activity found in the high-activity strain was surprising, and in an attempt to further understand these results the level of ambient illumination was reduced from the moderate levels normally used for testing. Under the low level of ambient illumination, mice of both strains with hippocampal destruction were more active then animals with neocortical lesions or the sham-operated control animals. These results highlight the need to understand lesion-induced changes in locomotor activity in terms of the genetic endowments of the animals and the conditions under which behavior is being evaluated.

Furthermore, even though heightened levels of activity have been found in many species after hippocampal damage, the motivational conditions of the animals being tested must also be considered. For example, Jarrard and Bunnell (1968) found that hippocampal lesions did not alter open-field activity in the hamster when tested under conditions of satiety. However, if the hamsters were deprived of food, the lesioned animals increased their activity in the open-field apparatus beyond that of control animals. The pattern of the hyperactivity in the hamster was different from that found in the rat after hippocampal lesions. In the hamster, activity actually *increased* over the testing sessions.

When activity is repeatedly measured beginning just after surgery and continuing over several months, systematic changes are observed. There is an initial increase which reaches a maximum about 1 week after the hippocampal destruction and then a decline to a stable level which is attained about 3 weeks postoperatively. This stable activity level of the animals with hippocampal lesions is greater than the activity level of control animals (L. Lanier and R.L. Isaacson, unpublished observations), and it appears to be permanent. Not all types of brain damage produce permanent hyperactivity. For example, the enhanced locomotor activity resulting from destruction of the frontal regions of the rat neocortex gradually becomes attenuated over time (Campbell *et al.*, 1971). Hyperactivity can be also found after lesions of the transitional cortex outside of the hippocampus itself. In the cat, Entingh (1971) found that damage to the entorhinal cortex, just below the ventral hippocampus, produces a hyperactivity. Similar lesions of the entorhinal area have been shown to produce a deficit in passive avoidance behavior (Van Hoesen *et al.*, 1972).

Despite the increases in exploratory activities found after hippocampal destruction, the lesioned animal fails to use the information gained from its locomotor excursions effectively. Kimble and Greene (1968) discovered that animals with bilateral hippocampal damage fail to use information derived from pretraining exploration of a Lashley III maze in subsequent acquisition training. While being trained to navigate the maze, animals with hippocampal destruction which had investigated the maze more actively than normal animals were no better off than animals which had not done so. The problem may be the assumption that increased locomotor activity implies a greater amount of "exploration." The term "exploration" implies an investigative attitude, an orientation toward environmental stimuli, and the processing of information derived from the activity. This implication probably is not justifiable in the case of animals with hippocampal damage. The fact is that such animals exhibit more locomotor activity, but the significance of this activity is, as yet, unknown.

Wimer *et al.* (1971) have made correlations between the relative size of the hippocampus and open-field locomotion. They found that the larger the hippocampus the smaller the amount of activity. This is a suggestive result, but so far Wimer *et al.* have examined only the size of the hippocampus and there may well be other anatomical correlates of the increased activity.

Distractibility

Animals with hippocampal destruction seem to be less distractible while performing goal-oriented behavioral acts. Early studies on the behavioral distractibility after hippocampal lesions indicated that these animals were less disturbed by the introduction of irrelevant stimuli into the middle of a runway while working for food rewards when hungry (Wickelgren and Isaacson, 1963; Raphelson *et al.*, 1965). A distinction must be made between distractibility and reactivity. "Distractibility" refers to the extent to which a goal-oriented set of actions is disrupted by an unexpected stimulus, whereas "reactivity" refers to the magnitude of the animal's reactions to the unexpected. Animals with hippocampal lesions are sometimes more reactive than intact animals to unexpected stimulation. For example, gerbils with hippocampal destruction respond more intensely to intense levels of auditory or visual stimulation in stabilimeter cages than normal animals (Ireland and Isaacson, 1968). The startle responses elicited by auditory stimulation are also increased by hippocampal destruction in the rat (Coover and Levine, 1972).

Recent research has stressed the importance of the ongoing behavioral sequence in determing the degree to which animals with hippocampal lesions will be distracted by novel or unexpected stimuli. Kaplan (1968) found that animals with hippocampal lesions are not influenced by extraneous stimulation in making approach responses only if they have been trained and are actively executing the learned response. Normal orientation to novel auditory or visual stimulation is found if the stimulus is presented when the lesioned animals are inactive (Hendrickson *et al.*, 1969). A related observation indicates that the animals with hippocampal lesions do not orient toward novel stimuli when performing a predominant response in a specific situation but have normal reactions to novel stimuli (which also habituate in a normal fashion) if their behavior is not dominated by some ongoing, prepotent response sequence (Crowne and Riddell, 1969).

There are several reports of decreased habituation by rats with damage to the hippocampus (e.g., Douglas and Isaacson, 1964; Roberts *et al.*, 1962; Teitelbaum and Milner, 1963). A similar deficit was found by Douglas and Pribram (1969) in monkeys. These animals show no signs of habituation to the repeated presentation of a distracting stimulus as measured by the speed with which the response is made. On the other hand, habituation *is* found if the number of actual responses toward the distracting stimulus is counted. These results point out an important difference between response and speed measures of distractibility and habituation. Apparently, they should be considered as independent processes, ones which are subject to separate processes of habituation. The speed measure (latency of response) is most likely to be affected by hippocampal destruction.

Alternation

The tendency for animals to alternate visits to the two goal boxes of a T-maze on consecutive trials without providing a reward for responses to either goal box has been called "spontaneous alternation." In a sense, it reflects an unlearned tendency of animals not to repeat visits to the same goal box regions on two consecutive opportunities. Animals with bilateral hippocampal destruction do not exhibit this spontaneous alternation behavior, as a rule. In a series of carefully controlled experiments, Douglas (1966) demonstrated that spontaneous alternation in normal animals arises from a tendency of the animal to visit alternately the *spatial locations* of the two goal boxes in two-choice T-mazes. The normal animal does not alternate the specific stimuli of the arms of the maze or the responses of turning to the right or to the left at the choice point. This is important because it suggests that the deficit produced by the hippocampal lesion is one which involves the spatial organization of the animal's environment. Specifically, Ellen and DeLoache (1968) have presented additional evidence that an inability to use spatial cues is found in animals with dorsal hippocampal lesions and this could result in the impaired spontaneous alternation performance. However, it must be pointed out that small electrolytic lesions of restricted regions of the hippocampus are rarely effective in altering spontaneous alternation. Usually, large, almost complete, bilateral lesions are required. The inability to use spatial location as a cue in learning tasks is a suggested consequence of septal lesions, as mentioned in the previous chapter.

Douglas (1974) believes that the close correlation found between the time of onset of behavioral alternation during development and the time of maturation of cells of the dentate gyrus implies a causal relationship. This is a fascinating correlation, and the presumption of a causal relationship may be correct. Furthermore, the work of Douglas and his associates makes it almost certain that the cholinergic systems of the brain are strongly associated with spontaneous alternation. Spontaneous alternation is abolished by scopolamine (Douglas and Isaacson, 1966; Meyers and Domino, 1964). Treatment with physostigmine can induce spontaneous alternation in rabbits at very early ages (Baisden et al., 1972).

Since animals with hippocampal destruction were impaired in the nonrewarded spontaneous alternation tests given in a T-maze, it was natural to ask whether they could be trained to exhibit other response alternation by the use of rewards. Jackson and Strong (1969) showed that animals could learn long sequences of response alternation in a two-bar operant situation. In their task, animals had to press first the right bar and then the left bar to obtain a reinforcement. Subsequently, the animals were trained to make longer strings of alternated responses on the two bars in order to obtain a reinforcement, i.e., R-L-R-L, etc. These authors found that the animals with hippocampal lesions could learn the alternation of lever presses more readily than normal animals. Using a discrete trial procedure, Means et al. (1970) found the same type of result. However, Buerger (1970) did not have success in training cats on an alternation problem in an operant chamber, unless these animals had had preoperative training in the task. However, his animals suffered relatively small lesions in the extreme ventral portions of the hippocampus. The damaged area included the entorhinal cortex as well as some portions of the amygdala.

Dalland (1970) reported that animals with limbic system lesions tended to perseverate their responses in a T-maze instead of alternating them. This result is related to the theory of Lash (1964). While a "response-inhibition" deficit cannot explain all of the behavioral debilities produced by hippocampal destruction, animals with hippocampal lesions may, in fact, tend to perseverate responses in some situations. This may be because the animals are not able to utilize information about the spatial location of the goal boxes as normal animals do and fall back on other sources of information. They must respond on the basis of less preferred cues, e.g., the stimuli in the arms of the T-maze or the stimulation produced by the responses themselves. Therefore, the results obtained by Dalland and Lash may have been correctly interpreted; the animals may have been basing their behavior on response-produced information in these T-maze studies. The problem is, however, that it should not be assumed that animals with hippocampal lesions will always, and in every case, rely on or perseverate to such information. On the basis of recordings made from single cells in the CA1 and CA4 areas of the hippocampus, O'Keefe and Dostrovsky (1971) have suggested that the hippocampus provides the animal with a spatial map of the environment. These authors found that eight of 76 single cells responded only when the animal was in a particular place on the recording platform and oriented in a particular direction. On this basis alone, it would suggest that approximately 10% of the cells from which recordings were made had special place and directional characteristics. Most of the cells from which recordings were obtained were not responsive to specific places or directions. Therefore, while the data of O'Keefe and Dostrovsky are suggestive, they do not prove the hippocampus to be responsible for creation of environmental maps.

Relations to the Autonomic Nervous System

Kaada (1951), in his classic study of the effects produced by limbic system stimulation, failed to find any effect produced by hippocampal stimulation on respiration or blood pressure in cat, dog, or monkey. These initial results of Kaada have been frequently supported (e.g., Koikegami et al., 1957; Koikegami and Fuse, 1952; Pampiglione and Falconer, 1956). On the other hand, some contrary observations were made by Votaw and Lauer (1963), who found that stimulation of the hippocampus in the anterior portions of the temporal lobe reduced respiration and heart rate. This initial depressive response was followed by increases in both measures. Recently, Kaada et al. (1971) returned to the investigation of the effects of hippocampal stimulation on heart rate and respiration in both awake and anesthetized animals. Some small and transient effects were found when the hippocampus was first stimulated, but these quickly habituated. Further stimulation did not alter heart rate or respiration. No stimulation-induced effects were found when the stimulation was applied during a CS which signaled shock or on the decrease in heart rate and respiration normally found when smoke was blown into the rabbit's nose. In addition, hippocampal afterdischarges failed to alter heart rate or respiration. Their conclusions support the original results obtained by Kaada (1951) in that the hippocampus remains one of the few "autonomically silent" regions of the limbic system.

On the other hand, some changes in heart rate responses to stimulation have been found after septal or hippocampal lesions. For example, Sanwald *et al.* (1970) found that heart rate habituation to a series of tones was decreased following septal or hippocampal lesions. Somewhat contrary to this result, Jarrard and Korn (1969) reported habituation of the heart rate in animals with hippocampal damage while they were engaged in a locomotor exploratory task even though their activity did not habituate. In another respect of their study, the heart rate of animals with hippocampal lesions increased after a single shock experience in a passive avoidance training task where the heart rate of animals with neocortical lesions and of normal animals decreased after shock. The heart rate effect found in the animals with hippocampal lesions was short-lived, however. By the second trial after the shock, identical heart rates were found in animals of all groups, despite the fact that the hippocampal-lesioned animals still exhibited impaired passive avoidance. Thus heart rate and behavior were not closely related in their study. Nevertheless, the heart rate response of the animals with hippocampal lesions on the first postshock trial was not only different in magnitude from that of the control animals but also different in nature.

Endocrine Relations

A number of studies have tried to determine relationships between the pituitary–adrenal hormones and the hippocampus, but such studies have not always been successful. Nakadate and deGroot (1963) found identical morning and afternoon levels of the 17-hydroxysteroids after fornix lesions in rats. This indicated that the circadian rhythms of the hormone release might have been altered by the lesion. Moberg *et al.* (1971) found a reduced circadian cycle in the measurements of corticosterone after section of the fornix and attributed this both to a rising of the lowest levels and to a decrease in the highest values. Some of the difficulties encountered by earlier investigators in trying to establish hippocampal–endocrine relationships may have come from the fact that the effect of hippocampal activity on the pituitary–adrenal axis depends on the activities of the animal and its past history. This is clearly shown by the opposite effects which can be produced by hippocampal stimulation when applied under different circumstances. Kawakami *et al.* (1968) stimulated the hippocampus under stressful and nonstressful conditions. Under the stressful condition the stimulation inhibited the level of corticosteroids, while under the nonstressful condition their release was facilitated. Thus, depending on the state of the animal, stimulation of the hippocampus could produce an increase or a decrease in the adrenal steroids.

Using a different approach, Pfaff *et al.* (1971) gave ACTH or corticosterone to adrenalectomized rats while recording the activity of single neurons (pyramidal) in the hippocampus. Corticosterone decreased hippocampal unit activity about 45 min after injection. On the other hand, ACTH increased hippocampal unit activity within 3–10 min after the injection. Data recently collected in my laboratory indicate that this same time course can be followed in intact animals anesthetized with urethane (Lanier, Lanthorn, Isaacson, in preparation). ACTH had a facilitatory effect on neurons in dorsal hippocampus shortly after injection, but it did not affect neurons more ventrally located in the hippocampus until 40–60 min after the injection. This increase was presumed to be due to the secondary release of corticosterone from the adrenal glands instigated by the ACTH injection. However, even though the pituitary and adrenal hormones can influence the activity of cells in the hippocampus, this does not mean that these cells are the mechanisms whereby the hormones produce their behavioral effects. Indeed, there is reason to believe that the effects of ACTH and vasopressin are produced through the action of these hormones on cells in the posterior thalamus and the reticular formation and not in the hippocampal formation (Van Wimersma Greidanus and deWied, 1969, 1971; Van Wimersma Greidanus *et al.*, 1973).

Studies of Learning and Memory— Avoidance Conditioning

The facilitation of two-way active avoidance conditioning and an impairment in the one-way active avoidance conditioning and passive avoidance problems after hippocampal damage are now reasonably well documented in several species. Olton (1973) points out that it is necessary to understand the cues used by subjects of different species in establishing avoidance responses. Spatial cues are important for rats in learning this problem. If rats with hippocampal destruction are deficient in the use of spatial cues in learning, this could help to explain the effect of the hippocampal destruction, as was pointed out for septal area lesions. For example, the intact animal may associate the locations of both sides of the two-way active avoidance chamber with painful shocks and therefore hesitate to approach either place. The hippocampal-lesioned animal, if it suffers from an inability to utilize information about the spatial locations of the goal boxes, is less likely to be able to make an association of a spatial area with the electrical shock. Consequently, the animal should experience less conflict about returning to a location in which shocks had been received and consequently establish the shuttle-box behavior more rapidly. The deficit in the one-way avoidance task should be due to the fact that the animal is less likely to establish an association between the location of the box into which it is placed and the punishing shocks. The location of the other "safe" compartment should also be less well established. A similar explanation which might hold for passive avoidance deficits could be adopted.

Also, as mentioned in the previous chapter, the inability to utilize information about spatial location could make the lesioned animal learn a different response than that of the intact animals. Animals with hippocampal damage, like those with septal lesions, may learn "to run" at the sound of the warning signal rather than to run to a particular place as intact animals may.

Isaacson et al. (1961) were the first to document the more rapid acquisition of two-way active avoidance tasks in rats. However, 20 years earlier Allen (1941) had shown that dogs with bilateral hippocampal destruction could acquire an olfactory discrimination, and many of his lesioned animals acquired the task more rapidly than the control animals. The study by Isaacson et al. (1961) actually stemmed from unpublished observations by Dr. Corneliu Giurgea and me to the effect that dogs with bilateral hippocampal destruction acquired a leg-lift avoidance response faster than normal animals.

Since these early studies, more rapid acquisition of a number of different types of problems has been found subsequent to hippocampal damage. Duncan and Duncan (1971) found that hippocampal destruction facilitated the learning of an operant avoidance task but impaired the learning of a visual discrimination problem in a T-maze task based on the avoidance of footshock. The failure to find a facilitation of learning in the T-maze avoidance task could be due to either an impairment in the ability of the animal to use the brightness cues or a difficulty with the spatial aspects of the T-maze, or both. Woodruff and Isaacson (1972) have found that animals with hippocampal lesions are sometimes deficient in acquiring brightness discrimination tasks in an operant situation, although most often the lesioned animals can learn a brightness discrimination in a T-maze at about the same rate as intact animals. However, the rate of learning does not tell the entire story, and there are reasons to believe that the animals with hippocampal lesions learn such problems in a different manner than control animals (Isaacson and Kimble, 1972). Using other techniques and species, faster acquisition of a nictitating membrane response has been found in rabbits (Schmaltz and Theios, 1972). Rabbits have also been shown to exhibit faster acquisition of the two-way active avoidance response and impaired passive avoidance behavior following hippocampal lesions (Papsdorf and Woodruff, 1970).

A deficit in passive avoidance tests subsequent to hippocampal destruction has been found in several species (e.g., Isaacson and Wickelgren, 1962; Nonneman and Isaacson, 1973; Papsdorf and Woodruff, 1970). However, the effect depends on the location and size of the lesion within the hippocampus, the specific requirements of the task (Snyder and Isaacson, 1965), and the strength of the tendency of the animal to make the approach response which is punished. The strength of the approach response is difficult to specify with precision. The tendency to make a response depends on the training given the animal in the task, the motivational circumstances (usually the amount of deprivation), and the value of the incentives provided. In 1966, Kimble et al. reported that animals with hippocampal lesions had to receive specific training in the to-be-punished approach response if a deficit was going to be found. This suggestion was given further support in an experiment by Stein and Kirkby (1967). However, Isaacson *et al.* (1966) did not find specific training to be necessary provided that sufficient motivation was used to induce the response. At that time, I believed that the important factor was the total behavioral tendency to make the approach response and not the training per se (Isaacson, 1967). The strength of the approach response can be manipulated through training *or* through adjustments in the motivation of the animals or the incentives used. The trick is to get the lesioned animal sufficiently disposed to make the particular response. Once this is achieved, punishments, lack of rewards, novel stimuli, and other events disturb the lesioned animals less than the normal animals.

Wishart and Mogenson (1970*b*) found that if experiences with passive avoidance procedures were given before surgery, hippocampal lesions did not produce animals with a passive avoidance deficit. This, of course, is in general support of the view that the effect of the hippocampal lesion somehow fixates the predominant behavioral dispositions of the animals. It also demonstrates that animals with hippocampal destruction are not categorically unable to inhibit responses.

Most often, exposing animals to a stimulus before training has been shown to decrease the ability of that stimulus to serve as a signal once training is started. Ackil *et al.* (1969) studied the effects of presenting a tone to animals before it was used as the CS in a two-way active avoidance task. Giving 30 exposures to the tone before conditioning retarded the learning of both normal animals and animals with neocortical lesions. Not only was the acquisition of the task impaired, but also the number of responses made during extinction was reduced. In other words, preexposure to the signal made learning more difficult and more fragile. The learning of the animals with hippocampal lesions, however, seemed unchanged by the preexposure to the CS. They learned the task quickly and were more resistant to extinction, whether or not they had received the pretraining exposure to the CS. The presentation of the tone before training did affect other behaviors of the animals with hippocampal destruction, however. For example, Ackil *et al.* recorded the locomotor activity of all animals as the tone was being presented before training in the shuttlebox. They also recorded locomotor activity on the day before training for groups of animals not exposed to the tone before training. The activity of animals with hippocampal lesions placed in the shuttlebox the day before training started, but not given the tone, was extremely high relative to that of all other groups. The activity of animals with hippocampal damage placed in the apparatus and given the 30-tone presentations was the same as found in the control groups.

Olton and Isaacson (1969) investigated the nature of the deficit found in animals with hippocampal destruction in the one-way active avoidance task. They found that this deficit could be greatly reduced if the animals were given a number of trials in which the CS was paired with the electrical footshock on the day before the training in the avoidance task was begun. If the CS and footshocks were given to the animals in a nonsystematic way, the animals were not helped when the one-way active avoidance training was begun. These results suggest that the lesioned animals have some difficulty in associating the CS with the painful events motivating behavior, but why this should be so in the one-way task yet not in the two-way task remains to be explained.

Learning in Appetitive Tasks

The performance of animals with hippocampal lesions engaged in acquiring tasks based on obtaining incentives like food or water, when hungry or thirsty, is sometimes different and sometimes the same as that of intact animals. One of the main goals of researchers is, therefore, to determine on which tasks the lesioned animals are impaired and from this information to formulate adequate theories of the behavioral characteristics altered by the lesions. Animals with hippocampal damage are not greatly different from normal animals in learning to press levers in operant chambers for food or water rewards when the rewards are provided after each lever press (continuous reinforcement). Their behavior does become unusual when certain types of reinforcement schedules are used by the experimenter, especially those in which the animal must wait between bar presses to obtain rewards, i.e., the DRL schedule. This reinforcement schedule was first used with animals with hippocampal lesions to test their ability to withhold responses by Clark (Van Hartesveldt) and Isaacson (1965). It was felt that if the lesioned animals suffered from a general inability to inhibit responses, they would perform poorly on the task.

The DRL Impairment

The impairment of animals with hippocampal lesions on DRL schedules has now been established in several species. The deficit has two aspects: a greatly exaggerated rate of response and a reduction in the ratio of reinforced responses to total responses (efficiency). Obviously these two characteristics are not entirely independent. High rates of response almost certainly will produce low efficiency scores, but there is some reason to doubt that the complete explanation of the deficit shown by animals with hippocampal damage is their higher rate of response. For example, certain drugs can alter the animals' rates of response without changing efficiency scores (Van Hartesveldt, 1974).

The DRL impairment is an example of a deficit which occurs when the lesioned animals are trained with one schedule of reinforcement and then transferred to another. This produces an uncertainty about the reinforcement contingencies in their training environment. When animals with hippocampal lesions are changed from one set of training contingencies to another, their behavior becomes greatly activated relative to that of normal animals. This has been found both for DRL schedules and for variable-interval schedules (Jarrard, 1965). This conclusion is based in part on the results obtained by Schmaltz and Isaacson (1966), who demonstrated that it was the *change* from the continuous reinforcement conditions to a partial or intermittent reinforcement schedule which was debilitating. Animals with hippocampal lesions entirely trained under DRL reinforcement contingencies, including those procedures used to establish the bar-press response in the first place, were not impaired. The DRL impairment is but one example of a more general behavioral anomaly which is found when the animals are subjected to alterations in the environment.

When training animals on a DRL schedule, usually no cue is given to signal the end of the delay period. Animals must depend on internal cues of some kind to determine the appropriate delay between responses. Pellegrino and Clapp (1971) found that when an external cue is provided to signal the end of the delay period, subjects with hippocampus or with amygdala lesions can perform adequately on the task. This result has been replicated by Van Hartesveldt and Walker (1974). In addition, these latter authors determined whether or not some extraneous behaviors could be used by the lesioned animals to help "time" their responses. They gave animals objects to manipulate, such as blocks of wood to gnaw during the delay period. These added objects did not help the rats with hippocampal lesions gauge the appropriate waiting interval on the DRL-20 task. The animals with hippocampal damage chewed the blocks of wood more than did the control animals, but they did so while maintaining extremely high response rates on the DRL task. Improvements were found only when a specific signal was given to indicate the end of the delay period.

The impaired DRL performance exhibited by animals with hippocampal destruction might be due to a heightened level of motivation. This hypothesis was investigated by Carey (1969). He compared the performance of animals with hippocampal lesions tested under a 23.5-hr water deprivation with those of normal animals at the same level of deprivation, or at 1 or 2 additional days of deprivation. He found that the response rates of the animals with hippocampal lesions were greater than those of the normal animals under all deprivation regimes. This strongly suggests that the behavioral alteration of the animals with hippocampal destruction is not due to increased thirst. Studying cats with hippocampal damage, Nonneman and Isaacson (1973) found that the rate of response under continuous reinforcement conditions was diagnostic for the degree of impairment suffered when the animals were shifted to the DRL schedule. Animals with hippocampal lesions having high response rates under CRF showed exaggerated response rates, ones well beyond those of normal animals when shifted to the intermittent schedule. Animals with lower response rates under CRF did not have as large increases when the schedule requirements were changed. On the other hand, the response rate under CRF was not a determinant of effective performance for normal cats. Regardless of their response rates under CRF, intact animals could adjust them downward to create the appropriate-length pauses required to obtain reinforcement.

Discrimination Learning

In most experiments, animals with hippocampal damage have been reported to have little trouble with the learning of visual discrimination problems. By and large, the early studies trained animals in a two-choice maze fashioned as a T or Y. As will be reported below, it is now clear that animals with hippocampal damage do not behave as do normal animals in such problems. Whether or not a substantial difference between normal and lesioned animals is found depends on several characteristics of the training situation. Beyond this, however, there is evidence that hippocampal lesions can affect visual discrimination learning even when tested in operant situations.

Woodruff and Isaacson (1972) found that bilateral destruction of the hippocampus greatly impaired the learning of a visual discrimination in an operant paradigm. Rats were trained to respond to the lever over which a small light was illuminated in a two-lever operant chamber. In this original study and a subsequent replication using a slightly modified procedure (Woodruff *et al.*, 1972), the animals with hippocampal damage failed to show any signs of learning of the discrimination problem over 10–20 days of training. These results were surprising in light of the older data, especially those from maze studies, which had revealed relatively rapid learning of visual discriminations by the animals with hippocampal damage.

Kimble (1961, 1963) studied the acquisition of simultaneous and successive brightness discrimination problems using a Y-maze. These names of the discrimination tasks refer to two conditions in which black and white cardboard inserts were placed in the two arms of the maze. In the simultaneous discrimination, the animals were confronted with a gray starting arm (the base of the Y) and, at the choice point, with one black arm and one white arm. These arms formed the top arms of the Y. A food reward was given at the end of either the black or the white arm, depending on the arbitrary designation of which was to be considered "correct" for a particular animal. The location of the white or black insert in the right or left arm of the Y was predetermined according to a quasi-random, Gellermann schedule (Gellermann, 1933). In the successive discrimination task, the animals were faced with a situation is which the starting stem was gray and both upper arms were either black or white. The animal had to learn to enter the right arm of the Y when both arms were white (follow the rule "right if both white") and to enter the left arm of the Y when both arms were black (follow the rule "left if both black") or vice versa. The stimulus situation as it might appear to an animal on two different trials is shown in Figure 13. About half of the rats were trained to go "right if both white, left if both black," while the other half were trained to go "right if both black, left if both white."

As a group, animals with hippocampal damage were impaired, relative to normal animals and to animals with brain damage restricted to the posterolateral neocortex, in the acquisition of the

SIMULTANEOUS DISCRIMINATION

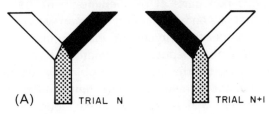

SUCCESSIVE DISCRIMINATION

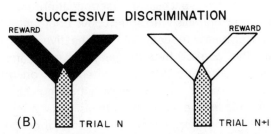

Figure 13. Schematic representation of simultaneous and successive discrimination tasks. In (A), the situation faced by animals on two different trials is shown. The start arm is gray. A black or a white insert is placed in the right or left arm on a nonsystematic basis. The animal is rewarded for approaching one of the colors. In (B), the successive discrimination as it could appear on two successive trials is shown. On any given trial, the two cross-arms are either black or white. The animal must turn right or left depending on the color of the two arms. From Isaacson and Kimble (1972).

successive discrimination. These same subjects, however, were not impaired in learning the simultaneous discrimination.

Complete understanding of Kimble's results depends on a more complete analysis of the data, and there is one additional factor of the experimental design to consider. All the animals in this study were trained on both the simultaneous discrimination and the successive discrimination problems. This was done in a balanced fashion. Some subjects learned the simultaneous discrimination as their first task, while the other subjects learned the successive discrimination first. Considering animals that learned the simultaneous problem first, there was little difference among the three experimental groups. All animals learned to approach the black arm more readily than they learned to approach the white arm. This suggests that all rats, whether lesioned or not, found the hypothesis "approach the darker arm" more compatible with their predispositions than the alternative hypothesis, "approach the lighter arm." This result is not surprising, since rats tend to approach the darker parts of new environments (Munn, 1950). The point is that rats enter a learning situation with predispositions which help or hinder them in solving the new task.

When the simultaneous discrimination was learned as the second task, i.e., after the animals had already learned the successive discrimination, there was a substantial difference between the normal animals and those with either neocortical or hippocampal damage.

Training on the successive discrimination task served to provide the normal animals with an effective orientation toward the simultaneous problem. Indeed, four of the five normal subjects started with the correct hypothesis, and, more important, *all* normal subjects attacked the problem while operating on a "brightness hypothesis." The previous training had served to disconfirm a "place (spatial) hypothesis." As a consequence, normal animals no longer needed to test the "food on the right" or "food on the left" hypothesis. They acted on hypotheses related to the brightness of the arms of the maze.

An individual analysis of the brain-lesioned animals failing to acquire the simultaneous discrimination within a few trials indicated the following: In the hippocampal-lesioned group there were two such animals: one rat required 33 trials and made 28 responses to the left goal box before learning; the other rat in this group requiring 33 trials to criterion performance made 24 responses to the right goal box in the presolution period. Of the animals with neocortical lesions failing to perform well in the simultaneous problem administered as the second task, one rat required 34 trials and made 33 responses to the left goal box prior to solution. Another rat required 15 presolution responses and made seven responses to the left goal box out of the first nine trials. Then it made six successive responses to the right goal box. Perhaps the most interesting subject was the animal with a neocortical lesion which required 27 presolution responses. This animal did not adopt a consistent position hypothesis. It made five responses to the right goal in the first seven trials and then began a series of 13 responses distributed between both arms of the maze, but only one of the responses was correct! This string of responses is understandable only if the animal were operating on an "approach the black arm" hypothesis, even though this hypothesis was wrong and consistently nonreinforced.

The animals with hippocampal damage which performed poorly were acting in accordance with a position hypothesis which the normal animals had eliminated during their previous training, despite the fact they had given up this strategy while solving the previous task. When starting their second problem, they returned to it and did so with vigor. The two most impaired animals with hippocampal lesions required more correct responses and more errors in attaining the correct solution than any animal with hippocampal lesions learning the problem without previous training.

For all animals, the successive discrimination problem is more difficult than simultaneous problems. Why the successive problem is more difficult can best be understood in terms of the type of hypothesis that must be held for the correct solution. The animals must learn "if both arms are white, go right," and "if both arms are black, go left," or vice versa. In addition, the animals must learn to suppress all forms of spatial and brightness hypotheses.

The successive discrimination task can be viewed in several ways. One way is to assume that the animal compares the two situations with which it is confronted on various trials. It may compare the effects of responses to the left and right arms of the Y, given on subsequent trials, when the arms of the maze are both white or both black. According to this view, the animal learns one complex problem. Another way of looking at this task, however, is to think of the problem as two separate tasks: a "white maze" and a "black maze." Taking this view, it would be anticipated that the animal could master one of these problems without doing very well on the other. This seems to be the case. Normal animals can perform quite well on one of the two problems (e.g., the white maze task) while performing at almost chance levels on the other (e.g., the black maze task). Furthermore, if the successive discrimination is analyzed as if it were two tasks, the performance of animals is "nonincremental" in each. That is, the animals make as many errors in the last half of the presolution trials as in the first half. This sort of nonincremental learning is found in the learning of the simultaneous discrimination, but is not seen in the successive discrimination task *unless* the data are considered on the basis of the black maze—white maze subdivisions.

Adopting the two-task orientation for learning of the successive discrimination problem, it is possible to determine the ease with which each task is acquired. Animals in all experimental groups learned one of the two tasks (i.e., white maze, black maze) with about the same number of correct and incorrect responses. The difference among the groups came about in the number of responses required to master the second task. Normal animals were only slightly slower in acquiring the second subproblem than the first. They did so while maintaining an adequate performance level on the first subproblem. For the subjects with hippocampal damage, however, the lesion limited their capacities. They were able to learn one of the two subproblems as rapidly as the normal animals but were seriously impaired in learning the second. A similar impairment was found to result from neocortical destruction alone. In order to clearly understand the nature of the deficit produced by hippocampal lesions in this situation, it becomes necessary to explain the effects of neocortical destruction as well. This problem will be discussed after considering the behavior of animals with hippocampal damage under conditions of frustration (p. 191).

In an experiment reported by Kimble and Kimble (1970), rats were trained in a brightness discrimination task to a criterion of nine correct responses in ten trials. A Y-maze was used and the rats were rewarded with water when they entered the illuminated arm. The other arm was dark and responses to it were not rewarded. The location of the correct, bright goal arm was varied according to a Gellermann schedule, once again. An animal was allowed 20 sec to drink after a correct choice and was detained in the goal box with no reward for 20 sec after an incorrect choice. Each rat was given 1 additional day of training after the day it reached criterion performance. Testing under no-reward, extinction conditions began the next day. During extinction, the water bottle was removed and metal covers were placed in both goal arms over the holes where the drinking tube had been inserted during acquisition training. The animals again received ten trials each day with a 10-min intertrial interval. If a rat did not enter either goal arm within 60 sec after being released from the start box, the trial was ended, and the trial was considered as an "extinction trial."

Using a traditional measure of learning, trials to the learning criterion, there were no differences among the groups of normal animals, animals with neocortical lesions, and animals with hippocampal and neocortical lesions. In fact, both brain-damaged groups took somewhat fewer trials to reach the acquisition criterion than did the normal animals. However, the tendency to exhibit "hypothesis behavior" (Krechevsky, 1935) was different among the groups. Kimble and Kimble defined two kinds of hypotheses. A spatial hypothesis was defined as a sequence of three or more consecutive responses to either the right or the left goal arm, provided that goal arm was both illuminated and nonilluminated on various trials during the response sequence. A brightness hypothesis was defined as a sequence of three or more consecutive responses to either the light or the dark arm of the maze, provided that the response sequence included responses to both the left and right arms. In this analysis, any given trial could be scored in accord with a spatial hypothesis (left or right), or a brightness hypothesis (light or dark), or no hypothesis.

The hypothesis behavior of the normal animals was characterized as consisting of many short series of trials in accord with one or the other hypothesis. The individual performances of the subjects can be seen in Figure 14. The mean number of hypotheses displayed by normal animals was 6.2 (median 6).

This is similar to the performance of the animals with lesions restricted to the neocortex, whose mean number of hypotheses was 5.9 (median 5.5). The hippocampally lesioned animals, however, could be characterized as evidencing fewer but longer hypotheses, making only 4.5 hypothesis runs (median 4) on the average. These animals with hippocampal damage tended to stay with a particular hypothesis almost 50% longer than the other animals: mean length 7.3 (median 5.5). As can be observed in Figure 14, the longer sequences of hypothesis-based responses occurred only when the subjects were acting on a place hypothesis and not

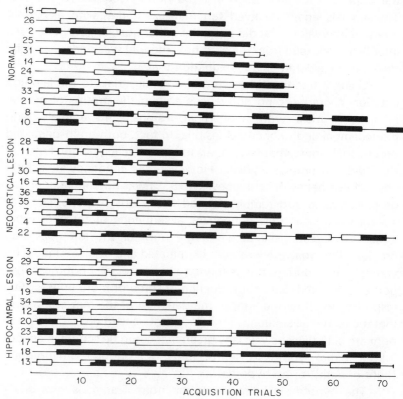

Figure 14. Number of trials on which normal animals, animals with neocortical lesions, and those with hippocampal lesions exhibited behaviors consistent with a spatial hypothesis (open rectangles), a brightness hypothesis (filled rectangles), or no defined hypothesis (straight line only) while learning a brightness discrimination task. Data from Kimble and Kimble (1970). Figure from Isaacson and Kimble (1972).

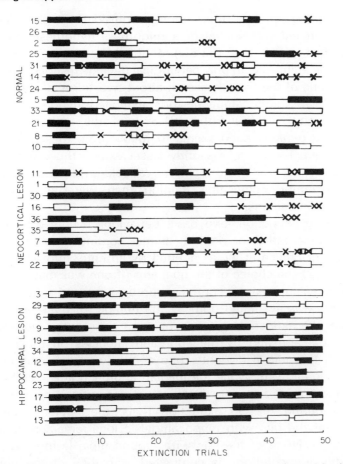

Figure 15. Number of trials on which the three groups given in Figure 14 exhibited behavior consistent with a spatial hypothesis, a brightness hypothesis or no defined hypothesis during extinction of the brightness discrimination. Designation of hypothesis is as in Figure 14. The symbol × indicates that the animal did not respond on a particular trial. Data from Kimble and Kimble (1970). Figure from Isaacson and Kimble (1972).

when acting on a brightness hypothesis. Not all of the animals with hippocampal damage evidenced this pattern, but the majority did: eight out of twelve of them produced hypothesis runs of ten or more trials during acquisition, whereas only one animal with neocortical damage and no normal animal did.

Another measure which distinguished among the groups was

the percentage of total trials during acquisition which could be included in either a spatial or a brightness hypothesis. For the normal rats, about half (53.8%) of the trials were "hypothesis trials." The animals with only neocortical damage responded on the basis of one of the hypotheses on about two-thirds of their trials. Animals with hippocampal lesions exhibited hypothesis-based behavior on over four-fifths (81.3%) of the trials. A simple descriptive generalization seems to follow from these data: the normal animals and, to a slightly lesser extent, those with neo-cortical lesions were much more variable in their hypothesis behavior during acquisition training than were animals with hippocampal damage.

During extinction, two basic behavioral events were mon-itored: (1) whether or not the animal continued to make any response or choice at all, as defined by an entry into either goal arm, and (2) the choice of the goal arm (if one was made).

The willingness to continue approaching and entering the goal arms was evaluated both by the number of trials necessary to attain the extinction criterion of three consecutive nonentries into a goal arm and by the approach latencies on those trials in which the animal did enter one of the two goal arms within the 60 sec allowed. While the median approach latencies for the normal animals and for those with neocortical damage in-creased during the 50 extinction trials, the median approach latency for the rats with hippocampal lesions remained virtually unchanged. None of the rats with hippocampal lesions reached the extinction criterion, as contrasted with 42% of the normal and 44% of the neocortically damaged animals.

Since all the animals were trained to approach the brighter arm of the Y-maze during acquisition, it might have been expected that a preponderant number of responses of all animals would be toward that arm during extinction. Actually, the hippocampally lesioned animals exhibited this tendency far more than did animals in either of the other two groups. The point is that while the choice behavior for both normal animals and those with neocortical lesions rapidly became more variable during extinction, that of the animals with hippocampal lesions was characterized by long strings of responses in accord with a brightness hypothesis, usually (but not always) consisting of approach responses to the brighter arm. Further analysis of these data has been published (Kimble and Kimble, 1970).

Of special significance is the fact that at the end of acquisition the animals with hippocampal lesions were now responding extensively in accord with the brightness hypothesis. The special attractiveness of the place hypothesis had been supplanted by the brightness hypothesis. During extinction, this acquired hypothesis was given up only with great reluctance. This suggests that the predominant hypothesis was held beyond normal limits of disconfirmation by animals with hippocampal damage and that the status of a "predominant hypothesis" can be achieved either through preexperimental, and possible genetic, influences or through the results of specific training. However, it should be remembered that animals with hippocampal damage also returned to a previously rejected place hypothesis when being trained in the simultaneous discrimination as their second task (Isaacson and Kimble, 1972). This leads to the conclusion that the perseveration of the acquired hypothesis is maintained during nonreinforcement in the same experimental environment, but that the initially predominant (spatial) hypothesis is reactivated when the testing procedures are changed. The animals with hippocampal lesions may suffer from both a perseveration of a hypothesis during conditions of nonreward and a decreased ability to transfer experiences between two different, yet similar, training paradigms.

Olton (1972) has extended our knowledge of the behavioral deficits following hippocampal destruction in discrimination tasks by pointing out that the ability to suppress a preferred response, as measured by the latency of the response, is less affected than is the ability to make the correct choice from two possible responses. In Olton's study, animals had to make a choice between two stimulus positions, and most animals initially responded to one or the other positions, i.e., acted on a place hypothesis. Both normal and brain-lesioned animals evidenced differential latencies of response to the positive and negative stimuli before they gave up consistently responding to their favorite place. The animals with hippocampal damage continued to respond toward the preferred place for many days after the differential latencies to the positive and negative places had first become evident. After the onset of differential latencies, control animals quickly began to respond to the side where the positive stimulus is presented. These results are an example of a dissociation of the overt, expressed behavior and presumptive knowledge about the environment held by the animals with hippocampal damage. The differential latencies to the two stimuli must reflect the fact that the animals know that the response to a particular place is less likely to produce a reward when the negative stimulus is there than when the positive stimulus is there. Despite this information, the animals with hippocampal damage perseverate the spatial hypothesis. This type of perseveration of overt behaviors is often found as a result of frustrating circumstances in normal animals, and the relationship between frustrating events and the effects of hippocampal damage will be discussed next.

Frustration

In our 1972 report, Kimble and I alluded to the possible usefulness of Maier's theory of frustration-induced behavior (Maier, 1949) in describing and explaining the effects of hippocampal destruction. We felt that since animals with hippocampal damage could give up some hypotheses as readily as intact animals, even though their selection of new hypotheses might be limited, their behavior could not be explained as a simple perseveration of learned responses or hypotheses. Animals with hippocampal damage seem to have sufficient flexibility in behavior under many circumstances, but lose it when the environment becomes uncertain or rewards are not obtained with accustomed regularity. This decrease in flexibility, coupled with other changes in the deportment of the lesioned animals, made us give serious consideration to Maier's frustration theory.

The title of Maier's book, *Frustration: The Study of Behavior Without a Goal*, made some readers think that the frustrated individual, whether human or nonhuman, was without normal goals. This is not correct. What Maier meant was that a particular behavioral act or episode in a specified environmental circumstance was not goal oriented (Maier, 1964). The behavior exhibited in the frustration-inducing situation was *not* based on normal motivational considerations and was a result of a fixation of a response (or hypothesis) when forced to make some response. It is important to recognize that Maier first observed fixated, perseverative behaviors when animals were presented with insoluble problems. The frustrated animals continued to exhibit the fixated behavior even when the problem was made soluble. In passing, Maier noted that there were considerable individual differences in the tolerance of animals to frustrating circumstances; some animals quickly adopted the fixated, nongoal directed behavior patterns whereas others required much longer exposure to the insoluble problems.

While there has been controversy about the notion of frustration-induced perseverative behaviors, it is the most useful conceptualization available for the results obtained by him and other investigators. (For a discussion of the alternative explanations, see Maier, 1964.) Taking this position, it may be useful to consider some of the points of similarity between frustration-instigated behaviors and the behaviors often exhibited by animals with hippocampal lesions.

Many animals with hippocampal damage exhibit long strings of inappropriate behaviors during the learning and reversal of discrimination problems. Not all the lesioned animals exhibit these behaviors. This is due in part to the nature of the hypothesis being tested by the animals but also to the individual tendencies of the animals to respond with fixated behaviors to the frustrations of the testing situation. The hippocampal lesion may tend to lower the threshold for frustration-induced effects, but in animals constitutionally resistant to frustration this reduction may not be great enough to induce the perseverative, non-goal-oriented behaviors. The lesion, then, could be thought of as affecting thresholds for frustration-induced behaviors, and, given some variability in the animals' tolerance to frustration, this would mean that the effects produced by the lesions would be reflected in the proportion of animals affected. The effect would be all-or-none for any particular animal, but some animals might not be influenced in a particular task. This is exactly what was found by Nonneman and Isaacson (1973) in their study of task-dependent behavioral changes induced by hippocampal lesions made early or late in life. In our study, the earliness of the lesion determined the proportion of animals affected in a particular task.

Maier also pointed out that the response which becomes fixated is not predictable from the responses learned in the past. This same result has been found in studies accomplished in my laboratory. We have been unable to predict the response to be fixated by a particular animal with hippocampal lesions during reversal training on the basis of the number of past responses or the number of reinforced responses made in accordance with a particular hypothesis. This suggests that at some point the animal changes its pattern of behavior from one which is goal-oriented or hypothesis-directed to one which is not goal-oriented. The perseverated response may not be the one to which the animal has been trained or the first one exhibited in the training situation.

There is evidence that the animals exhibiting fixated behaviors induced by insoluble problems often perseverate a response even though they "know better." Such animals perseverate responding to one side of a Lashley jumping stand after the problem has been made soluble while showing differential latencies of their responses depending on whether the positive or negative card was placed on the side to which they jump. These differential latencies indicate that the animals know the occasions when they will be reinforced and when they will not, but they respond with the fixated response in spite of this knowledge. As Olton has pointed out, and as discussed earlier, many times a similar distinction between "knowledge" and performance seems to be appropriate to animals with hippocampal lesions. Even more, animals with hippocampal damage continue to enter the compartment in which they have received an electrical shock in testing for the ability to withhold responses in the passive avoidance paradigm, despite vocalizations and other obvious manifestations of distress. It therefore appears as if the lesioned animals also know better, or know more, than they seem to on the basis of overt performance. A similar distinction between performance and information available is suggested by the improved performances on DRL schedules made possible by chloropromazine or by α-methyl-p-tyrosine in animals with hippocampal lesions. The animals do not *learn* to respond at lower rates under these drugs; rather, they respond efficiently as soon as they are placed on them.

Earlier, I pointed out the fact that in some experimental situations, including training on brightness discrimination problems, the effects of posterior neocortical lesions seem to resemble the effects of hippocampal destruction. While the neocortex of the rat (and maybe other species) may not be essential for learning visual discriminations, it may be presumed to be of some value or use to the animal. When it is destroyed, the animal should be handicapped and the problem less easily solved. To the extent that this occurs, the probability is increased that frustration-induced perseverative acts will occur in a group of animals. The reduction in threshold for the frustration response produced by the additional destruction of the hippocampus would potentiate this tendency. In some discrimination experiments, a maximal effect could be found after the neocortical lesion, alone, if the problem required a great amount of neocortical participation. Perhaps the fact that the neocortical damage inflicted in animals subjected to bilateral aspiration-produced lesions of the hippocampus is almost always somewhat greater than that produced in control animals is of significance. By and large, this is the case in experiments from my laboratory and many others despite firm intentions to make the neocortical lesions at least as large as those in our "hippocampal subjects." Histological evaluation almost always reveals that the lesions of the neocortex are greatest in the group with hippocampal lesions. If there is a correlation between the ease with which visual discrimination problems are solved and the amount of the neocortex destroyed (and this is by no means certain!), then the animals with hippocampal damage would be at a double disadvantage. My proposal is, however, that there is no one method by which frustration-induced perseveration of behavior is produced. It may occur from changes in environmental contingencies (e.g., an insoluble problem), the inability to use sensory information (neocortical damage), or the threshold of mechanisms responsible for the fixated behaviors (limbic damage). From these considerations, I believe it fair to say that the older view that hippocampal lesions do not impair the learning of simple visual discriminations is an oversimplification at best. It is certainly false for animals tested in operant situations and even has to be restricted to specific training conditions in nonoperant tasks (e.g., T- and Y-mazes). The analysis made by Isaacson and Kimble shows the importance of previous training and the hypotheses held by the individual animal in determining whether or not an impairment will be found.

Individual Differences in Learning Studies

In 1971, Thomas made explicit the puzzling effects which had been noted by many researchers investigating the effects of brain lesions on behavior. Thomas reported "all-or-none" effects on the retention of a maze problem produced by section of the fornix. Some animals were severely impaired and other animals unimpaired by what appeared to be exactly the same sort of brain damage. Why is it, Thomas asked, "That the same type of lesion will produce an impairment in one animal but not in the next?" Thomas suggested that the answer may be that some lesions produce abnormal activities in the tissue surrounding a lesion. There may be substantial differences in the behavioral effects of lesions that produce abnormal activities in cells around the site of the lesion and those that do not.

As mentioned above, it is likely that the animals could indeed respond quite differently to "identical" brain damage on the basis of individual differences in the macrostructure of the brain and regional differences in metabolic activity. These fine-grain differences could produce different responses to damage at the edge of a lesion, perhaps leading to an irritative focus of abnormal activity in one animal but not in another. However, this type of explanation will have to be extensively investigated, electrically and metabolically, before it can be accepted. On the other hand, Waxler and Rosvold (1970) found similar all-or-none effects in monkeys with a delayed response problem and suggested that the individual differences in lesion-produced effects may depend on the strategies used by the animal. This approach is similar to that of Isaacson and Kimble (1972), discussed above.

According to views which propose differences in strategies or the tendencies to use certain cues, the effects of past experiences should play an important role in determining the animal's attack on present environmental problems. The past may contribute special types of interference or assistance. If the effects of the past lead to inappropriate strategies, solution of the problem can be delayed and frustration become more likely.

My explanation of the all-or-none quality of behavioral deficiencies would be based on the factors which contribute to the animal's reactions to the frustrations of the task. These include the genetic tendencies to tolerate frustration as modified by interactions with past experiences, the changes in frustration tolerance induced by the brain damage, the abnormalities in the utilization of cues produced by the brain damage, the strategies used by the animal as it starts the problem, and possibly abnormal tissue reactions at the edge of the lesion.

Perseveration

Perseverative responding due to frustration or to brain damage does not develop immediately in those problems in which the lesioned animals show abnormal patterns of behavior, e.g., during reversals and extinction. It develops more or less slowly over the course of time and after the animals have found that successful performance is not quickly reached. This suggests that animals with hippocampal lesions develop a perseverative mode of responding secondary to the inability to solve the problem.

The surprising aspect is that while perseverative responding may be secondary to an inability to solve a particular problem, this inability could stem from a reduced ability to give up an inappropriate strategy or set of hypotheses. If the lesioned animal begins the problem on the wrong foot, it may keep with the inappropriate approach too long and a frustration-induced fixation of behavior could result. The sort of hypothesis perseverated could be one of several kinds, depending on the task. For example, Hirsh (1970) found that the changes observed in the behavior of the animals with hippocampal lesions were not identical. Some animals exhibited an enhanced alternation of responses, while others showed perseveration of responses. The point is that all of the animals studied by Hirsh did not perform in the same sort of perseverative fashion, even though they all perseverated in some way. In monkeys, Pribram *et al.* (1969) suggest that the animals with hippocampal lesions were faced with an inability to retain hypotheses pertaining to the problem before them in the face of distraction or disconfirmation, and this is one of the suggestions that Kimble and I have tried to emphasize in our analysis of the behavior of rats with hippocampal destruction.

The cues provided by the training apparatus are important determinants of perseverative tendencies. Cohen *et al.* (1971)

found that lesioned animals were impaired and exhibited perseveration in a T-maze if the arms of the maze were the same
color but not if they were of different colors. This would make sense
if the lesioned animals had difficulty using the spatial aspects
of the apparatus as a basis for solving the problem, as discussed
previously. When the arms of the maze were of the same color, the
problem would be more difficult for the animals with hippocampal
damage than for normal animals. If the animals do not solve the
problem, then they show perseveration in their behavior.

Animals with hippocampal lesions not only perseverate
presently favored hypotheses but also perseverate the hypotheses
which were acquired in the training situation prior to the change in
reinforcement contingencies which came to produce the frustration.
Winocur and Mills (1970) found that prior training interferes
with the performance of animals with hippocampal lesions when
the preceding tasks are related in some way to the current test problem. Training on unrelated tasks does not produce interference.
In other words, the impairment found in the hippocampal-
lesioned animals can be described as an inappropriate transfer of
strategies from one task to the next. The hypotheses formed in one
situation carry over into future situations which share some
similarity with it. The question of how similar the situations must
be for this transfer, and along what dimensions similarity is
critical, has yet to be investigated.

Douglas *et al.* (1969) found that monkeys with hippocampal
damage trained in a discrimination problem had more difficulty
when there was one positive cue presented along with several
negative cues than when only one positive cue and one negative
cue were presented. The more negative cues available, the greater
was the impairment. These data invite speculation as to the procedures whereby the animals form and reject hypotheses on the basis
of nonreward. However, the addition of negative (nonrewarded)
stimuli to the task produces another effect which could be the cause
of the behavioral deficit. With only two stimuli available, i.e., a rewarded stimulus and a nonrewarded stimulus, the animals obtain a
reward on about one-half of the training trials, before the problem is
learned. With four negative stimuli and one positive, the animal
receives a reward on only about 20% of its prelearning trials.
This difference in the frequency of reward may be of importance,

especially since the animals in that study had received prior training in the apparatus with close to 100% reward. This suggests that this type of experiment needs to be performed varying the number of stimuli from which choices can be made and also the proportion of reinforcements obtained throughout the training procedures. The frequency of reinforcement must be considered separately from the issue of how many negative instances are needed to disconfirm a particular hypothesis. Pribram *et al.* (1969) first proposed the relationship between the hippocampus and the rejection of hypotheses on the basis of negative consequences of behavior based on the hypotheses. Isaacson and Kimble (1972) suggested that this relationship might hold but only for well-established "hypothesis sets" rather than for individual hypotheses. A "hypothesis set" can be considered to be a collection of possible hypotheses all pertaining to some attribute of behavior, e.g., "go left," "go right"; "approach gray," "approach white," "approach black." In the example, one hypothesis set has to do with responses to places or to the turning responses made in the apparatus. Another hypothesis set has to do with making responses to the colors in different parts of the appartus. Kimble and I felt that there was ample evidence that animals with hippocampal lesions could give up a particular hypothesis as readily as normal animals but had trouble moving beyond hypotheses related to the attribute originally guiding behavior.

Regional Differences Within the Hippocampus

Several authors have undertaken the evaluation of behavioral changes resulting from lesions of the dorsal or ventral hippocampus or lesions of both. Several types of behaviors are altered in a similar fashion by dorsal and ventral lesions, whereas other behaviors are selectively influenced by dorsal or by ventral lesions. Still other behaviors do not seem to be changed by either dorsal or ventral lesions by themselves, but are influenced by lesions which involve *both* dorsal and ventral regions.

Nadel (1968) undertook the study of small electrolytic lesions of the dorsal or ventral hippocampus. In one part of this study, he examined the activities exhibited by animals in a relatively small chamber (12 by 8 inches) which was brightly illuminated by a fluorescent lamp on the top of the box. Nadel reported a small enhancement of "activity" after either type of lesion relative to intact control animals. However, the behaviors scored as "activity" by Nadel were all related to sniffing (rearing, walking, and sitting while sniffing). They were not locomotor activity as usually defined. In other tests made over 3 days in an automated chamber of somewhat larger dimensions (19 by 12 inches), both types of lesioned animals evidenced somewhat greater levels of activity. Several things should be said about these aspects of Nadel's study: (1) the chambers used for testing were small and probably did not measure the same kinds of activity called locomotor exploration measured by others; (2) the high values of illumination probably tended to suppress the activity of all animals, especially those with hippocampal damage; and (3) the lesions were quite small. From the published report, it is not possible to determine the postoperative time at which testing was undertaken.

Lanier and Isaacson (1974) have studied the locomotor activity of rats receiving dorsal, ventral, or combined dorsal—ventral lesions produced by aspirative techniques. During surgery, the hippocampus was exposed at its greatest dorsal—ventral extent through a slit made in the neocortex. Then either the dorsal or the ventral portion was removed as far as possible, in two groups, or the majority of it removed in a third group. Testing was done in a large open-field box measuring 4 by 4 ft. The results were straightforward: animals with near total destruction of the hippocampus and animals with lesions of the ventral hippocampus exhibited greater activity than did animals with lesions of the dorsal hippocampus. This is surprising, perhaps, in that the lesions of the dorsal hippocampus were complete, removing the fornix—fimbria complex and often causing massive degeneration within the hippocampal commissure system.

In this experiment, we began testing the animals almost immediately after surgery and continued to do so for many days. While the animals with almost complete or with ventral lesions of the hippocampus maintained their hyperactive state throughout testing, they showed the greatest activity levels about 6 days after surgery. At this time, the animals with dorsal hippocampal lesions also had their peak activity. The activity of the animals with dorsal hippocampal lesions decreased quickly after the peak at 6 days and became close to that of control animals. Therefore, while the time of testing after surgery is an important variable, only the ventral and near total hippocampal lesions produced permanently elevated levels of locomotor activity.

In Nadel's study, the acquisition of a conditioned emotional response was not affected by either the dorsal or the ventral lesions, although there appeared to be some slight enhancement of CER conditioning in the animals suffering from the dorsal lesions. The failure to find a deficit in the conditioned emotional response is at odds with the report of Brady (1958), who warned that his results should be cautiously accepted since the histology had not been completed at that time. As far as I know, the histology of the lesions has not yet been reported. Supporting Nadel's observation is the report of Hunt et al. (1957), who failed to find any CER deficit after hippocampal lesions in cats. Nadel found no passive avoidance deficit following either the dorsal or the ventral hippocampal lesions, but reported that the dorsal lesions produced a deficit in one-way active avoidance conditioning. The ventral lesions produced a slight facilitation in this same task.

Rabe and Haddad (1968) found that lesions of the dorsal hippocampus produced a hyperreactivity at the transition from a continuous to an intermittent reinforcement schedule, in this case a fixed-ratio schedule. The same sort of effect was produced by more extensive lesions of the hippocampus, including both dorsal and ventral portions. The subjects with dorsal hippocampal lesions, however, did not exhibit an increased resistance to extinction, whereas those with large lesions did. In a subsequent study (Rabe and Haddad, 1969), large lesions of the hippocampus were found to facilitate two-way active avoidance behavior, as would be expected. However, this result could not be duplicated by lesions restricted to either the dorsal or the ventral hippocampus. This result is somewhat surprising in view of the fact that Van Hoesen et al. (1972) found that lesions of the fimbria–fornix produced a facilitation of the two-way active avoidance task. Their investigation was aimed at trying to dissociate the effects of interrupting either the fimbria–fornix or the entorhinal input–output systems of the hippocampus. Accordingly, lesions were made in either the fimbria–fornix or the entorhinal region. Both types of lesions resulted in facilitated acquisition of the two-way active avoidance task. There were behavioral differences produced by the two lesions, however. The fimbria—fornix lesioned group received fewer shocks during acquisition than did the entorhinal-lesioned group. Their results substantiate the earlier report of Green et al. (1967) to the effect that the septal—hippocampal interconnections are important for the acquisition of active avoidance responses. Van Hoesen et al. found a passive avoidance deficit only after entorhinal lesions and not after the fimbria—fornix damage. A deficit in passive avoidance behavior was also reported by Entingh (1971) to follow entorhinal damage in cats.

Changes in the frequency of water lapping were observed to follow destruction of the posteroventral hippocampus but not the dorsal hippocampus (Holdstock, 1972). Despite the increase in the frequency of drinking, the posteroventral-lesioned animals did not actually consume more water than control animals. They initiated the lapping response more frequently even when they received electrical shocks from the drinking tube (a passive avoidance deficit). If the dorsal hippocampal lesion invaded the posterior septal area, behavioral changes like those found after the postero-ventral hippocampal lesion were obtained. This suggested grounds for a functional association of the two areas.

The differences between dorsal and ventral hippocampal contributions to behavior were approached in a different manner by Fried (1970, 1972). Earlier, Fried and Goddard had argued that effects produced by hippocampal destruction could be explained on the basis of a perseveration of response sets established before the removal of the hippocampus. Corroborative data were collected by Wishart and Mogenson (1970), who found that hippocampal lesions produced passive avoidance deficits only if approach training was given to the animals before the lesion. A much smaller passive avoidance deficit was found if the training in the approach response on which the passive avoidance response was based was given postoperatively. It was in this methodological and theoretical context that Fried investigated the difference in effects produced by dorsal and ventral lesions of the hippo-campus using "resistance to extinction" as the diagnostic response.

Three types of hippocampal lesions were studied: dorsal lesions, ventral lesions, and combined dorsal and ventral lesions.

These three types of lesions were studied in two training paradigms. In the first, training and extinction were both given postoperatively. In the second, the approach training was given preoperatively while the extinction training was given postoperatively. Animals with lesions in the dorsal hippocampus showed enhanced resistance to extinction under both training conditions. On the other hand, animals with ventral hippocampal lesions showed a resistance to extinction only when approach training had been given preoperatively and the extinction training given postoperatively. When both training and extinction testing were accomplished postoperatively, the animals with the ventral hippocampal lesions extinguished responding faster than did control animals. The combined lesion group evidenced the same performance as that group receiving only the ventral hippocampal lesions (Fried, 1972).

In a recent review, Jarrard (1973) summarized evidence for certain regional differentiation within the hippocampus based on the classical division of the hippocampus into the several CA areas. He argues that areas CA3 and CA4, as well as the interconnections of the septal area with these regions, play an important role in the inhibition of responses. Region CA1, Jarrard argues, is primarily concerned with the regulation of incentive motivation, particularly with regard to hunger and thirst. Considering activity and arousal, Jarrard believes that all regions of the hippocampus participate in the regulation of the activating mechanisms of the posterior hypothalamus and the brain stem reticular formation. This argument is based in part on the study by Grant and Jarrard (1968) in which chemical stimulation was applied to either the anterodorsal or posteroventral hippocampus. Drinking could be elicited only by cholinergic stimulation of field CA1 in the anterodorsal hippocampus. Increased locomotor activity could be elicited by cholinergic stimulation throughout the hippocampus. Monoaminergic stimulation did not elicit increased activity when applied anywhere in the hippocampus.

From this brief review of some of the research on functional differentiation in the hippocampus, it should be clear that there are contradictory reports in the literature about the behavioral contributions made by its different portions. These discrepancies may be due to a number of factors, including the exact location of the lesions. For example, it is difficult to avoid encroaching on the septal area with lesions of the fimbria—fornix. Lesions of the dorsal hippocampus can destroy different amounts of this fimbra— fornix complex as well as some portions of the hippocampal commissures. Damage to the entorhinal cortex or the ventral hippocampus can affect adjacent pyriform, periamygdaloid, and amygdala tissue in different degrees. However, lesions aimed at destoying dorsal or ventral hippocampal tissue may also differentially invade the superior and inferior portions of the hippocampus, as well as the dentate gyrus. This is because of the fact that the hippocampal formation of the rat rotates and bends at its most dorsal and ventral aspects. Therefore, subtotal destruction of the dorsal and ventral regions may produce quite different damage to the subdivisions of the hippocampus. Adequate evaluation of dorsal and ventral contributions to behavior must take the differential damage to these other hippocampal subdivisions into account. The training and testing conditions as well as the time after the brain damage that the animals are tested all contribute their influences to the types of behavioral consequences produced. That differences in function exist within the hippocampal complex is not to be doubted, but the trick will be to find the most useful basis for subdividing the system.

Electrical Rhythms of the Hippocampus

For over 20 years, the theta rhythms and other electrical activities of the hippocampus have been intensively studied. A complete review of these efforts will not be undertaken (see Bennett,1974; Black, 1974; Winson, 1974), but I would like to consider at least some of these studies since they relate to studies using lesion and stimulation techniques.

Before doing so, it is important to remember that the Greek letter names used to describe the electrical activity of the brain refer to the frequency of electrical rhythms and not to the brain areas from which the records are obtained. In common usage, delta rhythms are those of frequencies 3 Hz and below. Theta rhythms are those of frequencies between 4 and 8 Hz, while alpha frequencies are those between 8 and 12 Hz. All of these rhythms can be found in recordings made from the structures of the limbic system, the neocortex, and even in the midbrain and brain stem. Some confusions has been created in the recent literature due to the description of rhythmic activities as "theta rhythms" when the frequencies are not in the appropriate range. At times, recordings of 8 Hz and faster obtained from the hippocampus have been called "hippocampal theta" because of their mathematical and esthetic purity. To reduce confusion, it would be better to describe them simply as rhythmic activities and to designate the predominant frequency as closely as possible.

A number of theories have been offered for the behavioral correlates and effects of slow-wave activity in the hippocampus. In 1961, Morrell suggested that slow synchronous activity of the brain might be related to the "inscribing" of experiences by the nervous system. He based this suggestion, in part, on the obser- vation that these rhythms are found in the early stages of learning but disappear when the response has become well established. This view has been pursued more fully by Adey (1964) and by Elazar and Adey (1967), who have argued that hippocampal theta activity is related to the processing, storage, and recall of information. They asserted that the slow rhythms are important in some way for information entering into storage and also for its being retrieved from storage. This assertion served as the basis of an investigation by Bennet *et al.* (1971). These investigators, working with cats, used scopolamine hydrobromide to block theta rhythms of the hippocampus. Scopolamine also produces some behavioral effects which resemble those of hippocampal lesions. In the smallest amounts used (0.05 mg/kg), and at somewhat higher levels (0.075 mg/kg), the drug was effective in disrupting theta activity but not performances indicative of memory retrieval. Therefore, Bennett *et al.* concluded that the presense of the theta rhythm was not necessary for the retrieval of information. Bennett was led to conclude that the most prominent correlated behavioral activities associated with rhythmic slow activities in hippocampus are those of orienting toward and attending to stimuli in the en- vironment (Bennett, 1971), a view much like that proposed earlier by Grastyán *et al.* (1959). Taking a different approach, Van- derwolf (1969, 1971) has proposed that the rhythmic slow activity recorded from the dorsal hippocampus is related to the activation of motor systems necessary for voluntary actions. The rhythmic activities are supposed to indicate the activation of systems which couple motor behavior to the motivational states of the organism and to the incentives of the environment. In a related approach, Klemm (1970) has presented evidence that hippocampal theta-wave activities are related to changes in the electrical activity recorded from muscles. Komisaruk (1968, 1970) has related hippocampal theta activity to vibrissae twitching in rats, as well as other behaviors normally exhibited with similar frequencies of the musculature. However, rhythmic slow activity can be recorded from the hippocampus of rats which are swimming and not exhibiting vibrissae twitches (Whishaw and Vanderwolf, 1971). Gray (1971) has reported that the elimination of rhythmic slow activity in the hippocampus subsequent to septal lesions which did not produce a loss in vibrissae twitching. Gray has also noticed relatively fast rhythmic activities of about 7.5–8.5 Hz in rats that are remaining immobile and not making any voluntary movements. This result was observed by Bennett (1970), as well. Black (1972) points out still other exceptions to a categorical relationship between voluntary movements and fast rhythmic activities. In broadest perspective, it would appear that the most constant correlation of hippocampal theta activity in animals of several species is their orienting toward and attending to stimuli in the environment, although there is also an association of rhythmic activity of 6 Hz and higher with bodily movements in the rat, at least.

Not only do the amount and duration of rhythmic activity in the hippocampus change with alterations in the animal's environment, but its frequency is altered as well. Lopes DaSilva and Kamp (1969) found a change in theta frequency ranges from 4–5 Hz to 5–6 Hz when an animal which was pressing a pedal in an operant situation backed away from the pedal after a reinforcement. In a subsequent article, Kamp et al. (1971) found the same increase in hippocampal frequencies when a dog changed its behavior from turning around looking for a thrown stick to actually running after it. These authors interpret their results to indicate an increase in the frequency of hippocampal electrical activities when the animal alters its ongoing behavioral sequences, i.e., when it stops one pattern of behavior and begins another one.

The arrest of ongoing behavior patterns has been found to be associated with a desynchronization of electrical activities recorded from the hippocampus, while the initiation of behaviors has been associated with rhythmic slow activities. In a task presumed to require the inhibition of movement, Bennett and Gottfried (1970) found that the EEG from the cat hippocampus was dominated by desynchronized activity. Pond *et al.* (1970) recorded electrical rhythms from the hippocampus in free-roving animals. They found that normal eating produced irregular and desynchronized activity in the hippocampus. On the other hand, if feeding behavior was elicited by direct hypothalamic stimulation, rhythmic slow activity was produced in the hippocampus. Rhythmic activities have been found after stimulation of the posterior regions of the hypothalamus by a number of investigators, but Pond *et al.* found that stimulation of the hypothalamus without an appropriate goal object present produced rhythmic slow activity in the hippocampus, but the frequency was 1–2 Hz below that found when stimulation with the appropriate goal object was present. This is important since it shows that even though the hippocampus may be inhibited by the stimulation of the hypothalamus, as measured by changes in electrical rhythms, its activity can still be subject to modification by the environment.

In 1965, Stumpf suggested that the theta frequency recorded from the hippocampus might be useful as an indicator of reticular formation arousal. It may be a better indicator of arousal mediated by the posterior hypothalamus. Stimulation in this region is more likely to produce rhythmic slow activity in the hippocampus than is stimulation of the reticular formation, although both areas can produce these activities when electrically stimulated. The rhythmic slow activities are of a "purer" nature when produced by hypothalamic stimulation than by reticular formation stimulation. There also is a functional differentiation between the posterior and anterior hypothalamus in that it is only the stimulation of the posterior hypothalamus which produces rhythmic slow activities in the hippocampus. Stimulation of the anterior hypothalamus produces a desynchronization of the hippocampus and, in addition, a high-frequency rhythmic response in the amygdala and the olfactory bulb (Kawamura *et al.*, 1961).

There is little doubt that there are multiple systems through which other brain regions regulate electrical rhythms of the hippocampus. Torii (1961) identified two systems, each of which stood in a particular relationship to both hippocampal activity and regulation of the autonomic nervous system. The first was a system including the ventromedial tegmentum, the lateral hypothalamus, and the medial septal area. Electrical stimulation applied at 100 Hz to the structures of this system produced desynchronized activity in the hippocampus and parasympathetic effects in the autonomic nervous system. The second system involved the dorsolateral central gray and the periventricular hypothalamus. Stimulation in these areas produced rhythmic activities in the hippocampus and sympathetic responses in the autonomic nervous system. The basic distinction between lateral desynchronizing and medial synchronizing systems of the hypothalamus relative to hippocampal rhythms has been supported by recent work of Anchel and Lindsley (1972). They also were able to confirm the suggestion of Torii that the synchronizing influences reaching the medial (paraventricular) regions of the hypothalamus from the tegmentum were carried over the dorsal fasciculus of Schütz. The desynchronizing influences were thought by Torii to be reaching the hypothalamus over the mammillary peduncle.

Anchel and Lindsley reported that the rhythmic slow activities elicited by medial hypothalamic stimulation can be blocked by lesions of the dorsal fornix but that the desynchronization response is not affected by these lesions. Anchel and Lindsley suggest that input from the fibers of tegmental origin which pass through the dorsal fasciculus of Schütz and medial hypothalamus reach both the septal area regions presumably containing the theta rhythm pacemakers and the intralaminar nuclei of the thalamus. The existence of this anatomical pathway was suggested by Nauta (1958). The two branches of this ascending system could have opposite effects in their regions of termination, such as to produce slow rhythmic activities in the hippocampus and desynchronization in the neocortex. However, it must be emphasized that hippocampal slow waves and neocortical desynchronization are not always closely associated. In most, if not all, species, hippocampal slow-wave activity can occur with any type of neocortical activity.

Several investigators have found that the frequency of the theta rhythm is sensitive to the intensity (voltage) of the stimulation applied to the hypothalamus but less so to the frequencies used (e.g., Anchel and Lindsley, 1972; G. Karmos, personal communication, 1973). Depressants like sodium amylobarbital decrease the frequency of the theta rhythms (Gray and Ball, 1970). This would suggest that the frequencies recorded from the hippocampus could be used as an indicator of the level of activity found in the medial hypothalamus. It is of theoretical interest that the frequencies are often fastest as an animal begins an approach response but quickly become slower as the behavior progresses. This suggests, by inference, that posterior hypothalamic activity is greatest at the beginning of a response sequence but becomes reduced as the act continues.

Despite the fact that stimulation of the lateral aspects of the posterior hypothalamus can produce a desynchronized hippocampal state, the electrical rhythms recorded from the hippocampus do not seem to stand in any particular or necessary relationship with rewarding effects produced by electrical stimulation of the same hypothalamic area or of the septal area. Pond and Schwartzbaum (1970) found no difference between the types of hippocampal EEG patterns found after rewarding or aversive stimulation of the hypothalamus or the midbrain. Rhythmic slow activities in the hippocampus were produced by both types of stimulation and were related to the intensity of the stimulation rather than its affective qualities. Ball and Gray (1971) stimulated the septal area and could get either rhythmic slow activities or desynchronization from the hippocampus by using different frequencies of stimulation. The different frequencies of stimulation were not related to the behavioral effects produced by the stimulation, since the animal would depress a lever to obtain stimulation at all frequencies used. Ito and Olds (1971) found that stimulation in a rewarding area of the lateral hypothalamus produced inhibitory effects on the activity of single cells in the hippocampus (but an excitatory effect on activity of cells in the cingulate cortex).

From these studies, several points of contradiction with the studies indicating separable systems of the hypothalamus related to hippocampal rhythms may be seen. Stimulation of the lateral hypothalamus—medial forebrain bundle area can, at times, produce rhythmic slow activities in the hippocampus and not desynchronization. This may be due to the fact that Pond and Schwartzbaum as well as Ball and Gray used rats instead of cats. There may be less segregation of the two types of tegmental and hypothalamic systems in the rat, or perhaps the smallness of the rat brain makes it impossible to stimulate one or the other of the systems selectively. In addition, the dissociation of rewarding and punishing effects is not correlated with a similar difference in hippocampal electrical rhythms. Perhaps both types of affective responses produced a common physiological effect beyond their hedonic aspects.

In recent review articles, Winson (1972, 1974) has pointed out that there is no good reason to believe that behaviors correlated with hippocampal rhythmic slow activities should be the same in all species. He concludes that the only firm correlate of hippocampal slow-wave activity across species is the stage of paradoxical sleep. Otherwise, he concludes, theta rhythms are found in relation to different kinds of behaviors in different species. Rhythmic slow activities are frequently found to be correlated with activity in the rat but not in the cat. The tentative suggestion offered by Winson is that hippocampal slow waves are related to certain species-typical behaviors which are of survival value to the species, e.g., exploration and sniffing in the rat, flight in rabbit, and stalking in the cat. When these behaviors are dominant, the hippocampal recordings are predominantly slow and rhythmic. This may indicate that behavior is being organized and regulated by other systems of the brain and the hippocampus is being subjected to strong inhibitory regulation.

The Conditioning of Hippocampal Slow Waves

One way to study the significance of the rhythmic slow-wave activity of the hippocampus is to explore its conditioning to various signals. Black and his associates have been successful in conditioning rhythmic slow activity (4–7 Hz) and a desynchronized state in the same dogs. This was accomplished using both food and brain stimulation as rewards. Black et al. (1970) demonstrated rhythmic slow activity conditioning in curarized dogs, as well. This would indicate that the conditioning of the rhythmic slow activities of the hippocampus need not be mediated via bodily activities. Black et al. have also investigated the physiological and behavioral states which might be related to electrical activities of the hippocampus. They found that desynchronization of the neocortex can be associated with any type of electrical activity in the hippocampus. This implies that even if pathways of tegmental origin pass through the medial hypothalamus to reach the theta-pacemaking cells of the septal area and the intralaminar nuclei, producing opposite effects in each, this ascending system cannot be the sole determinant of the electrical rhythms in hippocampus and neocortex. Heart rate was not associated with the type of electrical activity found in the hippocampus but rather with the actual motor activity being exhibited by the animal. The main behavioral correlate of hippocampal slow activity discovered was locomotor movement. When the hippocampus evidenced a desynchronized state, the animals were likely to be standing still (Black, 1972). When the animals were taught to make an active conditioned response, there were increases in rhythmic slow activity. When the animals were trained to inhibit overt responses, a much decreased level of rhythmic slow activities was obtained. In a related experiment, Holmes and Beckman (1969) found that rhythmic slow activity was a good indicator of whether or not a cat would run a simple runway for a food reward when signaled to do so.

Movements are not essential for the occurrence of rhythmic slow activities from the hippocampus, since they can be conditioned in animals immobilized under curare. Using a related approach, Black has tried to make animals be immobile and yet produce rhythmic slow activities in the hippocampus. The animals had to do both in order to be rewarded. This was possible for lower frequencies but not for the higher frequencies in the "slow range" (Black and DeToledo, 1971).

Overall, rhythmic slow activities are found in recordings made from the hippocampus during periods of approach responding, active orientation, and when animals are engaged in a behavior sequence requiring locomotor activities. Desynchronized activity in the hippocampus seems to be correlated with the suppression of movement and an arrest of ongoing behavioral sequences.

Electrical Seizure Activity

The hippocampus is thought of as an area of the brain especially prone to seizure activity. Almost any physical or chemical disturbance will lead to a series of epileptiform afterdischarges.

The afterdischarges may spread beyond the hippocampus to involve other regions of the limbic system or may remain confined to the hippocampus. Once begun, seizures or afterdischarges initiated in the hippocampus seem to propagate throughout the extent of the structure. The propagation of these seizures to other structures, if it does occur, is quite different depending on the site of initiation of the seizures, especially its dorsal or ventral aspects (Elul, 1964).

Woodruff et al. (1973a) have found that the seizure-prone nature of the hippocampus is dependent on projections to it from the pontine portions of the brain stem. In rabbits, a section through the brain stem ahead of the pons makes the hippocampus no more prone to seizure activity than the posterior neocortex.

The hippocampus also can influence the mechanisms of the brain responsible for general bodily seizures. Adler (1972) has reported that small lesions in the dorsal hippocampus were more effective in altering the threshold for total body convulsions produced by flurothyl gas than lesions in the amygdala, the septal area, or the olfactory tubercule. The effects produced by the hippocampal destruction were biphasic. At 1 week, the threshold for the seizures was raised approximately 10% while at 15 weeks postoperatively the threshold had been reduced by about 17%.

Using rats, Van Hartesveldt and Vernadakis (1972) studied two aspects of convulsive behavior produced by transcorneal electrical stimulation in animals with extensive hippocampal destruction. They measured the thresholds for indicators of minimal seizures, which included small twitching movements, and for maximal clonic effects, including bodily extension and paddling movements of the back feet. Lesions of the neocortex overlying the hippocampus with or without concomitant hippocampal damage produced a lowered threshold for the minimal seizures, but only destruction of the hippocampus lowered the threshold for the maximal convulsions. The durations of the maximal convulsions were also increased by the hippocampal damage.

When afterdischarges are produced in the hippocampus, there is a change in the type of effect produced by the hippocampus on hypothalamic units. Earlier, the fact that stimulation of the hippocampus facilitated neuronal firing in the anterior hypo-

thalamus was mentioned. During afterdischarges in the hippocampus, the effect on anterior hypothalamic neurons changes
from a predominantly excitatory effect found under normal
conditions to a condition in which excitatory and inhibitory
effects on cellular activity are equally likely (Kinnard et al., 1970).

Seizures and Memory

In 1972, I examined the possibility that the human memory
deficits reported to follow temporal lobe surgery may be related to
seizure activities of temporal lobe origin. This form of seizure was
the "presenting complaint" of most of the patients involved
(Isaacson, 1972b). The deficit reported to follow temporal lobe
destruction in man is a loss of memory for events intervening
between the time of surgery and extending to the span of immediate
memory. In general, the amnesic syndrome which results from
medial temporal lobe destruction is not associated with losses in
attention, skills, or intelligence. Reasoning and perception seem
unaffected. Memories of the remote past likewise seem unaffected,
but new memory formation is impaired from the time of surgery
onward.

In considering the temporal lobe memory deficit, it should be
emphasized that the memory debility found after medial destruction
of the temporal lobe is not an all-or-none phenomenon nor is the
brain damage without other, albeit relatively minor, behavioral
consequences. Some patients need to be reminded to shave and to
eat. Sometimes there is a disturbance of gait and coordination with
a loss of sensitivity in the extremities. It is possible that these
disturbances in sensory and motor functions were present before
the temporal lobe surgery and merely became more noticeable with
time.

The disease processes responsible for human temporal
lobe surgery may have interacted with the surgical lesion to
produce behavioral changes which would not be found after a
surgical lesion in a normal brain. The majority of patients in whom a
disturbance of recent memory has been reported were suffering
from epileptic disorders so severe as to prohibit normal life
activities and to justify the surgery. The only patients with severe
memory disturbances after surgery who were not epileptic were

cases D.C. and M.B. of Scoville (Scoville and Milner, 1957). These two people had grossly impaired adjustments to their environment, were diagnosed as psychotic, and had experienced a series of insulin and electroconvulsive shock treatments. In addition, spike discharges from the temporal lobes had been found at the time of operation in one of them (case D.C.). Could the process causing the epileptic condition be related to the recent memory losses?

The nature of the lesion responsible for most cases of temporal lobe epilepsy is not fully established. In general, the mesial portions of the temporal lobes will often show sclerotic regions at autopsy, especially in those cases in which the seizures began early in life (Falconer et al., 1964). The damaged area is not limited to the hippocampus, but often extends to include the amygdala and other portions of the temporal lobe. The view that the primary cause of the epileptic zone is a herniation of the temporal lobe into the incisura of the tentorium at birth which in turn causes ischemic damage due to compression of the anterior choroidal artery and branches of the posterior cerebral artery, as proposed by Earle et al. (1953), has not been universally accepted.

An "epileptogenic focus" refers to a group of cells thought to be responsible for production of abnormal electrical patterns recorded from brain tissue. The cells in an epileptogenis focus are more excitable than normal cells and have the capability of generating autonomous paroxysmal discharges.

An observable convulsion or seizure may not result if the epileptogenic focus remains restricted to the immediate area of the focus. Even though cells in the area of the focus function in an aberrant fashion, without the spread of the discharges to other regions behavioral manifestations of the seizure will not be seen. It is believed that seizure discharges must propagate into the extrapyramidal motor nuclei before motor signs occur. For the other types of seizures, discharges must propagate to other, probably subcortical, regions.

Epileptogenic foci can be artificially created by the direct application of many different compounds and procedures, including the application of aluminum hydroxide gel, penicillin, other antibiotics, cobalt powder, conjugated estrogens, pentylene-tetrazol (Metrazol), and by local freezing. The mechanism by which penicillin acts to create an epileptogenic focus is largely unknown, but abnormal electrical discharges have been established in a number of species by its topical application. The exact length of time the penicillin-induced epileptiform activity will last is unknown, but it appears that at least some components of a neocortical focus last over a period of months in rats. When recording from the hippocampus at prolonged times after penicillin injection, definite epileptiform activity can frequently be observed (Schmaltz, 1971). Spike discharges occur singly, in bursts, or in trains which last over periods of 10–20 sec or longer. In about half of the animals studied, spiking was not observed but bursts of high-voltage fast activity could be recorded against a relatively normal background. Thus it appears that a single application of penicillin can produce anomalies in the neocortex and the hippocampus of the rat which will extend over a period of months, at least.

Behavioral Consequences of Artificial Epileptogenic Foci

The behavioral effects of the applications of agents which cause epileptogenic foci in the brain have received some attention, but most studies have investigated behavioral alterations produced by neocortical foci. For example, Kraft et al. (1960) found that irritative lesions of the striate area of monkeys induced by aluminum hydroxide injections produced a greater impairment in two visual tasks than did surgical extirpation of tissue (Wilson and Mishkin, 1959). The retention of visual problems learned before the application of the epileptogenic agent was unaffected (Henry and Pribram, 1954; Chow and Obrist, 1954). Stamm and Pribram (1960) reported impaired acquisition of a delayed alternation problem with epileptogenic lesions of the prefrontal cortex of monkeys, but observed no deficit on previously acquired problems. Chow (1961) found visual performance to be disrupted when electrically induced afterdischarges were present bilaterally in the temporal lobe neocortex. Interestingly, unilateral temporal lobe afterdischarges and electrical shocks delivered to the occipital areas failed to interfere with the animals' performance.

From several studies, it is clear that penicillin injected into the hippocampus can produce profound behavioral effects which are quite different from those found after surgical destruction of the same areas. In some ways, results obtained from the application of penicillin into the hippocampal area resemble the deficits reported at the human level.

Probably the most dramatic results were those obtained by Schmaltz (1971). In his work, a two-way active avoidance task was used. This shuttlebox task is one in which the performance of animals with bilateral destruction of the hippocampus by aspiration is enhanced. Schmaltz found that penicillin injected unilaterally into the rat hippocampus greatly impaired the animals in learning the task.

Equally interesting was the observation that animals with the impaired performance due to penicillin injection showed better performance during the last five trials each day than during the first five. The animals apparently were able to learn something about the problem within each day's training session but started the next day's training as if this previous training had not taken place. This inability to carry over the effects of training from one day to the next suggested an inability to consolidate the memories from the past into a form useful on subsequent days. Significant impairments were obtained with unilateral injections of penicillin into hippocampus; however, the effect is much more pronounced when a unilateral injection of penicillin is combined with the ablation of the contralateral hippocampus.

Nakajima (1969) has found impairment in the learning and relearning of a shock-motivated spatial discrimination in a T-maze following the injection of actinomycin D into the hippocampus. The learning impairment is similar to that produced by electrolytic lesions of hippocampus, but the electrolytic lesion fails to influence retention as measured by relearning on the following day. The actinomycin-injected animals, on the other hand, showed impaired retention of the problem when tested by relearning. This deficit is suggestive of a memory impairment of events occurring beyond the training period.

Olton (1970) confirmed the observations of Schmaltz and extended them by considering the effects of pencillin injections into different brain regions in otherwise intact animals and in animals with bilateral aspirative destruction of the hippocampus. He used an avoidance training paradigm similar to that used by

Schmaltz. Penicillin injections into the septal area or into the entorhinal cortex failed to produce the same debilitating effects as did injections into the hippocampus. In animals with bilateral destruction of the hippocampus, the rate of active avoidance learning was improved and was not altered by penicillin introduced into the septal area. Penicillin injections into entorhinal cortex, on the other hand, offset the improvement in performance produced by hippocampal destruction. This was interpreted as suggesting that the interaction between the hippocampus and adjacent entorhinal cortex is of greater significance than the hippocampus–septal area interaction.

Hamilton and Isaacson (1970) studied the effect of penicillin implantation into a variety of brain stem locations. When behavior in the two-way active avoidance tasks was studied, locations in the ventral tegmental area were especially effective in disrupting learning. Drug implantation sites in the reticular formation produced slight, if any, debilitating effects. Penicillin application to many other regions, e.g., mammillary bodies, caudate nucleus, midline thalamus, and the dorsomedial thalamic nucleus, failed to disrupt the avoidance behavior. After the avoidance training had been completed, the animals were tested in a visual discrimination task for food reward. All of the animals were able to learn this visual discrimination problem. Therefore, the debilitation was specific to the avoidance task and did not carry over to the visual discrimination problem. Animals with penicillin implanted into one hippocampus with the contralateral hippocampus surgically removed, the most impaired preparation studied by Schmaltz and Olton, were also studied in this task. No deficit in their behavior was observed.

Even though Hamilton and I did not find any effect from reticular formation implantation of the epileptogenic drugs, Kesner and Conner (1972) were able to show effects of reticular formation electrical stimulation on the retention of a punishing event using a response suppression paradigm. Amnesic effects were found in animals tested a minute later but not in animals tested a day afterward. These authors also found that hippocampal stimulation failed to affect retention of the footshock when measured a minute afterward, but amnesia was found in animals tested 24 hr later. The stimulation of the reticular formation and the hippocampus had produced opposite effects. These results suggest independent and parallel systems of memory, long-term and short-term retention of the noxious event.

The results obtained by Hamilton and Isaacson (1970) testing animals in the visual discrimination task have been confirmed by Woodruff and Isaacson (1972) and by Woodruff et al. (1973b). In the latter study, daily injections of penicillin were made into the hippocampus, but even this failed to impede the acquisition or retention of the discrimination.

This line of research has led us to several possible conclusions. One is that the epileptic condition induced in the hippocampus, coupled with a unilateral lesion, does indeed produce some kind of an amnesic effect but that this effect is limited to avoidance tasks. The work with appetitive tasks would seem to rule out a more general deficit in mnemonic functions. If this were to be the case, it would have to imply that the verbal memories disturbed in the human after temporal lobe surgery rely on processes similar to those used by the rat during avoidance conditioning. On the other hand, the avoidance deficits found after penicillin injections into the hippocampus may not be due to any changes in memory or retrieval but due to some aspect of function related to performance in some unknown way which mimics a memory deficit. Another possible basis for the memory deficits found in the amnesic patients relates to the exaggerated proactive effects commonly found both in man and in animals after hippocampal damage. This approach will be discussed in greater detail in the next chapter.

Summary and Reflections

Overall, the studies of hippocampal contributions to behavior have been suggestive of some kind of inhibitory function. Most of the theories put forward have stressed behavioral inhibition in one way or another. The nature of the inhibitory influence varies according to the theory: inhibition in sensory systems, motor responses, cognitive acts, or whatever. Yet each theorist seems to have to use some form of suppressive influence to explain the behavioral changes produced by lesions or stimulation. Despite the fact that there are serious differences among investigators with regard to the nature of inhibitory effects ascribed to the hippocampus, it is significant that there is this core of agreement. It suggests that there are some common characteristics seen by different observers which just escape unequivocal description at the present time.

Beyond this agreement on an impairment to suppress behavioral sequences, most investigators also agree that animals with hippocampal damage are especially prone to initiate and continue responses. All animals can be considered to contain energy stored in a more or less unstable fashion. The appropriate signal can release great amounts of this stored energy in the form of motoric or autonomic reactions. It is as if the animals with hippocampal lesions had a greater amount of energy available waiting to be released by opportunities to respond. Not only is it released easily, but the released energy also is maintained during the execution of the goal-directed act. This metaphor is based on observations of the rapid acquisition of certain problems, the lesser distractibility, the greater resistance to extinction, difficulties during reversal training, and the inability to withhold responses in passive avoidance and DRL tasks. But the energy metaphor is weak. It does not provide any insight as to the neural mechanisms involved in the actions of the lesioned animals which suggest greater responsiveness.

There is, however, almost a uniform acceptance of the view that the influences of the hippocampus are exerted on hypo-thalamic systems. This is based in part on the hippocampal–hypothalamic connections which have been so strongly em-phasized by neuroanatomists and also on the fact that many similar effects can be produced by stimulation and lesions of hypothalamic regions and other limbic regions. Electrophysiolog-ical studies have also shown a strong, and possibly dual, ef-fect of the hypothalamus on the hippocampus. But what is the nature of this interrelationship between the hippocampus and the hypothalamus and what significance does it have for behavior? What sorts of hypothalamic systems fall under the regulation of the limbic system and under what conditions do they come under the influence of the hippocampus?

Information about the neurochemical systems of the brain and the brain mechanisms served by them may give us insight into hypothalamic–hippocampal relationships. It is clear that the hippocampus is closely related to both adrenergic and cholinergic subsystems of the brain. Destruction of this structure seems to make the animals more reactive to amphetamine and drugs that reduce effective norepinephrine levels which seem to mitigate the lesion effects, at least on some tasks. However, animals with lesions of the hippocampus are also overly responsive to anti-cholinergic drugs. Furthermore, there are substantial similarities between the effects of hippocampal destruction and the systemic administration of anticholinergics. Some of the strongest parallels between the effects of hippocampal destruction and anticholinergic drug administration come from the studies using avoidance conditioning. They include the facilitation of two-way active avoidance conditioning and impairments in the one-way active avoidance problems (Suits and Isaacson, 1968). It is of some interest also that both amphetamine and scopolamine enhance the acquisition of two-way active avoidance problems (e.g., Barrett et al., 1973). It appears that the drugs have affected the animals' tendencies to initiate the required response rather than produced an enhanced amount of learning. On the other hand, it is likely that the sudden shift from a certain drugged state to a nondrugged state produces such a new condition for the animals that performance deteriorates. Barrett et al. (1972) have shown that this deterioration of performance can be reduced by gradually reducing drug dosages over time.

Other studies concerned with the effect of anticholinergic drugs on the behavior of animals have found that animals with hippocampal lesions were less responsive to the anticholinergic drugs than were control animals (Warburton, 1969a,b). According to this suggesion, the drug produces its effect by modifying the activities of the hippocampus. If this is so, lesions of the hippo-campus should decrease the behavioral effects of cholinergic drugs. Data opposed to such a view are reported by Clark (1970). In her study of exploratory activity, animals with hippocampal lesions were more responsive to scopolamine than were normal animals.

The administration of scopolamine to animals with hippo-campal lesions produces hyperreactive and hyperactive animals. At times, in the laboratory, we have not been able to handle them because of their heightened reactivity. However, it has not been possible to improve the performance of animals with extensive hippocampal lesions in tasks by enhancing the cholinergic system with physostigmine either in spontaneous alternation tasks (unpublished observations) or in the DRL task (Van Hartesveldt, 1974). In studies of spontaneous alternation, R. J. Douglas (personal communication) has found that physostigmine administration will enhance alternation rates in intact animals but not in animals with nearly complete hippocampal destruction.

Therefore, we have a situation in which the reduction of cholinergic activities will drastically influence the behavior of the lesioned animals but the enhancement of cholinergic activity is not of observable benefit. In contrast, changes in the norepinephrine system in either direction produce easily discernible effects.

These results suggest that the influences of the hippocampus play on and help regulate neural (both cholinergic and adrenergic) subsystems of the brain, although the types of regulation of these other subsystems must be quite different.

But what model can be generated to account for the regulatory influences of the hippocampus and other regions of the limbic system on behavior? A model will be proposed in the next chapter which may provide a context for the data which have been assembled in the many studies reviewed in the preceding chapters.

Chapter 6

THE GRAVEN IMAGE, LETHE, AND THE GURU

In this final chapter, I will suggest a way of looking at the limbic system as it may function with regard to behavior. It must be recognized that the limbic system does not do its work independently of other "systems" of the brain. This implies that no reasonable theory of the activity of the limbic system can be developed until a more general framework for the brain's activities has been achieved. This accomplishment is not likely in the foreseeable future.

Yet, the human mind needs a theoretical structure for understanding the diverse facts of nature and of science. Most people need, and indeed some *must* have, a conceptual framework for thinking about the brain and for guiding their research. It is because of such a need that telephone switchboard theories, computer-analogy theories, and holographic models have been advocated. All are but metaphors taken from other contexts and applied to brain activities. There is nothing wrong with metaphors so long as they are not confused with fact.

The Triune Brain

Paul MacLean (1970) has suggested that neural and behavioral distinctions can be made among three types of systems found in the brains of mammals. This differentiation is based in part on comparative anatomy, neurochemistry, and evolutionary theory. MacLean's basic divisions of the brain are a protoreptilian brain, a paleomammalian brain, and a neomammalian brain. The protoreptilian brain is thought to represent a fundamental core of the nervous system, consisting of systems in the upper spinal cord and parts of the midbrain, diencephalon, and basal ganglia. The paleomammalian brain is, in essence, the limbic system. The neomammalian brain refers to the neocortical developments, so prominent in primates.

These three divisions must be considered as speculative, since there is no evidence that any reptile ever had a brain very much like the "reptilian core brain" of mammals. Furthermore, the brains of all living forms of reptiles have sectors of "general cortex" which may be homologous to the neocortex as well as parts which may be homologous to the limbic system in mammals. MacLean's "reptile brain," the core of the mammalian brain, must be considered as a prototypic or hypothetical "reptile brain" and not as the actual neural apparatus of any species, living or dead. It does not really matter whether or not there ever were animals with protoreptilian brains or with paleomammalian brains. The significance of the triune brain approach relates to the usefulness of describing behavioral functions in terms of more or less specific anatomical systems. In this sense, the triune brain model deserves serious consideration as a metaphor for the hierarchical structures of the brain as it relates to behavior.

MacLean considers the protoreptilian brain as responsible for stereotyped behaviors based on "ancestral learning and ancestral memories"; it plays a crucial role in the establishment of home territories, the finding of shelter and food, breeding, and other activities necessary for the survival of the species and the individual. The paleomammalian or limbic brain is thought to be nature's tentative first step toward providing self-awareness, especially awareness of the internal conditions of the body. To MacLean, it is still a "visceral brain" (see MacLean, 1949), but it also has some role related to neocortical formations more generally. It is thought to be able to override the ancestral basis of behavior found in the protoreptilian brain. The elaboration of information arising from inside the person or animal is thought to provide a necessary component of, or context for, significant memories. All memories, according to MacLean's view, depend on a mixture of information from the inner and outer worlds. The hippocampus is thought to be an especially good place for such mixtures to occur. It receives "internal information" from the septal area and "external information" from sensory systems projecting to nearby transitional cortical areas (MacLean, 1972).

The role of the neocortex is not greatly discussed in MacLean's writings, but he seems to consider it to be responsible for the cold (nonemotional) and fine-grain analysis of the external environment. It operates "unhindered by signals and noise generated in the internal world." Its ability to make fine discriminations is emphasized, and it is thought to have a predilection for dividing things into smaller and smaller units.

My own thoughts about the function of the "three brains in one" agree fairly well with MacLean's analysis as it relates to the protoreptilian brain. With regard to the role of the limbic system and the neocortex, however, there are great differences. Basically, I consider the limbic system as regulating the protoreptilian brain, primarily in an inhibitory fashion, and I assume the neocortex to have more interesting duties than the fine-grain analysis of the external world. I suspect that it is responsible for the generation of expectancies about the future. If the limbic system does indeed act to inhibit the ancient memories of the protoreptilian brain, then it is acting to produce forgetfulness. It is acting as the river (or goddess) of forgetting—Lethe. If the neocortex does look to the future, it is acting as a neural Guru. From these considerations, the title of the chapter came about.

Animals with Predominantly Protoreptilian Brains

Living animals with a variety of types of nervous systems exhibit remarkable adjustments to their environments. For that matter, single-celled animals have extraordinary adjustive capacities. They survive and propagate, often doing so in the context of environmental changes which require structural or behavioral modifications. The nervous system develops to make these same types of adjustments possible for animals made up of many diverse kinds of cells. The development of the nervous system adds no unique quality to basic animal life, but it does allow larger populations of highly specialized cells to operate synergistically to achieve ends advantageous to the group. The amoeba exhibits many forms of behavior which might be thought to depend on the nervous system (see Isaacson and Hutt, 1971). Four basic behavioral principles are exemplified in the behavior of this single-celled animal: responses depend on the conditions of stimulations; responses habituate and change with repeated stimulation; the state of the internal environment determines the reaction produced by the stimulation; and several stimuli acting at the same time can produce responses different from those produced by any one of the stimuli alone. Even without a nervous system, the amoeba can make specialized adjustments to its environment, taking the internal and external environments into consideration.

Learning and memory are possible for animals made up of relatively few cells (see McConnell and Jacobson, 1973). These animals make adjustments suited to their specialized patterns of behavior and their ecological circumstances. It might be argued, however, that animals with no nervous system or a meager one would be less intelligent than those with more elaborate coordinating systems. This difference in intelligence could be reflected in the ability to learn new tasks, however, it is doubtful that comparisons in learning abilities can be made among animals of different species. Historically, the comparative study of differences in the intelligence of animals came to naught because the behavioral capabilities of animals of various species cannot readily be compared owing to the specialized character of species-typical behaviors. Furthermore, each species has its own way of analyzing the world in which its members live. The comparison of intellectual abilities among existing species cannot reveal evolutionary trends, since all living forms are highly specialized and, by definition, successful.

If it is true that animals with the most meager of nervous systems are capable of complex adjustments to the world and of modifying their behavioral patterns according to the demands of the environment, it is likely that these fundamental aspects of animal behavior could easily be served by the protoreptilian brain described by MacLean. According to such a view, the basic operations necessary for life *and* for many of the adjustments required by changes in the environment, including learning and memory, could be accomplished by the neural apparatus of portions of the basal ganglia, hypothalamus, brain stem, and spinal cord.

If there is some universality in the abilities of animals relative to adjustments to a changing environment, these should be found in the behavior of many species. Consider the learning of simple behaviors in the fish as a point of departure. Conditioned responses of different sorts have been readily formed to visual and auditory stimuli (Froloff, 1925), water temperature, small changes in the salinity of the water (Bull, 1928), and water currents (Sears, 1934). Discriminations among stimuli can also be made by some fish, and Reeves (1919) was able to train them to discriminate between blue and red-orange lights. Higher-order conditioning can also be established, at least by goldfish. For example, fish trained to approach a disk for food can be trained to approach the disk when a chemical is added to the water (Sanders, 1940). Active avoidance learning is rapidly acquired by fish and toads (Behrend and Bitterman, 1963; Crawford and Langdon, 1966).

Not only can fish learn many types of problems readily but their learning is also often marked by *sudden* improvements in performance. In a study using sharks, Aronson *et al.* (1967) found a rapid reduction in errors over the first few trials in their learning to strike targets for food reward. Invertebrates (Morrow and Smithson, 1969) can learn simple problems quite readily with their relatively limited neurological apparatus, and their learning, also, is often characterized by abrupt, steplike reductions in the number of errors made.

Lesions of the forebrain of fish are without drastic effects on their performance in learning various problems; e.g., such lesions do not disrupt learning to discriminate a colored patch of paper from others. Sears (1934) found that goldfish were able to acquire a conditioned response to light after a large part of the optic lobes had been damaged and, in addition, that these lesions did not disturb the retention of the discrimination when the fish were tested 3 days postoperatively.

The neural mechanisms responsible for the rapid learning and long-term memory are not limited to whatever forebrain tissue that exists in fish. Nevertheless, there are some differences in the performance of fish relative to mammals. These differences include observations that fish extinguish learned responses more quickly if small food rewards are used in training than if large rewards are used (Gonzales and Bitterman, 1967). Just the opposite is true for mammals. Fish also extinguish partially reinforced responses more rapidly than continuously reinforced responses, again a result opposite to that found in mammals (Wodinsky and Bitterman, 1959, 1960). This suggests that the learning mechanisms of the fish brain are associated with the number, frequency, and magnitude of primary rewards. They are little affected by the variables often thought to be associated with "expectations" held about the environment. It is commonly held that mammals extinguish more rapidly after training with large rather than with small rewards because of the greater disruptive effects produced when the expected reward is no longer furnished. The effectiveness of partial reward schedules during extinction is also related to changes in what the animals have come to expect in previous training sessions.

Reporting work in his laboratory, Beritoff (1971) states that the retention of "images" of the place where food had been eaten or where schock had been received on only one occasion was only of a very short duration, roughly 10 sec, in fish. The memory of conditioned responses was maintained for long periods of time. Forebrain lesions in fish reduced the time during which these animals could act on the "images" of the place of food or punishment, reducing it to a period of 4–5 sec. This might mean that one form of short-term memories relating to places of interest in the environment could be facilitated by neural systems of forebrain origin. This need not be a specific effect of the forebrain, however, but due to some general facilitatory effect of the forebrain on lower brain stem systems.

More Complicated Forms of Learning and Memory

It has been suggested that the ability to form learning sets is a quality which distinguishes more highly developed brains from the less developed (Harlow, 1959). However, there are several reasons to doubt this conclusion. For example, Mackintosh and Mackintosh (1964) have shown that learning sets can be formed in the octopus. Nevertheless, this is not a critical point since the capacity of the octopus to establish learning sets could mean only that alternate neural mechanisms related to learning sets have evolved in these animals, independent of the evolutionary development of the neural mechanisms of mammals used to achieve the same environmental goals. Gonzales *et al.* (1967) did not find evidence for learning set formation over a number of discrimination problem reversals in fish. Pigeons, on the other hand, have been shown to have the ability to form learning sets, as have chickens (Plotnick and Tallarico, 1966).

However, the entire question of the meaning of differences in learning set tasks is open to serious question because of the different abilities of various species to respond to sensory stimulation, the difficulty in controlling the degree of original learning, and various aspects of the training environment which could help or hinder members of a particular species. For these reasons, Warren (1973) doubts that learning set performance can be used to evaluate the intellectual superiority of one species over another.

When animals are tested with multiple reversals of a discrimination task, they are trained to make a discrimination between two stimuli. After this is mastered, the significance of the two stimuli is reversed so that responses to the formerly correct stimuli are not rewarded and those to the formerly negative stimulus are. This reversal procedure can be repeated indefinitely and the time required to master each reversal recorded. In his original studies, Bitterman and his colleagues were unable to show any improvements in the learning of multiple reversals by goldfish or by mouthbreeders. Representatives of several mammalian groups have been shown to learn reversal problems with greater and greater ease. The improvement in the acquisition of successive reversals by mammals was correlated with an apparant reduction in the memory of the animal for the previously learned problem. The inference might be made that the improved performance on subsequent reversal problems was due to the rapid forgetting which occurs after learning many similar reversals, i.e., a proactive inhibition effect. On the other hand, the goldfish and mouthbreeders, which fail to show improvements in the acquisition of reversal problems, may have trouble in forgetting the previous problem. Therefore, it would be tempting to conclude that the formation of learning sets is related to the ability to forget past events as a function of prior learning. This forgetting system could be more effective in mammals than in fish. The inference would be that the development of a complex forebrain, namely the limbic system and the neocortex, results in an increased ability to forget.

Unfortunately, this analysis and the inferences drawn from it may not be of particular value. Bitterman (1972) has found that the apparent inability of the goldfish to show improvement in the successive reversal paradigm is linked to procedural variables and not to some basic behavioral capacities of the species. By modifying the apparatus used in testing the animals, improvements over repeated reversals were found and they were of a magnitude equal to those found in birds and mammals. Therefore, neither learning set formation nor the more rapid acquisition of successive reversals offers a basis for determining behavioral capacities related to the elaboration of limbic or neocortical mechanisms.

It is also unlikely that measures of response inhibition can be used for this purpose. A technique to investigate passive avoidance behavior in goldfish was perfected by Riege and Cherkin (1971). The animals were trained to swim against currents of water flowing from a "well." After this approach response had become established, the animals were given an electrical shock at the well. The animals were tested at various postshock times to determine the effect of this shock on the approach response.

The fish showed retention of the effects of the electrical shock (as reflected in substantially increased approach latencies) *immediately* afterward but not when tested 1 min afterward. When tested 2 min after the shock, some memory was present. Their approach latencies were longer when tested 4 min after the shock and at all subsequent times. Thus the retention curve for the punishing effect of the shock was complex: an immediate period of retention which dissipated in about 1 min only to be followed by a second more permanent phase beginning at 2–4 min after the shock and persisting well beyond.

A similar biphasic curve has been reported for mice in a passive avoidance task by Irwin *et al.* (1964). In this study, the period of poorest retention was at 5 min after shock. Cherkin (1971) has also found a biphasic retention curve for the chick.

A number of suggestions have been made to account for

the biphasic retention curves, including (1) that there is a deficit in the retrieval processes at the intermittent, short-latency period (Klein and Spear, 1970) and (2) that fear requires time to be incubated in memory (Pinel and Cooper, 1966). It seems that the two aspects of the obtained retention curves could also be explained on the basis of two independent memory processes: a short-term memory component and a long-term memory component. If this interpretation were made, it could be assumed that the goldfish has both memory mechanisms available to it, although its short-term (image) memory decays more rapidly than in mammalian species.

The remarkable fact which arises from these studies is that at least some forms of learning and memory seem to be quite adequate in animals having very little beyond protoreptilian brain mechanisms. At least, this would indicate that the basic mechanisms of the less complicated animals are adequate to maintain many forms of learning and memory.

Fish seem to be dominated by primary rewards and the frequency of their application to a greater extent than are animals with more forebrain tissue. They seem to pay little heed to the uncertainties of the environment. Their "images" of places in their environment fade quickly, but established conditioned responses tend to remain indefinitely.

Surprisingly little work has been done on the permanence of memory in animals with meager forebrain tissue. It might be expected that they would have strong and stable forms of memory since fish and amphibians tend to live in environments that change more slowly than those above the water. However, the apparent stability of the sea environment may be more apparent than real—especially to the species that populate the ocean. The question as to the permanence of memories in any animal is an empirical question to be resolved by observation and experimentation.

In studies by Georgian workers at the Physiological Laboratory at Tbilisi (summarized by Beritoff, 1971), long-term retention of conditioned responses has been demonstrated in fish, even those with lesions of the forebrain. After forebrain destruction, retention of previously established responses was demonstrated. As mentioned before, after the forebrain lesions the animals could not seem to remember the location of a place where they had been fed even for a few seconds (poor "image memory") and would quite readily approach a location in which they had received a punishing electrical shock. This latter effect might appear to represent a deficiency in passive avoidance abilities, but it also could be due to a reduced ability to remember, for any protracted period of time, the *places* where either favorable or unfavorable events have happened.

Beritoff believes that as the neocortex and forebrain develop there is little change in the permanency of "memories" for conditioned reflexes but a large change in the ability of animals to hold "images" of rewards and punishments. Image memory for Beritoff pertains to things learned in one trial, and in which the location of the reward is important. The older portions of the brain are thought to be able to mediate fear responses (emotional memory) for limited periods of time, but long-range retention of punishing events is thought to depend, also, on the development of the neocortex.

Beritoff's conclusions come from the study of animals which have only small amounts of forebrain tissue beyond the systems of the reptilian brain complex. These studies suggest that the protomammalian brain can subserve the ability to learn and remember habits formed through conditioning just as well as more complicated forebrains. The failure of the protoreptilian brain, if it should be called that, lies on holding memories formed on a one-time association for longer than the briefest periods. This could reflect a lack in flexibility, an inability to adjust quickly to new information, and a reliance on habitual ways of responding.

These tentative conclusions from the basis of neurally simpler organisms need not apply to the functions of the reptilian core brain of advanced animals. In all likelihood, there are substantial functional differences in the protoreptilian core brain of mammals and the same neural core in fish, living reptiles, and amphibians. At best, they are hints as to functions that might be subserved by the reptilian core brain in mammals.

Huston and Borbély (1973) have investigated the learning capacities of rats which have had most of the forebrain destroyed by aspiration. The lesions included all of the neocortex, most of the limbic system, and much of the striatum. The thalamus and hypothalamus were left more or less intact. Behaviors were trained by the use of rewarding electrical stimulation of the hypothalamus. These authors were able to condition simple movements of the head or tail by operant procedures. This means that the movements became more frequent when they were followed by the stimulation of the hypothalamus. Most of the "thalamic animals," those without damage to the diencephalon, were able to demonstrate conditioning but were unaffected by extinction procedures. Once they had been conditioned, they persisted in the learned movements even in the absence of rewards. The animals could be induced to stop making the acquired movements, however, by training them to make a different response. Thus these lesioned animals retained the capacity to stop making responses but not through nonreward only. These authors also found that in the beginning the hypothalamic stimulation tended to produce forward locomotion in the animals. Once a response had been established in the animals through conditioning, however, the stimulation would frequently elicit the conditioned response. The conditioned response could also be evoked by noises or by touching the animals.

Animals with little more than the diencephalon left tend to be hyperactive in a cyclic fashion. Periods of activity alternate with periods of inactivity even though the normal day—night cycle is abolished (Borbély et al., 1973). Amphetamine-produced increases in activity can be observed in the animals as well as an increased stereotypy of behavior. (This suggests that the dopaminergic innervation of the basal ganglia may not be an essential aspect of the neural systems responsible for stereotyped behavior patterns.)

The Limbic System and the Paleomammalian Brain

As has been seen in the earlier chapters of the book, the extrahypothalamic portions of the limbic system exert regulatory influences on the hypothalamus and midbrain. Therefore, it is possible that the best way to conceptualize the limbic system is as a regulator of the reptilian core brain. On the basis of behavioral analysis, this regulation seems to be inhibitory in nature. Stimulation of the limbic system often produces a suppression of ongoing behaviors, and lesions made within it often seem to "release" various activities. Each limbic system structure may be sensitive to characteristic conditions under which this regulation becomes manifest. This would mean that each of the limbic system structures is highly specialized, tuned to specific changes of the internal or external environment. Each has its own unique contribution to make to the guidance of behavior, and indeed subportions of each structure may have independent effects. The hypothesis is that however specialized the structures of the limbic system may be, their end-product is the regulation and suppression of activities in the protoreptilian core brain. What kinds of evidence would support such a view?

The effects of destruction of the hippocampus and the septal area have been difficult to characterize in general terms and, accordingly, interpretations have been varied. Among the characteristics shared by animals suffering destruction of either the septal or the hippocampal areas are overly energetic responsiveness to changes in reward schedules, resistance to extinction in certain tasks, more rapid acquisition of certain types of avoidance tasks, and more rapid acquisition of certain simple behavioral problems. Effects of lesions of the amygdala are even more varied but include a potentiation of behaviors guided by positive incentives and a decrease in the ability to initiate behaviors based on punishing environmental events.

Animals with hippocampal or septal damage tend to initiate responses faster and more frequently than do intact animals. This has been found both in conditioning situations and in naturally occurring, species-typical behavior (e.g., Glickman et al., 1970). It would seem that limbic system damage frees some "starting mechanism," perhaps in the reptilian core brain, from normal regulation.

One of the behavioral characteristics which marks limbic system damage is an unusual transfer of experiences. Schmaltz and Isaacson (1968), for example, demonstrated that animals with hippocampal lesions were impaired on the acquisition of a DRL-20 schedule if presented after the animals had been trained on a continuous reinforcement schedule. The animals that were trained on a DRL-20 schedule without prior continuous reinforcement experience were not impaired on the DRL-20 task. Therefore, the previous learning under continuous reinforcement conditions produced a debilitating effect in later training on the delay schedule.

The impairment on the DRL task may have been caused by the animals' overresponsiveness to the uncertainties of obtaining reinforcement. Their behavior seemed excessively energized, their reactions too extreme for efficient performance.

In one way, this type of deficit can be interpreted as a "failure of forgetting," since the effects of the continuous reinforcement schedule carried over and interfered with performance on the new task. The animals with hippocampal damage were unable to overthrow the habitual way of responding.

If the limbic system plays a critical role in the suppression of "protoreptilian habits," then limbic system destruction should interfere with the development of learning sets. Large lesions of the temporal lobe, including the associated limbic structures, in primates do interfere with object-discrimination learning sets (Riopelle *et al.*, 1953). Schwartzbaum and Poulos (1965) have found that lesions of the amygdala produce impaired formation of learning sets as measured by repeated reversals of a discrimination problem.

In the preceding chapter, attention was given to the difficulties of animals with hippocampal damage being trained on simultaneous and successive discrimination tasks (pp. 178–188). Normal animals showed a positive transfer of training between the two tasks. Training on the successive discrimination facilitated the acquisition of the simultaneous discrimination problem. Damage to the brain, on the other hand, prevented this positive transfer. Animals with cortical lesions *and* animals with hippocampal destruction were both adversely affected. With either type of lesion, there was very little difference between the behavior of the animals learning the task originally and those learning it after having learned the successive discrimination.

The benefit on the simultaneous task derived by the normal animals from prior training on the successive discrimination task probably has to do with the elimination of inappropriate hypotheses. For example, when an animal begins training in a T- or Y-maze there are many different hypotheses which could be tested. One has to do with simple spatial positions of a potential reward. The rewards could be located in the right or in the left goal box. This is the first hypothesis tested by most animals. Training in the successive discrimination causes the normal animals to consider this hypothesis as unlikely, since it did not produce consistent rewards. Afterward, when the animal is trained in the simultaneous discrimination task this hypothesis is not often tested by normal animals. Furthermore, during the training in the successive discrimination problem, the animals have had to learn to pay attention to the colors of the walls of the maze. This selective attention to wall color helps the animals to learn the simultaneous problem, too. These benefits of prior training are lost on the animals with either neocortical or hippocampal destruction.

Other information was gained from the analysis of the transfer effects obtained on the successive discrimination task from prior training on the simultaneous discrimination task. Positive transfer was found in normal animals. Positive transfer effects were also exhibited by animals with neocortical destruction. Animals with hippocampal damage not only failed to show positive transfer but even evidenced negative transfer effects.

In large part, this negative transfer seemed to result from the fact that the animals with hippocampal damage learned only one component of the problem. Totally successful performance required the learning of two components of the task, but although the animals with hippocampal damage learned one of them as well as the control animals, they were greatly impaired in acquiring the other.

In one sense, this may be another instance in which the animals with hippocampal damage are impaired by what has been learned previously. In this case, the prior learning of one aspect of a problem interferes with learning another aspect of the same problem.

The more general conclusion seems to be that specific training in a particular situation produces changes in the animals which are difficult to overcome and which persist into the future, disturbing the acquisition of new behaviors and the alteration of hypotheses in the light of changed environmental circumstances. This carryover from the past is a type of negative transfer of training and may also be considered to be a case of abnormally strong proactive interference.

Proactive Interference

From their study of amnesic patients, Warrington and Weiskrantz (1973) conclude that verbal associations from the past adversely influence the retrieval of new information. As has been mentioned, the past affects the present behaviors of animals with hippocampal damage in atypical ways, and indeed Weiskrantz (1971) has suggested that proactive interference could serve as an explanation for the behavioral deficits found in man and in other animals after such destruction.

The data obtained by Warrington and Weiskrantz were of two kinds. The first demonstrated that the amnesic patients with recent memory problems could be greatly improved by giving them additional information when being tested for the retention of verbal information. In one technique, this involved giving the subjects the first two letters of the to-be-remembered words. The improvements that were found suggested that the patients were able to store the information and that their problem was in the retrieval of the words. The second kind of data came from the analysis of the errors made by the amnesic patients. Warrington and Weiskrantz found that the patients had many more words from lists learned previously intruding into their retention tests. Taken together, the implication is that the patients had difficulty with the retrieval of acquired information due to a failure to suppress adequately the words learned under similar circumstances in the past. On the other hand, experimental rats and cats are often taught only one task after surgery, although monkeys may serve in quite a few different experimental paradigms. In any event, the laboratory animal is exposed to a limited number of training procedures and consequently should have fewer sources of proactive interference in most experimental studies.

It is of interest that Warrington and Weiskrantz found that the "intrusion errors" made by their subjects were words which had appeared in former lists. The intrusions were not simply frequently occurring words in the English language. This suggests that the proactive interference was restricted, to some extent at least, to words occurring under the circumstances of testing. Is there evidence that there is a similar limitation of the interfering effects found in nonhuman animals?

Riddell et al. (1971) reported the effects of training animals in three different problems in an operant situation. The animals were trained to make a lever-press response at one end of the box. This response allowed the animals to make responses on two pigeon keys at the other end of the box. All animals were first trained to make a brightness discrimination and then a position discrimination. Finally, they were given training in a response alternation task. All training was given postoperatively for the lesioned animals.

The animals with hippocampal lesions were impaired in learning the alternation response but not in learning the other two problems. Since other experiments have shown that animals with hippocampal damage are not impaired in learning alternation problems in an operant setting, (e.g., Means et al., 1970; Jackson and Strong, 1969), there is presumptive evidence that the prior experiences had negatively affected performance in this problem. It could well be asked why the training in the brightness discrimination had not affected performance in the position problem. My hunch would be that the "place hypothesis" is very prominent in rats, as demonstrated by Kimble and Kimble (1970), and that it is one which the animals quickly adopt under conditions of uncertainty.

In another study, Winocur and Mills (1970) found negative transfer in the behavior of normal animals when they were trained preoperatively on a brightness discrimination task and post-operatively on pattern discrimination. This interference was considerably exaggerated in animals with hippocampal destruction. These authors also investigated the question of how general the interference would be. To do so, they tested animals in an operant task with all responses rewarded (CRF), an active avoidance task (one-way), and a simultaneous brightness discrimination task, using different orders of testing for different groups of animals. All testing was done postoperatively. They found that the animals with hippocampal damage acquired the tasks at the same rates regardless of the order in which they were experienced. This implies that the transfer effects found in animals with hippocampal damage are restricted to tasks similar to ones experienced in the past.

Thus, even though the evidence is not overwhelming, there are suggestions that the abnormal transfer effects are situation specific in animals with hippocampal damage and that the generality of the effects is more restricted than in normal animals.

There is evidence that the deficit found in animals with limbic system damage are not due to a failure of a retention of information, but rather to an interference with the expression of the knowledge in behavior. This evidence includes the effects of chlorpromazine on the performance of lesioned animals on the DRL-20 task (e.g., Van Hartesveldt, 1974) and the observation that animals with hippocampal lesions often change from a period of response fixation to perfect performance on discrimination problems or their reversal (Nonneman and Isaacson, 1973). It is as if the lesioned animals have the information at hand for the correct solution but cannot bring this information into play relative to their overt behavioral acts.

These facts represent further points of similarity between the effects of a form of limbic system damage in man and other animals. This has been reflected in the analysis of proactive, interfering effects, but one other aspect of the hippocampal lesion syndrome must not be forgotten: the energizing of behavioral acts. Hippocampal lesions in nonhuman animals do produce hyperactivity (as measured by locomotion in open fields), overresponsiveness to changes in operant schedules, failure to inhibit the initiation of responses under some conditions, and a greater willingness to initiate behavioral acts. These changes have not been reported to occur in man after temporal lobe surgery as correlates of the recent memory disturbances. This possible discrepancy could be related to additional psychological compensatory mechanisms found in the human or to the fact that disease processes had intervened in the human before surgery, or both.

Inferred Characteristics of the Reptilian Core Brain

One of my basic assumptions is that lesions of the limbic system act to remove the mechanisms of the protoreptilian core brain from certain regulatory influences normally supplied by the damaged regions. The lesion technique does not reveal the activities of the pure protoreptilian brain, of course, since regulation can still occur through the remaining limbic system structures and from the neocortex. What the lesion techniques may reveal is the nature of those circumstances under which a particular region of the limbic system does exert its influences. Over the years, most of my own research has been directed toward understanding the circumstances under which the hippocampus acts to regulate the activities of other brain regions. In essence, these seem to be conditions of uncertainty. Life becomes uncertain when old patterns of responding fail to produce the anticipated rewards, when old habits fail to pay off. By turning things around, the hippocampus can be seen as a mechanism which suppresses the activity in the protoreptilian core brain when the unexpected happens. This suppression prevents the animal from continuing in its old ways of responding and from overreacting in general.

An animal with damage to the amygdala, on the other hand, reveals quite a different sort of behavioral syndrome. It is slow to initiate new responses and seems characterized by a reduction in reactive quality. Both the joys and disasters of life seem reduced. This suggests that the role of the amygdala under normal conditions is to accentuate the conditions of arousal and activation of the hypothalamic systems when external conditions are appropriate. In some ways, the amygdala contributions seem opposed to those of the hippocampus. However, because of the diversity of functions found within the amygdala system, this could at best be a description of the contributions played by certain portions of the amygdala and not by "the amygdala" as an entity. Lesions in some portions of the amygdala produce behavioral effects quite similar to those of the hippocampus.

Considering the hippocampus, septal area, and cingulate region as "entities" is no more justifiable than considering the amygdala as a unified structure or system. Each of the limbic structures, including the hypothalamus itself, is a complex set of subsystems in terms of anatomical relationships with other brain regions and in terms of behavioral functions. We should talk about limbic systems, not a limbic system. Different portions of each of the limbic areas act synergistically with each other and in a similar fashion on the hypothalamus and protoreptilian brain. Other portions act in different, and sometimes opposing, ways. The ultimate aim of each, however, can be considered as changing the activities or the character of activities in the protoreptilian brain complex.

Lesions or stimulation of the limbic system can produce an intensification or reduction of activities in systems representative of activities of the protoreptilian core brain. These effects are mediated by changes in activities in or related to the hypothalamus. Accordingly, most or all of the activities of the hypothalamus should be capable of modification by manipulations of the limbic system.

Returning to the characteristics of the protoreptilian core brain inferred from studies of the limbic system, a picture emerges of a neural system which reacts to changes in the environment by increasing or decreasing the intensity of the predominant response sequence. Modifications of behavior are possible, of course, but these tend to be made on the basis of the establishment of new responses. Suppression of response on the basis of nonreward or punishment is difficult. Some subportions of the limbic system act to suppress established responses, while others intensify them. In the intact animal, the net effect of all of these systems on behavior is probably the resultant, at the hypothalamic level, of the total amount of facilitating and inhibiting influences.

The greatest change which occurs as a correlate of increased forebrain tissue is the ease with which rapid and, perhaps, temporary associations can be achieved. Earlier in this chapter, the proposal of Beritoff that the temporary "image" of the place of food or of punishment could be held only briefly by fish and for an even briefer period by fish with forebrain damage was noted. The limbic system makes possible the supression of the traditional ways of responding in order to allow behavioral modifications based on newly acquired information. It may not do so only by the force of its own activities but in conjuction with those systems arising with the development of the neocortical mantle. Indeed, since both the limbic system and the neocortex become elaborated in mammals a close association of the two may be presumed.

In a series of studies, Olds and his colleagues (summarized in Olds, 1973) have shown that single neurons in the hippocampus can reflect the formation of temporary associations in their activity. Some cells have been found which respond when the animal anticipates a food reward but not when the animal anticipates a water reward. However, this specificity of response was not an absolute characteristic of a particular cell. When conditions were modified, the same cell might signal the other type of reward, e.g., water, but not food. Thus these hippocampal cells responded selectively to the anticipation of one reward but were not categorically linked to food, water, or the act of anticipation itself. It was a temporary marriage of convenience. This led Olds to think of some of the cells in the hippocampus as acting to represent stimuli in the environment in a temporary fashion. These facts are of interest but are open to other inter-pretations, including those which would suggest that the cells are being influenced or driven from other brain regions. These other regions could provide the actual locations of cells holding some temporary representation of anticipated rewards. Nevertheless, Olds' work does reveal that many cells of the hippocampus are influenced by conditions indicative of the formation of new and temporary associations.

Data from another experiment from Olds' laboratory (Hirano *et al.* (1970) stimulate a different line of thought. Cells were found in the hippocampus whose activity was changed during condition-ing, but which did not return to former patterns of responding during extinction. Olds (1972) suggests that these cells might be indicating a memory for the task on which the animals were trained despite the extinction of the behavioral response. On the other hand, the activity of hippocampal cells which maintain their conditioned form of response during extinction might also suggest that they are actively suppressing the behavioral manifestation of the learned response when it no longer leads to reward. In his 1972 paper, Olds presents the data from a hippocampal cell (Fig. 5, Olds, 1972) which are of special interest. It did not show differen-tial activity to the two signals used in the conditioning procedure except during the extinction phase of the experiment. Working with Olds, Segal (1972) has found units in the hippocampus which maintain changed discharge rates acquired during conditioning despite changes in the significance of the conditioned stimulus for the animal.

These observations would be compatible with the view that the limbic system is responsible for the suppression of previously learned behavioral sequences. As such, it can be viewed as the mechanism which is directed toward the elimination of influences from the past, i.e., from the stored memories of the protoreptilian brain.* The limbic brain thus fulfills the role of Lethe. It provides the

---

* A puzzling problem is presented by the data of Poletti *et al.* (1973). They have found that the vast majority of hypothalamic neurons influenced by hippocampal stimula-tion are changed toward greater rates of response. This includes cells in the lateral hypothalamus. It might be expected on the basis of behavioral and physiological evaluation that hippocampal stimulation would have produced largely inhibitory effects, especially on cells of the lateral hypothalamus but at least on some regions of the hypothalamus.

basis of forgetting of chronic memories, the graven images of the protoreptilian brain, and opens the way for new, temporary associations. It does so in collaboration with the neocortical systems, which have their own role to play in behavior.

The Neocortex: The Guru

While it is presumptuous to suggest that the functions of any brain region are understood at all well, it is especially so in connection with the systems of the neocortex. The neocortex presents the neuroscientist with his greatest challenge.

It may be best to consider first the behaviors for which the neocortex is not essential. Lesions of the primary sensory areas of the neocortical surface do not produce a complete loss of sensory experience. Lesions of the primary auditory neocortex do not alter auditory thresholds for frequency or intensity (e.g., Diamond and Neff, 1957). Destruction of the primary visual areas does not eliminate some forms of pattern discriminative capacities, even in primates (Humphrey and Weiskrantz, 1967). Similar results have been found for the somatosensory system.

From the point of view of motor activities, the primary motor areas of the neocortex impose a rapidly conducting system controlling fine-grain movements of the extremities on a reasonably effective motor apparatus largely based in subcortical and brain stem regions. The most obvious result of damage to the primary motor cortex of mammals is a loss of the rapid, fine-grain movements of the digits.

The neocortex, then, seems to be especially capable of the quick and efficient processing of information which has too many fine details to be easily handled by the mechanisms in lower brain regions. Its adjustive contributions are those which require a delicacy beyond the capabilities of the lower centers.

The neocortex may speed up the processing of information, at least of some types of information. Gerbrandt *et al.* (1970) have shown that stimulation of the inferior temporal neocortex can alter the activity in the visual areas of the neocortex of a bored and disinterested monkey to the extent that the neural reactions are comparable to those obtained from the animal when it is paying keen attention. By implication, this inferior temporal neocortex can be thought of as regulating the excitability and processing time of the primary sensory systems.

Whether or not an animal pays attention to visual stimulation depends on the possibility that the stimulation will influence its life in important ways. Wilson *et al.* (1972) have shown that the inferior temporal neocortex is involved in making this determination. Lesions in the anterior portions of the inferior temporal neocortex changed monkeys such that they responded on the basis of the number of past rewards associated with a stimulus instead of the stimulus most recently associated with rewards. It is as if some ability to hold recent reward associations in mind was decreased in favor of a more habitual association of a stimulus with reward. The associations of rewards with stimuli interferes with the learning to respond to stimuli presently being rewarded due to a change in reinforcement conditions. This reliance on the more established way of responding found after inferior temporal lesions may pose a handicap, of a proactive nature, in problems in which new adjustments are required to the visual environment. With the neocortical lesion, reliance on the past can interfere with the flexibility of behavior required in circumstances of change.

But surely, it might be said, the great neocortical mantle does more than provide additional speed and precision in information processing. Surely it must be involved in those aspects of behavior valued most by educators: knowledge, learning, and memory. Since these are the "highest" attributes of man, they should be subserved by the "highest" neural machinery of the brain.

Unfortunately, there is precious little evidence for such a view. What evidence there is shows a remarkable retention of previously learned information after brain damage. The search for the location of the engram has not been successful. The memory engrams of the brain are everywhere or nowhere.

Karl Lashley developed his theories of "mass action" and "equipotentiality" because of failures to find specific locations within the brain which, when destroyed, eliminated the memories of previously learned problems. In maze studies, he found the greater the amount of neocortex destroyed the greater the loss in retention in rats. The location of the lesions *per se* was not critical, which indicated that the information was diffusely stored.

The storage of any information in neocortical sites can be questioned. The amount of the deficit in retention of a pre-operatively learned problem following neocortical insult depends on the length of the postoperative recovery period and treatments given the animals in this period. Treatments which produce greater "arousal," whether they be environmental or chemical, tend to act to reduce the usual deficits and facilitate recovery. Moreover, if steps are taken to control for the "distortions" of the sensory world produced by damage to the primary sensory areas, often no loss in retention is found at all after surgery (Bauer and Cooper, 1964). This suggests that memories may *not* be localized uniquely in the neocortex at all. Furthermore, there is a strong possibility that the real problem faced by the rat after destruction of the visual neocortex is the retrieval of previously learned information. Meyer (1972) has suggested that destruction of the posterior neocortex produces a condition in which the *access* to previously acquired knowledge is disturbed. This hypothesis was tested by LeVere and Morlock (1973). They trained animals postoperatively in the same visual habit learned preoperatively or its reversal. If memories of the preoperatively learned problem were destroyed by the neocortical damage, the animals should learn the two problems equally well. They did not. It took much longer for the animals trained on the reversal task to learn the problem than those retrained on the original problem, a result compatible with Meyer's hypothesis.

The one well-established characteristic that separates man from other animals is his use of language. This capability is closely related to certain neocortical areas, especially regions of the left hemisphere. Damage to this neocortical area in man produces one or more of the several speech and language abnormalities that have been documented in the clinical literature. With language and the messages communicated by language, man becomes free from domination by his environment.

Of the many benefits given to us by the ability to use language, one may be of special significance. This is the ability to institute changes in perspective, beliefs, and activities quickly on a permanent or temporary basis. Information can be received and stored in a twinkling of an eye, and its influence can be brief or lasting depending on a number of factors. Spoken or written language conveys information in a very rapid manner. Indeed, through his own implicit verbal abilities it would appear that man can originate new organizations of the knowledge which he has acquired in the past.

Language serves as both the message and the vehicle by which messages are received. One of the tricks used by memory experts is to memorize a list of words or a series of visual objects to be used as points of reference with which new material can be associated. For example, a person might memorize a list of words each of which begins with a different letter of the alphabet, e.g., APPLE, BANJO, CART. Given a new list, an association is made between the new words and the previously memorized list. If the new list contains the words DRUM, KING, CHAIR, it could be combined with the previous list by the person thinking of an APPLE sitting on a DRUM, a KING playing a BANJO, and CHAIR sitting on a mobile CART. Whether or not images of the words need to be involved in this method of temporary retention of verbal material is an unresolved question. In any case, the fact that a previously learned set of words can be used to facilitate retention of new words provides an additional dimension for the retention of new verbal materials. It provides another technique by which information can be quickly stored and used.

With language, man can override the demands both of his internal environment and of the outer world. He can reject the feelings of thirst and hunger in favor of abstract goals, sometimes ones of his own creation. Thus we have martyrs who will starve to death to further their own "salvation" or the "salvation" of others. Man can reject the directions provided by the world and the people around him. He can, in short, be free from internal and external factors which shape the destinies of those animals without language.

To exercise this freedom, man must override and suppress the well-learned and genetically determined behaviors which are presumed to be properties of the protoreptilian core brain. Therefore, the neocortical mechanisms must overcome the habits and memories of the past, either indirectly by activating some portions of the paleomammalian brain, or by a more direct control process. In short, the neocortex too is profoundly concerned with suppressing the past.

My suggestion is that the neocortical systems use the paleomammalian brain mechanisms to accomplish this suppression of previously learned behaviors as required to alter behavior. For the neocortical systems to "gain control" of the organism, the past must give up its domination of behavior.

The protoreptilian brain looks to the past. It learns and remembers but is poor at forgetting. The neocortical brain looks to the future, either to tomorrow, next week, next year, or to heavenly rewards. The neocortex is the brain of anticipation. It prepares for, anticipates, and predicts the future. All religious leaders, the gurus, have pleaded with man to give up his old ways and images of the past. The sin of excessive "attachment" to things, places, even roles, is excoriated in the wisdom of East and West alike. In the triune brain metaphor, this means that the graven images of the protoreptilian brain must be overcome.

It is paradoxical that this most delicate and yet dominating neocortical brain is the one responsible for our longest and most elaborate memories, ones even longer than those subserved by the protoreptilian brain. By the use of language, we can store the memories of the past. We build libraries and repositories of information which can extend our knowledge of the past for thousands of years, far beyond the life span of the protoreptilan brain. The neocortical contribution of language enables us to forecast the future and to anticipate conditions hours, weeks, years, and centuries from the present. It is this extension of time, both forward and backward, which represents the singular advance produced by the neocortex.

REFERENCES

Ackil, J. E., Mellgren, R. L., Halgren, C., and Frommer, G. P. (1969). Effects of CS preexposures on avoidance learning in rats with hippocampal lesions. *Journal of Comparative and Physiological Psychology* **69**:739–747.

Adey, W. R. (1964). Neurophysiological correlates of information transaction and storage in the brain. In Stellar, E., and Sprague, J. M. (eds.), *Progress in Physiological Psychology*, Vol. 1, Academic Press, New York, pp. 1–43.

Adey, W. R., and Meyer, M. (1952). An experimental study of hippocampal afferent pathways from prefrontal and cingulate areas in the monkey. *Journal of Anatomy* **86**:58–74.

Adler, M. W. (1972). The effect of single and multiple lesions of the limbic system on cerebral excitability. *Psychopharmacologia* **24**:281–230.

Ahmad, S. S., and Harvey, J. A. (1968). Long-term effects of septal lesions and social experience on shock-elicited fighting in rats. *Journal of Comparative and Physiological Psychology* **66**:596–602.

Allen, W. F. (1941). Effect of ablating the pyriform–amygdaloid areas and hippocampi on positive and negative olfactory conditioned reflexes and on conditioned olfactory differentiation. *American Journal of Physiology* **132**:81–92.

Anchel, H., and Lindsley, D. B. (1972). Differentiation of two reticulohypothalamic systems regulating hippocampal activity. *Electroencephalography and Clinical Neurophysiology* **32**:209–226.

Anden, N-E., Dahlström, A., Fuxe, K., Larsson, K., Olson, L., and Ungerstedt, U. (1966). Ascending monoamine neurons to the telencephalon and diencephalon. *Acta Physiologica Scandinavica* **67**:313–326.

Andersen, P., Blackstad, T. W., and Lömo, T. (1966). Location and identification of excitatory synapses on hippocampal pyramidal cells. *Experimental Brain Research* **1**:236–248.

Angevine, J. B., Jr. (1970). Critical cellular events in the shaping of the nervous system. In Schmitt, F. O. (ed.), *The Neurosciences: Second Study Program,* Rockefeller University Press, New York, pp. 62–71.

Aronson, L. R., Aronson, F. R., and Clark, E. (1967). Instrumental conditioning and light–dark discrimination in young nurse sharks. *Bulletin of Marine Science* **17**:249–256.

Bagshaw, M. H., and Benzies, S. (1968). Multiple measures of the orienting reaction and their dissociation after amygdalectomy in monkeys. *Experimental Neurology* **20**:175–187.

Bagshaw, M. H., and Pribram, J. D. (1968). Effect of amygdalectomy on stimulus threshold of the monkey. *Experimental Neurology* **20** :197–202.

Bagshaw, M. H., and Pribram, K. H. (1965). Effect of amygdalectomy on transfer of training in monkeys. *Journal of Comparative and Physiological Psychology* **59** :118–121.

Bagshaw, M. H., Kimble, D. P., and Pribram, K. H. (1965). The GSR of monkeys during orienting and habituation and after ablation of the amygdala, hippocampus, and inferotemporal cortex. *Neuropsychologia* **3** :111–119.

Bagshaw, M. H., Mackworth, N. H., and Pribram, K. H. (1972). The effect of resections of the inferotemporal cortex or the amygdala on visual orienting and habituation. *Neuropsychologia* **10**:153–162.

Baisden, R. H. (1973). Behavioral effects of hippocampal lesions after adrenergic depletion of the septal area. Unpublished Ph.D. dissertation, University of Florida.

Baisden, R. H., Isaacson, R. L., Woodruff, M. L., and Van Hartesveldt, C. (1972). The effect of physostigmine on spontaneous alternation in infant rabbits. *Psychonomic Science* **26**:287–288.

Ball, G. G. (1972). Self-stimulation in the ventromedial hypothalamus. *Science* **178**:72–73.

Ball, G. G., and Gray, J. A. (1971). Septal self-stimulation and hippocampal activity. *Physiology and Behavior* **6**:547–549.

Bandler, R. J., Jr., and Flynn, J. P. (1972). Control of somatosensory fields for striling during hypothalamically elicited attack. *Brain Research* **38**:197–201.

Barker, D. J. (1967). Alterations in sequential behavior of rats following ablation of midline limbic cortex. *Journal of Comparative and Physiological Psychology* **64**:453–460.

Barker, D. J., and Thomas, G. J. (1965). Ablation of cingulate cortex in rats impairs alternation learning and retention. *Journal of Comparative and Physiological Psychology* **60**:353–359.

Barker, D. J., and Thomas, G. J. (1966). Effects of regional ablation of midline cortex in alternation learning by rats. *Physiology and Behavior* **1**:313–317.

Barrett, R. J., and Ray, O. S. (1969). Attenuation of habituation by electroconvulsive shock. *Journal of Comparative and Physiological Psychology* **69** :133–135.

Barrett, R. J., Leith, N. J., and Ray, O. S. (1972). Permanent facilitation of avoidance behavior by *d*-amphetamine and scopolamine. *Psychopharmacologia* **25** : 321–331.

Barrett, R. J., Leith, N. J., and Ray, O. S. (1973). A behavioral and pharmacological analysis of variables mediating active-avoidance behavior in rats. *Journal of Comparative and Physiological Psychology* **82**:489–500.

Barrett, T. W. (1969). Studies of the function of the amygdaloid complex in *Macaca mulatta*. *Neuropsychologia* **7**:1–12.

Bauer, J. H., and Cooper, R. M. (1964). Effects of posterior cortical lesions on performance of a brightness discrimination task. *Journal of Comparative and Physiological Psychology* **58**:84–92.

Beatty, W. W., and Schwartzbaum, J. S. (1968*a*). Enhanced reactivity to quinine and saccharin solutions following septal lesions in the rat. *Psychonomic Science* **8**:483–484.

Beatty, W. W., and Schwartzbaum, J. S. (1968*b*). Commonality and specificity of behavioral dysfunctions following septal and hippocampal lesions in rats. *Journal of Comparative and Physiological Psychology* **66**:60–68.

Behrend, E. R., and Bitterman, M. E. (1963). Sidman avoidance in the fish. *Journal of the Experimental Analysis of Behavior* **54**:700–703.

Bennett, T. L. (1970). Hippocampal EEG correlates of behavior. *Electroencephalography and Clinical Neurophysiology* **28**:17–23.

Bennett, T. L. (1971). Hippocampal theta activity and behavior—A review. *Communications in Behavioral Biology* **6**:37–48.

Bennett, T. L. (1974). Hippocampal theta activity and processes of attention. In Isaacson, R. L., and Pribram, K. H. (eds.), *The Hippocampus: A Comprehensive Treatise*, Plenum Press, New York, in press.

Bennett, T. L., and Gottfried, J. (1970). Hippocampal theta activity and response inhibition. *Electroencephalography and Clinical Neurophysiology* **29**:196–200.

Bennett, T. L., Nunn, P. J., and Inman, D. P. (1971). Effects of scopolamine on hippocampal theta and correlated discrimination performance. *Physiology and Behavior* **7**:451–454.

Berger, B. D., Wise, C. D., and Stein, L. (1971). Norepinephrine: Reversal of anorexia in rats with lateral hypothalamic damage. *Science* **172**:281–284.

Beritoff, J. S. (1965). *Neural Mechanisms of Higher Vertebrate Behavior*, Little, Brown, Boston.

Beritoff, J. S. (1971). *Vertebrate Memory: Characterisitics and Origin*, Plenum Press, New York.

Bishop, M. P., Elder, S. T., and Heath, R. G. (1963). Intracranial self-stimulation in man. *Science* **140**:394–396.

Bitterman, M. E. (1972). Comparative studies of the role of inhibition in reversal learning. In Boakes, R. A., and Halliday, M. S. (eds.), *Inhibition and Learning*, Academic Press, New York.

Black, A. H. (1972). The operant conditioning of central nervous system electrical activity. In Bower, G. H. (ed.), *The Psychology of Learning and Motivation*, Vol. 6, Academic Press, New York.

Black, A. (1974). Hippocampal electrical activity and behavior. In Isaacson, R. L., and Pribram, K. H. (eds.), *The Hippocampus: A Comprehensive Treatise*, Plenum Press, New York, in press.

Black, A. H., and DeToledo, L. (1971). The relationship among classically conditioned responses: Heart rate and skeletal behavior. In Black, A. H., and Prokasy, W. F. (eds.), *Classical Conditioning II; Current Research and Theory*, Appleton-Century-Crofts, New York.

Black, A. H., Young, G. A., and Batenchuk, C. (1970). The avoidance training of hippocampal theta waves and its relation to skeletal movement. *Journal of Comparative and Physiological Psychology* **70** : 15–24.

Blackstad, T. W. (1956). Commissural connections of the hippocampal region in the rat, with special reference to their mode of termination. *Journal of Comparative Neurology* **105** : 417–538.

Blackstad, T. W. (1958). On the termination of some afferents to the hippocampus and fascia dentata: An experimental study in the rat. *Acta Anatomica* **35** : 202–214.

Blackstad, T. W., Walberg, F., and White, L. E. (1965). Early stages of terminal axonal degeneration in the fascia dentata. *Journal of Ultrastructure Research* **12** : 236.

Blanchard, R. J., and Blanchard, D. C. (1972). Effects of hippocampal lesions on the rat's reaction to a cat. *Journal of Comparative and Physiological Psychology* **78** : 77–82.

Blanchard, R. J., and Fial, R. A. (1968). Effects of limbic lesions on passive avoidance and reactivity to shock. *Journal of Comparative and Physiological Psychology* **66** : 606–612.

Blass, E. M., and Hanson, D. G. (1970). Primary hyperdipsia in the rat following septal lesions. *Journal of Comparative and Physiological Psychology* **70** : 87–93.

Bliss, T. V. P., and Lömo, T. (1970). Plasticity in a monosynaptic cortical pathway. *Journal of Physiology* **207** : 61P.

Bonvallet, M. and Bobo, E. G. (1972). Changes in phrenic activity and heart rate elicited by localized stimulation of amygdala and adjacent structures. *Electroencephalography and Clinical Neurophysiology* **32** : 1–16.

Borbély, A. A., Huston, J. P., and Baumann, I. R. (1973). Body temperature and behavior in chronic brain-lesioned rats after amphetamine, chlorpromazine, and γ-butyrolactone. *The Pharmacology of Thermoregulation* Basel, Karger, pp. 447–462.

Bower, G. H., and Miller, N. E. (1958). Rewarding and punishing effects from stimulating the same place in the rat's brain. *Journal of Comparative and Physiological Psychology* **51** : 669–674.

Boyd, E. S., and Gardner, L. C. (1967). Effect of some brain lesions on intracranial self-stimulation in the rat. *American Journal of Physiology* **213** : 1044–1052.

Brady, J. V. (1958). The paleocortex and behavioral motivation. In Harlow, H. F., and Woolsey, C. N. (eds.), *Biological and Biochemical Bases of Behavior,* University of Wisconsin Press, Madison, pp. 193–235.

Brady, J. V., and Nauta, W. J. (1955). Subcortical mechanisms in control of behavior. *Journal of Comparative and Physiological Psychology* **48** : 412–420.

Breglio, V., Anderson, C., and Merrill, H. K. (1970). Alteration in footshock threshold by low-level septal brain stimulation. *Physiology and Behavior* **5** : 715–719.

Bresnahan, E., and Routtenberg, A. (1972). Memory disruption by unilateral low level, sub-seizure stimulation of the medial amygdaloid nucleus. *Physiology and Behavior* **9** : 513–525.

Brobeck, J. R. (1964). Mechanisms of the development of obesity in animals with hypothalamic lesions. *Physiological Reviews* **26** : 541–559.

Brown, G. E., and Remley, N. R. (1971). The effects of septal and olfactory bulb lesions in stimulus reactivity. *Physiology and Behavior* **6** : 497–501.

Brown, G. E., Harrell, E., and Remley, N. R. (1971). Passive avoidance in septal and anosmic rats using quinine as the aversive stimulus. *Physiology and Behavior* **6**:543–546.

Brutkowski, S., and Mempel, E. (1961). Disinhibition of inhibitory conditioned responses following selective brain lesions in dogs. *Science* **134** : 2040–2041.

Buddington, R. W., King, F. A., and Roberts, L. (1967). Emotionality and conditioned avoidance responding in the squirrel monkey following septal injury. *Psychonomic Science* **8** : 195–196.

Buerger, A. A. (1970). Effects of preoperative training on relearning a successive discrimination by cats with hippocampal lesions. *Journal of Comparative and Physiological Psychology* **72** : 462–466.

Bull, H. (1928). Studies on conditioned responses in fish. *Journal of the Marine Biological Association* **15** : 485–533.

Bunnell, B. N. (1966). Amygdaloid lesions and social dominance in the hooded rat. *Psychonomic Science* **6** : 93–94.

Burkett, E. E., and Bunnell, B. N. (1966). Septal lesions and the retention of DRL performance in the rat. *Journal of Comparative and Physiological Psychology* **62**:468–472.

Butter, C. M., Mishkin, M., and Rosvold, H. E. (1963). Conditioning and extinction of a food-rewarded response after selective ablations of frontal cortex in rhesus monkeys. *Experimental Neurology* **7**:65–75.

Butters, N., and Rosvold, H. E. (1968). Effect of septal lesions on resistance to extinction and delayed alternation in monkeys. *Journal of Comparative and Physiological Psychology* **66**:389–395.

Campbell, B. A., Vallantine, P., II, and Lynch, G. (1971). Hippocampal control of behavioral arousal: Duration of lesion effects and possible interactions with recovery after frontal cortical damage. *Experimental Neurology* **33** : 159–170.

Campbell, C. B. G., and Hodos, W. (1970). The concept of homology and the evolution of the nervous system. *Brain, Behavior, and Evolution* **3**:353–367.

Campenot, R. B. (1969). Effect of amygdaloid lesions upon active avoidance acquisition and anticipatory responding in rats. *Journal of Comparative and Physiological Psychology* **69**:492–497.

Carder, B. (1971). Effects of septal stimulation on active avoidance in rats. *Physiology and Behavior* **6**:503–506.

Cardo, B. (1960). Action de lesions thalamiques et hypothalamiques sur le conditionnement de fruite et la differenciation tonale chez le rat. *Journale de Physiologie (Paris)* **52**:537–553.

Carey, R. J. (1969). Motivational and reinforcement scheduling factors in the effect of hippocampal injury on operant behavior. *Physiology and Behavior* **4**:959–961.

Carey, R. J. (1971). Quinine and saccarin preference–aversion threshold determinations in rats with septal ablations. *Journal of Comparative and Physiological Psychology* **76** : 316–326.

Carlson, N. R. (1970). Two-way avoidance behavior of mice with limbic lesions. *Journal of Comparative and Physiological Psychology* **70** : 73–78.

Carlson, N. R., and Cole, J. R. (1970). Enhanced alternation performance following septal lesions in mice. *Journal of Comparative and Physiological Psychology* **73**:157–161.

Carlson, N. R., and Norman, R. J. (1971). Enhanced go, no-go single-lever alternation of mice with septal lesions. *Journal of Comparative and Physiological Psychology* **75**:508–512.

Carlson, N. R., Carter, E. N., and Vallante, M. (1972). Runway alternation and discrimination of mice with limbic lesions. *Journal of Comparative and Physiological Psychology* **78**:91–101.

Carlton, P. (1969). Brain-acetylcholine and inhibition. In Tapp, J. T. (ed.), *Reinforcement and Behavior*, Academic Press, New York and London, pp. 285–325.

Casey, K. L. (1966). Unit analysis of nociceptive mechanisms of the awake squirrel monkey. *Journal of Neurophysiology* **29**:727–750.

Chalmers, B. M., and Holdstock, T. L. (1969). Effects of atropine on heart rate and hippocampal EEG following septal stimulation in rats. *Psychonomic Science* **16**:145–147.

Cherkin, A. (1971). Biphasic time course of performance after one-trial avoidance training in the chick. *Communications in Behavioral Biology* **5**:379–381.

Chi, C. C., and Flynn, J. P. (1971). Neural pathways associated with hypothalamically elicited attack behavior in cats. *Science* **171**:703–706.

Chow, K. L. (1961). Effect of local electrographic afterdischarges on visual learning and retention in monkey. *Journal of Neurophysiology* **24**:391–400.

Chow, K. L., and Obrist, W. D. (1954). EEG and behavioral changes on application of $AL(OH)_3$ cream on preoccipital cortex of monkeys. *AMA Archives of Neurology and Physchiatry* **72**:80–87.

Clark, C. V. H., and Isaacson, R. L. (1965). Effect of bilateral hippocampal ablation on DRL performance. *Journal of Comparative and Physiological Psychology* **59**:137–140.

Clark, C. V. H. (1970). Effect of hippocampal and neocortical ablation on scopolamine-induced activity in the rat. *Psychopharmacologia* **17**:289–301.

Clody, D. E., and Carlton, P. L. (1969). Behavioral effects of lesions of the medial septum of rats. *Journal of Comparative and Physiological Psychology* **67**:344–351.

Cohen, J. S., Laroche, J. P., and Beharry, E. (1971). Response perseveration in the hippocampal lesioned rat. *Psychonomic Science* **23**:221–223.

Coover, G. D., and Levine, S. (1972). Auditory startle response of hippocampectomized rats. *Physiology and Behavior* **9**:75–77.

Corman, C. D., Meyer, P. M., and Meyer, D. R. (1967). Open-field activity and exploration in rats with septal and amygdaloid lesions. *Brain Research* **5**:469–476.

Cowan, W. M., Raisman, G., and Powell, T. P. S. (1965). The connexions of the amygdala. *Journal of Neurology, Neurosurgery, and Psychiatry* **28**:137–151.

Cox, V. C., and Valenstein, E. S. (1965). Attenuation of aversive properties of peripheral shock by brain stimulation. *Science* **149**:323–325.

Cox, V. C., and Valenstein, E. S. (1969). Distribution of hypothalamic sites yielding stimulus-bound behavior. *Brain, Behavior, and Evolution* **2**:359–376.

Coyle, P. (1969). Cat parahippocampal unit discharge patterns during limbic stimulation. *Brain Research* **15**:175–183.

Cragg, B. G. (1965). Afferent connexions of the allocortex. *Journal of Anatomy (London)* **99**:339–357.

Crawford, F. T., and Langdon, J. W. (1966). Escape and avoidance responding in the toad. *Psychonomic Science* **6** : 115–116.

Crosby, E. C., Humphrey, T., and Lauer, E. W. (1962). *Correlative Anatomy of the Nervous System*, Macmillan, New York.

Crowne, D. P., and Riddell, W. I. (1969). Hippocampal lesions and the cardiac component of the orienting response in the rat. *Journal of Comparative and Physiological Psychology* **69** : 748–755.

Dahlström, A., and Fuxe, K. (1964). Evidence for the existence of monoamine-containing neurons in the central nervous system. 1. Demonstration of mono-amines in the cell bodies of brainstem neurons. *Acta Physiologica Scandinavica* **62**: Suppl. 232.

Dalby, D. A. (1970). Effect of septal lesions on the acquisition of two types of active avoidance behavior in rats. *Journal of Comparative and Physiological Psychology* **73** : 278–283.

Dalland, T. (1970). Response and stimulus perseveration in rats with septal and dorsal hippocampal lesions. *Journal of Comparative and Physiological Psychology* **71** : 114–118.

Deagle, J. H., and Lubar, J. F. (1971). Effect of septal lesions in two strains of rats on one-way and shuttle avoidance acquisition. *Journal of Comparative and Physiological Psychology* **77** : 277–281.

DeFries, J. C., and Hegmann, J. P. (1970). Genetic analysis of open-field behavior. In Lindzey, G., and Thiessen, D. D. (eds.), *Contributions to Behavior-Genetic Analysis: The Mouse as a Prototype*, Appleton-Century-Crofts, New York, pp. 23–56.

de Groot, J. (1959). *The Rat Forebrain in Stereotaxic Co-ordinates*. North Holland Publishers, Amsterdam.

Delgado, J. M. R., Roberts, W. W., and Miller, N. E. (1954). Learning motivated by electrical stimulation of the brain. *American Journal of Physiology* **179** : 587.

DeOlmos, J. S. (1972). The amygdaloid projection field in the rat as studied by the cupric-silver method. In Eleftheriou, B. E. (ed.), *The Neurobiology of the Amygdala*, Plenum Press, New York.

Deutsch, J. A., and Howarth, C. I. (1963). Some tests of a theory of intracranial self-stimulation. *Psychological Review* **70** : 444–460.

Diamond, I. T., and Neff, W. D. (1957). Ablation of temporal cortex and discrimination of auditory patterns. *Journal of Neurophysiology* **20** : 300–315.

DiCara, L. V. (1966). Effect of amygdaloid lesions on avoidance learning in the rat. *Psychonomic Science* **4** : 279–280.

Domesick, V. B. (1969). Projections from the cingulate cortex in the rat. *Brain Research* **12** : 296–320.

Domesick, V. B. (1970). The fasciculus cinguli in the rat. *Brain Research* **20** : 19–32.

Domesick, V. B. (1972). Thalamic relationships of the medial cortex in the rat. *Brain, Behavior, and Evolution* **6** : 457–483.

Donovick, P. J. (1968). Effects of localized septal lesions on hippocampal EEG activity in behavior in rats. *Journal of Comparative and Physiological Psychology* **66** : 569–578.

Donovick, P. J., and Burright, R. G. (1968). Water consumption in rats with septal lesions following two days of water deprivation. *Physiology and Behavior* 3:285–288.

Donovick, P. J., and Schwartzbaum, J. S. (1966). Effects of low-level stimulation of the septal area on two types of discrimination reversal in the rat. *Psychonomic Science* 6:3–4.

Donovick, P. J., Burright, R. G., and Gittelson, P. L. (1969). Bodyweight and food and water consumption in septal lesioned and operated control rats. *Psychological Reports* 25:303–310.

Douglas, R. J. (1966). Transposition, novelty, and limbic lesions. *Journal of Comparative and Physiological Psychology* 62:354–357.

Douglas, R. J. (1967). The Hippocampus and Behavior. *Psychological Bulletin* 67:416–422.

Douglas, R. J. (1974). The development of hippocampal function. In Isaacson, R. L., and Pribram, K. H. (eds.), *The Hippocampus*, Plenum Press, New York, in press.

Douglas, R. J., and Isaacson, R. L. (1964). Hippocampal lesions and activity. *Psychonomic Science* 1:187–188.

Douglas, R. J., and Isaacson, R. L. (1966). Spontaneous alternation and scopolamine. *Psychonomic Science* 4:283–284.

Douglas, R. J., and Pribram, K. H. (1969). Distraction and habituation in monkeys with limbic lesions. *Journal of Comparative and Physiological Psychology* 69:473–480.

Douglas, R. J., Barrett, T. W., Pribram, K. H., and Cerny, M. C. (1969). Limbic lesions and error reduction. *Journal of Comparative and Physiological Psyhology* 68:437–441.

Duncan, P. M. (1971). The effect of temporary septal dysfunction on conditioning and performance of fear responses. *Journal of Comparative and Physiological Psychology* 74:340–348.

Duncan, P. M., and Duncan, N. C. (1971). Free-operant and T-maze avoidance performance by septal and hippocampal-damaged rats. *Physiology and Behavior* 7:687–693.

Dunsmore, R., and Lennox, R. (1950). Stimulation and strychninization of supracallosal anterior cingulate gyrus. *Journal of Neurophysiology* 13:207–214.

Eager, R. P., Chi, C. C., and Wolf, G. (1971). Lateral hypothalamic projections to the hypothalamic ventromedial nucleus in the albino rat: Demonstration by means of a simplified ammoniacal silver degeneration method. *Brain Research* 20:128–132.

Earle, K. M., Baldwin, M., and Penfield, W. (1953). Incisural sclerosis and temporal lobe seizures produced by hippocampal herniation at birth. *Archives of Neurology and Psychiatry* 69:27–42.

Eclancher, F. S., and Karli, P. (1971). Compartement d'agression interspécifique et comportement alimentaire du rat: Effets de lésions des noyaux ventromédians de l'hypothalamus. *Brain Research* 26:71–79.

Egger, M. D., and Flynn, J. P. (1962). Amygdaloid suppression of hypothalamically elicited attack behavior. *Science* 136:43–44.

Eichelman, B. S., Jr. (1971). Effect of subcortical lesions on shock-induced aggression in the rat. *Journal of Comparative and Physiological Psychology* **7**: 331–339.

Elazar, Z., and Adey, W. R. (1967). Spectral analysis of low frequency components in the electrical activity of the hippocampus during learning. *Electroencephalography and Clinical Neurophysiology* **23**:225–240.

Eleftheriou, B. E., Elias, M. F., and Norman, R. L. (1972). Effects of amygdaloid lesions on reversal learning in the deermouse. *Physiology and Behavior* **9**:69–73.

Elias, M. F., Dupree, M., and Eleftheriou, B. E. (1973). Differences in spatial discrimination reversal learning between two inbred mouse strains following specific amygdaloid lesions. *Journal of Comparative and Physiological Psychology* **83**:149–156.

Ellen, P., and Deloache, J. (1968). Hippocampal lesions and spontaneous alternation behavior in the rat. *Physiology and Behavior* **3**:857–860.

Ellen, P., and Powell, E. W. (1962*a*). Effects of septal lesions on behavior generated by positive reinforcement. *Experimental Neurology* **6**:1–11.

Ellen, P., and Powell, E. W. (1962*b*). Temporal discrimination in rats with rhinencephalic lesions. *Experimental Neurology* **6**:538–547.

Ellen, P., Wilson, A. S., and Powell, E. W. (1964). Septal inhibition and timing behavior in the rat. *Experimental Neurology* **10**:120–132.

Elliot Smith, G. (1910). Some problems relating to the evolution of the brain. *Lancet* **1**:1–6, 147–153, 221–227.

Ellison, G. D. (1968). Appetite behavior in rats after circumsection of the hypothalamus. *Physiology and Behavior* **3**:221–226.

Ellison, G., and Flynn, J. P. (1968). Organized aggressive behavior in cats after surgical isolation of the hypothalamus. *Archieves Italienne de Biologie,* **106**: 1–20.

Ellison, G. D., Sorenson, C. A., Jacobs, B. L. (1970). Two feeding syndromes following surgical isolation of the hypothalamus in rats. *Journal of Comparative and Physiological Psychology* **70**:173–188.

Elul, R. (1964). Regional differences in the hippocampus of the cat. II. Projections of the dorsal and ventral hippocampus. *Electroencephalography and Clinical Neurophysiology* **16**:489–502.

Entingh, D. (1971). Perseverative responding and hyperphagia following entorhinal lesions in cats. *Journal of Comparative and Physiological Psychology* **75**: 50–58.

Epstein, A. N. (1960). Reciprocal changes in feeding behavior produced by intrahypothalamic chemical injections. *American Journal of Physiology* **199**: 969–974.

Faillace, L. A., Allen, R. P., McQueen, J. D. and Northrup, B. (1971). Cognitive deficits from bilateral cingulotomy for intractable pain in man. *Diseases of the Nervous System* **32**:171–175.

Falconer, M. G., Serafetinides, E. A., and Corsellis, J. A. N. (1964). Etiology and pathogenesis of temporal lobe epilepsy. *Archives of Neurology* **10**:233–248.

Fallon, D., and Donovick, P. J. (1970). Septal lesions, motivation, and secondary reinforcement: Lesion induced somatomotor inhibition. *Journal of Comparative and Physiological Psychology* **73**:150–156.

Fedio, P., and Ommaya, A. K. (1970). Bilateral cingulum lesions and stimulation in man with lateralized impairment in short-term verbal memory. *Experimental Neurology* **29** : 84–91.

Feindel, W., and Gloor, P. (1954). Comparison of the electrographic effects of stimulation of the amygdala and brain stem reticular formation in cats. *Electroencephalography and Clinical Neurophysiology* **6** : 389–402.

Finch, D. M., Surwit, R. S., and Johnson, R. R. (1968). The effects of amygdalectomy on shock-induced fighting behavior in rats. *Psychonomic Science* **10** : 369–370.

Fisher, A. E. (1969). The role of limbic structures on the central regulation of feeding and drinking behavior. *Annals of the New York Academy of Sciences* **157** : 894–901.

Flaherty, C. F., and Hamilton, L. W. (1971). Responsivity to decreasing sucrose concentrations following septal lesions in the rat. *Physiology and Behavior* **6** : 431–437.

Flaherty, C. F., Capobianco, S., and Hamilton, L. W. (1973). Effect of septal lesions on retention of negative contrast. *Physiology and Behavior,* **11** : 625–631.

Flynn, J. (1967). The neural basis of aggression in cats. In Glass, D. H. (ed.), *Neurophysiology and Emotion*, Rockefeller University Press, New York, pp. 40–60.

Foltz, E. L. (1959). Modification of morphine withdrawal by frontal lobe cingulum lesions. In von Bogaert, L., and Radermeker, J. (Eds.), *First International Congress of Neurological Sciences*, Pergamon, London.

Foltz, E. L., and White, L. E., Jr. (1957). Experimental cingulumotomy and modification of morphine withdrawal. *Journal of Neurosurgery* **14** : 655–673.

Foltz, E. L., and White, L. E. Jr. (1962). Pain "relief" by frontal cingulumotomy. *Journal of Neurosurgery* **19** : 89–100.

Fonberg, E. (1973). The normalizing effect of lateral amygdalar lesions upon the dorsomedial amygdalar syndrome in dogs. *Acta Neurobiologiae Experimentalis* **33** : 449–466.

Fonberg, E., and Delgado, J. M. R. (1961). Avoidance and alimentary reactions during amygdalar stimulation. *Journal of Neurophysiology* **24** : 651–664.

Fonberg, E., Brutkowski, S., and Mempel, E. (1962). Defensive conditioned reflexes and neurotic motor reactions following amygdalectomy in dogs. *Acta Biologiae Experimentalis* **12** : 51–57.

Freeman, W. J., and Patel, H. H. (1968). Extraneuronal potential fields evoked in septal region of cat by stimulation of fornix. *Electroencephalography and Clinical Neurophysiology* **24** : 444–457.

French, J. D., Hernandez-Peon, R., and Livingston, R. B. (1955). Projections from cortex to cephalic brain stem (reticular formation) in monkey. *Journal of Neurophysiology* **18** : 74–95.

Fried, P. A. (1970). Pre- and post-operative approach training and conflict resolution by septal and hippocampal lesioned rats. *Physiology and Behavior* **5** : 975–979.

Fried, P. A. (1972). The effect of differential hippocampal lesions and pre- and post-operative training on extinction. *Revue Canadienne de Psychologie* **26** : 61–70.

Froloff, J. (1925). Bedingte Reflexe bei Fischen. *Pflügers Archives Gesamte Physiologie* **220** : 339–349.

Fuller, J. L., Rosvold, H. E., and Pribram, K. H. (1957). The effect on affective and cognitive behavior in the dog of lesions of the pyriform—amygdala—hippocampal complex. *Journal of Comparative and Physiological Psychology* 50 : 89–96.

Fuxe, K., Hamberger, B., and Hökfelt, T. (1968). Distribution of noradrenaline nerve terminals in cortical areas of the rat. *Brain Research* 8 : 125–131.

Fuxe, K., Hökfelt, T., and Ungerstedt, U. (1970). Morphological and functional aspects of central monoamine neurons. *International Review of Neurobiology* 13 : 93–126.

Galef, B. G. (1970). Aggression and timidity: Responses to novelty in feral Norway rats. *Journal of Comparative and Physiological Psychology* 70 : 370–381.

Gallistel, C. R. (1964). Electrical self-stimulation and its theoretical implications. *Psychological Bulletin* 61 : 23–24.

Gallistel, C. R. (1969). Self-stimulation: Failure of pretrial stimulation to affect rats' electrode preference. *Journal of Comparative and Physiological Psychology* 69 : 722–729.

Gardner, L., and Malmo, R. B. (1969). Effects of low-level septal stimulation on escape: Significance for limbic–midbrain interactions in pain. *Journal of Comparative and Physiological Psychology* 68 : 65–73.

Gellermann, L. W. (1933). Chance orders of alternating stimuli in visual discrimination experiments. *Journal of Genetic Psychology* 42 : 206–208.

Gellhorn, E. (1970). The emotions and the ergotropic and trophotropic systems. *Psychologische Forschung* 34 : 48–94.

Genton, C. (1969). Etude, par la technique de Nauta, des degenerescences consecutive à une lesion electrolytique de la region septal chez le mulst sylvestre (*Adopemus sylvaticus*). *Brain Research* 14 : 1–23.

Gerbrandt, L. K., Spinelli, D. N., and Pribram, K. H. (1970). The interaction of visual attention and temporal cortex stimulation on electical activity evoked in striate cortex. *Electroencephalography and Clinical Neurophysiology* 29 : 146–155.

Girgis, M. (1972). The distribution of acetylcholinesterase enzyme in the amygdala and its role in aggressive behavior. In Eleftheriou, B. E. (ed.), *The Neurobiology of the Amygdala*, Plenum Press, New York.

Gittelson, P. L., and Donovick, P. J. (1968). The effects of septal lesions on the learning and reversal of a kinesthetic discrimination. *Psychonomic Science* 13 : 137–138.

Gittelson, P. L., Donovick, P. J., and Burright, R. G. (1969). Facilitation of passive avoidance in rats with septal lesions. *Psychonomic Science* 17 : 292–293.

Glass, D. H., Ison, J. R., and Thomas, G. J. (1969). Anterior limbic cortex and partial reinforcement effects on acquisition and extinction of a runway response in rats. *Journal of Comparative and Physiological Psychology* 69 : 17–24.

Glick, S. D., Greenstein, S., and Zimmerberg, B. (1972). Facilitation of recovery by α-methyl-p-tyrosine after lateral hypothalamic damage. *Science* 177 : 534–535.

Glickman, S. E., Higgins, T., and Isaacson, R. L. (1970). Some effects of hippocampal lesions on the behavior of Mongolian gerbils. *Physiology and Behavior* 5 : 931–938.

Gloor, P., Vera, C. L., and Sperti, L. (1963). Electrophysiological studies of hippocampal neurons. I. Configuration and laminar analysis of the "resting" potential gradient, of the main-transient response to perforant path, fimbrial and mossy fiber volleys, and of "spontaneous" activity. *Electroencephalography and Clinical Neurophysiology* 15 : 353–378.

Goddard, G. V. (1964a). Functions of the amygdala. *Psychological Bulletin* **62** : 89–109.

Goddard, G. V. (1964b). Amygdaloid stimulation and learning in the rat. *Journal of Comparative and Physiological Psychology* **58** : 23–30.

Goddard, G. V. (1969). Analysis of avoidance conditioning following cholinergic stimulation of amygdala in rats. *Journal of Comparative and Physiological Psychology* **68** : 1–18.

Goddard, G. V., McIntyre, D. C., and Leech, C. K. (1969). A permanent change in brain function resulting from daily electrical stimulation. *Experimental Neurology* **25** : 295–330.

Gold, R. M. (1967). Aphagia and adypsia following unilateral and bilaterally asymmetrical lesions in rats. *Physiology and Behavior* **2** : 211–220.

Gold, R. M. (1970). Hypothalamic hyperphagia produced by parasagittal knife cuts. *Physiology and Behavior* **5** : 23–25.

Gold, R. M., and Proulx, D. M. (1972). Bait-shyness acquisition is impaired by VMH lesions that produce obesity. *Journal of Comparative and Physiological Psychology* **79** : 201–209.

Gold, R. M., Quackenbush, P. M., and Kapatos, G. (1972). Obesity following combination of rostrolateral to VMH cut and contralateral mammillary area lesion. *Journal of Comparative and Physiological Psychology* **79** : 210–218.

Gollender, M. (1967). Eosinophil and avoidance correlates of stress in anterior cingulate cortex lesioned rat. *Journal of Comparative and Physiological Psychology* **64** : 40–48.

Gollender, M., Law, O. T., and Isaacson, R. L. (1960). Changes in the circulating eosinophil level associated with learned fear: Conditioned eosinopenia. *Journal of Comparative and Physiological Psychology* **53** : 520–523.

Gonzales, R. C., and Bitterman, M. E. (1967). Partial reinforcement effect in the goldfish as a function of amount of reward. *Journal of Comparative and Physiological Psychology* **64** : 163–167.

Gonzalez, R. C., Behrend, E. R., and Bitterman, M. E. (1967). Reversal learning and forgetting in bird and fish. *Science* **158** : 519–521.

Gotsick, J. E. (1969). Factors affecting spontaneous activity in rats with limbic system lesions. *Physiology and Behavior* **4** : 587–593.

Gotsick, J. E., and Marshall, R. C. (1972). Time course of the septal rage syndrome. *Physiology and Behavior* **9** : 685–687.

Grant, L. E., and Jarrard, L. E. (1968). Functional dissociation in hippocampus. *Brain Research* **10** : 392–401.

Grastyán, E. (1968). Commentary. In Gellhorn, E. (ed.), *Biological Foundations of Emotion,* Scott-Foresman, Evanston, Ill., pp. 114–127.

Grastyán, E., Lissák, K., Madarász, I., and Donhoffer, H. (1959). Hippocampal electrical activity during the development of conditioned reflexes. *Electroencephalography and Clinical Neurophysiology* **11** : 409–429.

Gray, J. A. (1971). Medial septal lesions, hippocampal theta rhythm and the control of vibrissal movement in the freely moving rat. *Electroencephalography and Clinical Neurophysiology* **30** : 189–197.

Gray, J. A., and Ball, G. G. (1970). Frequency-specific relation between hippocampal theta rhythm, behavior and amobarbital action. *Science* **168** : 1246–1248.

Green, R. H., and Schwartzbaum, J. S. (1968). Effects of unilateral septal lesions on avoidance behavior discrimination reversal and hippocampal EEG. *Journal of Comparative and Physiological Psychology* **65** : 388–396.

Green, R. H., Beatty, W. W., and Schwartzbaum, J. S. (1967). Comparative effects of septo-hippocampal and caudate lesions on avoidance behavior in rats. *Journal of Comparative and Physiological Psychology* **64** : 444–451.

Greene, E. G. (1968). Cholinergic stimulation of the medial septum. *Psychonomic Science* **10** : 157–158.

Greene, E. (1971). Comparison of hippocampal depression and hippocampal lesion. *Experimental Neurology* **31** : 313–325.

Greene, E., Saporta, S., and Walters, J. (1970). Choice bias from unilateral hippo-campal or frontal lesions in the rat. *Experimental Neurology* **29** : 534–545.

Grossman, S. P. (1960). Eating or drinking elicited by direct adrenergic or cholinergic stimulation of the hypothalamus. *Science* **132** : 301–302.

Grossman, S. P. (1966). The VMH: A center for affective reactions, satiety or both. *Physiology and Behavior* **1** : 1–10.

Grossman, S. P. (1969). A neuropharmacological analysis of hypothalamic and extrahypothalamic mechanisms concerned with the regulation of food and water intake. *Annals of the New York Academy of Sciences* **157** : 902–917.

Grossman, S. P. (1970). Avoidance behavior and aggression in rats with transections of the lateral connections of the medial or lateral hypothalamus. *Physiology and Behavior* **5** : 1103–1108.

Grossman, S. P. (1971). Changes in food and water intake associated with an interruption of the anterior or posterior fiber connections of the hypothalamus. *Journal of Comparative and Physiological Psychology* **75** : 23–31.

Grossman, S. P. (1972). Aggression, avoidance and reaction to novel environments in female rats with ventromedial hypothalamic lesions. *Journal of Comparative and Physiological Psychology* **78** : 274–283.

Grossman, S. P., and Grossman, L. (1970). Surgical interruption of the anterior or posterior connections of the hypothalamus: Effects on aggressive and avoidance behavior. *Physiology and Behavior* **5** : 1313–1317.

Grossman, S. P., and Grossman, L. (1971). Food and water intake in rats with parasagittal knife cuts medial or lateral to the lateral hypothalamus. *Journal of Comparative and Physiological Psychology* **74** : 148–156.

Gurowitz, E. M., Rosen, A. J., and Tessel, R. E. (1970). Incentive shift performance in cingulectomized rats. *Journal of Comparative and Physiological Psychology* **70** : 476–481.

Hall, E. (1972). Some aspects of the structural organization of the amygdala. In Eleftheriou, B. E. (ed.), *The Neurobiology of the Amygdala,* Plenum Press, New York.

Hamilton, G., and Isaacson, R. L. (1970). Changes in avoidance behavior following epileptogenic lesions on the mesencephalon. *Physiology and Behavior* **5** : 1165–1167.

Hamilton, L. W. (1972). Intrabox and extrabox cues in avoidance responding: Effect of septal lesions. *Journal of Comparative and Physiological Psychology* **78** : 268–273.

Hamilton, L. W., McCleary, R. A., and Grossman, S. P. (1968). Behavioral effects of cholinergic septal blockade in the cat. *Journal of Comparative and Physiological Psychology* **66** : 563–568.

Han, P. W. (1967). Hypothalamic obesity in rats without hyperphagia. *Transactions of the New York Academy of Science* **30** : 229–243.

Hara, K., and Myers, R. E. (1973). Role of forebrain structures in emotional expression in opposum. *Brain Research* **52** : 131–144.

Harlow, H. F. (1959). The development of learning in the rhesus monkey. *American Scientist* **47** : 459–479.

Harrison, J. M., and Lyon, M. (1957). The role of the septal nuclei and components of the fornix in the behavior of the rat. *Journal of Comparative Neurology* **108** : 121–137.

Harvey, J., and Hunt, H. F. (1965). Effect of septal lesions on thirst in the rat as indicated by water consumption and operant responding for water reward. *Journal of Comparative and Physiological Psychology* **59** : 49–56.

Heath, R. G., and Mickle, W. A. (1960). Evaluation of seven years' experience with depth electrode studies in human patients. In Ramey, E. R., and O'Doherty, D. S. (eds.), *Electrical Studies of the Unanesthetized Brain*, Hoeber, New York, pp. 214–242.

Heatherington, A. W., and Ranson, S. W. (1942). Hypothalamic lesions and adiposity in the rat. *Anatomical Record* **78** : 149–172.

Heimer, L., and Larsson, K. (1964). Drastic changes in the mating behavior of male rats following lesions in the junction of the diencephalon and mesencephalon. *Experientia* **20** : 1–4.

Heimer, L., and Larsson, K. (1966–1967). Impairment of mating behavior in male rats following lesions in the preoptic–anterior hypothalamic continuum. *Brain Research* **3** : 248–263.

Heimer, L., and Nauta, W. J. H. (1969). The hypothalamic distribution of stria terminals in the rat. *Brain Research* **13** : 289.

Heller, A. (1972). Neuronal control of brain serotonin. *Federation Proceedings* **31** : 81–90.

Henke, P. G., Allen, J. D., and Davison, C. (1972). Effect of lesions in the amygdala on behavioral contrast. *Physiology and Behavior* **8** : 173–176.

Hendrickson, C. W., Kimble, R. J., and Kimble, D. P. (1969). Hippocampal lesions and the orienting response. *Journal of Comparative and Physiological Psychology* **67** : 220–227.

Henry, C. E., and Pribram, K. H. (1954). Effect of aluminum hydroxide implantation on cortex of monkey on EEG and behavior performance. *Electroencephalography and Clinical Neurophysiology* **6** : 693–694.

Herrick, C. J. (1926). *Brains of Rats and Men*, University of Chicago Press, Chicago.

Herrick, C. J. (1948). *The Brain of the Tiger Salamander, Ambystoma tigrinum*, University of Chicago Press, Chicago.

Hess, W. R. (1949). *Das Zwischenhirn*, Schwabe, Basel.

Hirano, T., Best, P., and Olds, J. (1970). Units during habituation, discrimination learning, and extinction. *Electroencephalography and Clinical Neurophysiology* **28** : 127–135.

Hirsh, R. (1970). Lack of variability or perseveration: Describing the effect of hippocampal ablation. *Physiology and Behavior* **5** : 1249–1254.

Hjorth-Simonsen, A. (1971). Hippocampal efferents to the ipsilateral entorhinal area: An experimental study in the rat. *Journal of Comparative Neurology* **142** : 417–438.

Hjorth-Simonsen, A. (1973). Some intrinsic connections of the hippocampus in the rat: An experimental analysis. *Journal of Comparative Neurology* **147** : 145–162.

Hjorth-Simonsen, A., and Jeune, B. (1972). Origin and termination of the hippocampal perforant path in the rat studied by silver impregnation *Journal of Comparative Neurology* **144** : 215–231.

Hoebel, B. G. (1969). Feeding and self-stimulation. *Annals of the New York Academy of Sciences* **157** : 758–777.

Hoebel, B. G. (1971). Feeding : Neural control of intake. *Annual Review of Physiology* **33** : 533–568.

Hoebel, B. G., and Teitelbaum, P. (1966). Weight regulation in normal and hypothalamic hyperphagic rats. *Journal of Comparative and Physiological Psychology* **61** : 189–193.

Hoebel, B. G., and Thompson, R. D. (1969). Aversion to lateral hypothalamic stimulation caused by intragastric feeding or obesity. *Journal of Comparative and Physiological Psychology* **68** : 536–543.

Holdstock, T. L. (1967). Effect of septal stimulation in rats on heart rate and galvanic skin response. *Psychonomic Science* **9** : 37–38.

Holdstock, T. L. (1970). Plasticity of autonomic functions in rats with septal lesions *Neuropsychologia* **8** : 147–160.

Holdstock, T. L. (1972). Dissociation of function within the hippocampus. *Physiology and Behavior* **8** : 659–667.

Holloway, F. A. (1972). Effects of septal chemical injections on asymptotic avoidance performance in cats. *Physiology and Behavior* **8** : 463–469.

Holmes, J. E., and Beckman, J. (1969). Hippocampal theta rhythm used in predicting feline behavior. *Physiology and Behavior* **4** : 563–565.

Horvath, F. E. (1963). Effects of basolateral amygdalectomy on three types of avoidance behavior in cats. *Journal of Comparative and Physiological Psychology* **56** : 380–389.

Hothersall, D., Johnson, D. A., and Collen, A. (1970). Fixed-ratio responding following septal lesions in the rat. *Journal of Comparative and Physiological Psychology* **73** : 470–467.

Hudspeth, W. J., and Wilsoncroft, W. E. (1969). Retrograde amnesia: Time dependent effects of rhinencephalic lesions. *Journal of Neurobiology* **2** : 221–232.

Humphrey, N. K., and Weiskrantz, L. (1967). Vision in monkeys after removal of the striate cortex. *Nature* **215** : 595–597.

Hunt, H. F., Diamond, I. T., Moore, R. Y., and Harvey, J. A. (1957). Some effects of hippocampal lesions on conditioned avoidance behavior in the cat. In *Proceedings XVth International Congress of Psychology,* **8** : 203–204.

Huston, J. P. (1971). Relationship between motivating and rewarding stimulation of the lateral hypothalamus. *Physiology and Behavior* **6** : 711–716.

Huston, J. P., and Borberly, A. A. (1973). Operant conditioning in forebrain ablated rats by use of rewarding hypothalamic stimulation. *Brain Research* **50** : 467–472.

Ibata, Y., Desiraju, T., and Pappas, G. D. (1971). Light and electron microscopic study of the projection of the medial septal nucleus to the hippocampus of the cat. *Experimental Neurology* **33** : 103–122.

Ireland, L., and Isaacson, R. L. (1968). Reactivity in the hippocampectomized gerbil. *Psychonomic Science* **12** : 163–164.

Irwin, S., Laksner, S., and Curtis, A. (1964). Direct demonstration of consolidation of one-trial learning. *Federation Proceedings* **23** : 2.

Isaacson, R. L. (1967). Comment. *Psychonomic Science* **7** : 8.

Isaacson, R. L. (1972*a*). Neural systems of the limbic brain and behavioral inhibition. In Boakes, R., and Halliday, J., (eds.), *Inhibition and Learning,* Academic Press, New York.

Isaacson, R. L. (1972*b*). Hippocampal destruction in man and other animals. *Neuropsychologia* **10** : 47–64.

Isaacson, R. L., and Hutt, M. L. (1971). *Psychology: The Science of Behavior,* 2nd ed., Harper and Row, New York.

Isaacson, R. L., and Kimble, D. P. (1972). Lesions of the limbic system: Their effects upon hypotheses and frustration. *Behavioral Biology* **7** : 767–793.

Isaacson, R. L., and Wickelgren, W. O. (1962). Hippocampal ablation and passive avoidance. *Science* **138** : 1104–1106.

Isaacson, R. L., Douglas, R. J., and Moore, R. Y. (1961). The effect of radical hippocampal ablation on acquisition of avoidance response. *Journal of Comparative and Physiological Psychology* **54** : 625–628.

Isaacson, R. L., Olton, D. S., Bauer, B., and Swart, P. (1966). The effect of training trials on passive avoidance deficits in the hippocampectomized rat. *Psychonomic Science* **5** : 419–420.

Ito, M., and Olds, J. (1971). Unit activity during self-stimulation behavior. *Journal of Neurophysiology* **34** : 263–273.

Jackson, W. J., and Strong, P. M. (1969). Differential effects of hippocampal lesions upon sequential tasks and maze learning by the rat. *Journal of Comparative and Physiological Psychology* **68** : 442–450.

Jacobs, H. L., and Sharma, K. N. (1969). Taste versus calories: sensory and metabolic signals in the control of food intake. *Annals of the New York Academy of Sciences* **157** : 1084–1111.

Jarrard, L. E. (1965). Hippocampal ablation and operant behavior in the rat. *Psychonomic Science* **2** : 115–116.

Jarrard, L. E. (1968). Behavior of hippocampal lesioned rats in home cage and novel situations. *Physiology and Behavior* **3** : 65–70.

Jarrard, L. E. (1973). The hippocampus and motivation. *Psychological Bulletin* **79** : 1–12.

Jarrard, L. E., and Bunnell, G. N. (1968). Open-field behavior of hippocampal-lesioned rats and hamsters. *Journal of Comparative and Physiological Psychology* **66** : 500–502.

Jarrard, L. E., and Korn, J. H. (1969). Effects of hippocampal lesions on heart rate during habituation and passive avoidance. *Communications in Behavioral Biology* **3** : 141–150.

Johnson, D. A., and Thatcher, K. (1972). Differential effects of food deprivation on the fixed ratio behavior of normal rats and rats with septal lesions. *Psychonomic Science* **26** : 45–46.

Johnson, D. A., Poplawsky, A., and Bieliauskas, L. (1972). Alterations of social behavior in rats and hamsters following lesions of the septal forebrain. *Psychonomic Science* **26** : 19–20.

Johnston, J. B. (1923). Further contributions to the study of the evolution of the forebrain. *Journal of Comparative Neurology* **36** : 143–192.

Jonason, K. R., and Enloe, L. J. (1971). Alterations in social behavior following septal and amygdaloid lesions in the rat. *Journal of Comparative and Physiological Psychology* **75** : 286–301.

Kaada, B. R. (1951). Somatomotor, autonomic and electrocorticographic responses to electrical stimulation of rhinencephalic and other structures in primates, cat and dog. *Acta Physiologica Scandinavica* **24** : 83 (Suppl.).

Kaada, B. R., Rasmussen, E. W., and Kveim, O. (1962). Impaired acquisition of passive avoidance behavior by subcallosal, septal, hypothalamic and insular lesions in rats. *Journal of Comparative and Physiological Psychology* **55** : 661–670.

Kaada, B. R., Feldman, R. S., and Langfeldt, T. (1971). Failure to modulate autonomic reflex discharge by hippocampal stimulation in rabbits. *Physiology and Behavior* **7** : 225–231.

Kamp, A., Lopes DaSilva, F. H., and Storm Van Leeuwen, W. (1971). Hippocampal frequency shifts in different behavioural situations. *Brain Research* **31** : 287–294.

Kant, K. J. (1969). Influences of amygdala and medial forebrain bundle on self-stimulation in the septum. *Physiology and Behavior* **4** : 777–784.

Kaplan, J. (1968). Approach and inhibitory reactions in rats after bilateral hippocampal damage. *Journal of Comparative and Physiological Psychology* **65** : 274–281.

Kawakami, M., Seto, K., Terasawa, E., Yoshida, K., Miyamoto, T., Sekiguchi, M., and Hattori, Y. (1968). Influence of electrical stimulation of lesion in limbic structure upon biosynthesis of adrenocorticoid in the rabbit. *Neuroendocrinology* **3** : 337–348.

Kawamura, H., Nakamura, Y., and Tokizane, T. (1961). Effect of acute brain stem lesions on the electrical activities of the limbic system and neocortex. *Japanese Journal of Physiology* **11** : 565–575.

Keene, J. J. (1973). Opposite medial thalamic unit responses to rewarding and aversive brain stimulation. *Experimental Neurology* **39** : 19–35.

Keene, J. J., and Casey, K. L. (1970). Excitatory connection from lateral hypothalamic self-stimulation sites to escape sites in medullary reticular formation. *Experimental Neurology* **28** : 155–166.

Keene, J. J., and Casey, K. L. (1973). Rewarding and aversive brain stimulation: opposite effects on medial thalamic units. *Physiology and Behavior* **10** : 283–287.

Kelsey, J. E., and Grossman, S. P. (1969). Cholinergic blockade and lesions in the ventro-medial septum of the rat. *Physiology and Behavior* **4** : 837–845.

Kelsey, J. E., and Grossman, S. P. (1971). Nonperseverative disruption of behavioral inhibition following septal lesions in rats. *Journal of Comparative and Physiological Psychology* **75** : 302–311.

Kemble, E. D., and Beckman, G. J. (1969). Escape latencies at three levels of electric shock in rats with amygdaloid lesions. *Psychonomic Science* **14** : 205–206.

Kemble, E. D. and Beckman G. J. (1970). Vicarious trial and error following amygdaloid lesions in rats. *Neuropsychologia* **8** : 161–169.

Kemble, E. D., Levine, M. S., Gregoire, K., Koepp, K., and Thomas, T. T. (1972). Reactivity to saccharin and quinine solutions following amygdaloid or septal lesions in rats. *Behavioral Biology* **7** : 503–512.

Kent, M. A., and Peters, R. H. (1973). Effects of ventromedial hypothalamic lesions on hunger-motivated behavior in rats. *Journal of Comparative and Physiological Psychology* **83** : 92–97.

Kenyon, J., and Krieckhaus, E. E. (1965). Decrements in one-way avoidance learning following septal lesions in rats. *Psychonomic Science* **3** : 113–114.

Kesner, R. P., and Conner, H. S. (1972). Independence of short- and long-term memory : A Neural system analysis. *Science* **176** : 432–434.

Killeffer, F. A., and Stern, W. E. (1970). Chronic effects of hypothalamic injury— Report of a case of near total hypothalamic destruction resulting from removal of a craniopharyngioma. *Archives of Neurology* **22** : 419–429.

Kim, C., Choi, H., Kim, J. K., Chang, H. K., Park, R. S., and Kang, G. (1970). General behavioral activity and its component patterns in hippocampectomized rats. *Brain Research* **19** : 379–394.

Kim, C., Choi, H., Kim, J. K., Kim, M. S., Huh,M. K., and Moon, Y. B. (1971*a*). Sleep pattern of hippocampectomized cat. *Brain Research* **29** : 223–236.

Kim, C., Kim, C. C., Kim, J. K., Kim, M. S., Chang, H. K., Kim, J. Y., and Lee, I. G. (1971*b*). Fear response and aggressive behavior of hippocampectomized house rats. *Brain Research* **29** : 237–251.

Kimble, D. P. (1961). The effect of bilateral hippocampal damage on cognitive and emotional behavior in the rat. Ph.D. dissertation, University of Michigan.

Kimble, D. P. (1963). The effects of bilateral hippocampal lesions in rats. *Journal of Comparative and Physiological Psychology* **56** : 273–283.

Kimble, D. P. (1968). Hippocampus and internal inhibition. *Psychological Bulletin* **70** : 285–295.

Kimble, D. P., and Gostnell, D. (1968). Role of cingulate cortex in shock avoidance behavior of rats. *Journal of Comparative and Physiological Psychology* **65** : 290–294.

Kimble, D. P., and Greene, E. G. (1968). Absence of latent learning in rats with hippocampal lesions. *Psychonomic Science* **11** : 99–100.

Kimble, D. P., and Kimble, R. J. (1970). The effect of hippocampal lesions on extinction and "hypothesis" behavior in rats. *Physiology and Behavior* **5** : 735–738.

Kimble, D. P., Kirkby, R. J., and Stein, D. G. (1966). Response perseveration interpretation of passive avoidance deficits in hippocampectomized rats. *Journal of Comparative and Physiological Psychology* **61** : 141–143.

King, F. A. (1958). Effects of septal and amygdala lesions on emotional behavior and conditioned avoidance responses in the rat. *Journal of Nervous and Mental Diseases* **126** : 57–63.

King, F. A., and Meyer, P. M. (1958). Effects of amygdaloid lesions upon septal hyperemotionality in the rat. *Science* **128** : 655–656.

King, R. B., Schricker, J. L., and O'Leary, J. L. (1953). An experimental study of the transition from normal to convulsoid cortical activity. *Journal of Neurophysiology* **16** : 286–298.

Kinnard, M. A., Poletti, C. E., and MacLean, P. D. (1970). Preoptic unit responses to hippocampal stimulation. *Federation Proceedings* **29** : 792.

Klein, S. B., and Spear, N. E. (1970). Forgetting by the rat after intermediate intervals (Kamin effect) as retrieval failure. *Journal of Comparative and Physiological Psychology* **71** : 165–170.

Klemm, W. R. (1970). Correlation of hippocampal theta rhythm, muscle activity, and brain stem reticular formation activity. *Communications in Behavioral Biology* **3** : 147–151.

Kling, A. J., Orbach, J., Schwarz, N., and Towne, J. (1960). Injury to the limbic system and associated structures in cats. *Archives of General Psychiatry* **3** : 391–420.

Klüver, H., and Bucy, P. C. (1939). Preliminary analysis of the temporal lobes in monkeys. *Archives of Neurology and Psychiatry* **42** : 979–1000.

Koikegami, H. (1963). Amygdala and other related limbic structures; experimental studies on the anatomy and function. I. Anatomical researches with some neurophysiological observations. *Acta Medica et Biologica (Niigata)* **10** : 161–277.

Koikegami, H., and Fuse, S. (1952). Studies on the functions and fiber connections of the amygdaloid nuclei and periamygdaloid cortex. Experiment on the respiratory movements. *Folia Psychiat. Neurol. Japon.* **5** : 188–197.

Koikegami, H., Dodo, T., Mochida, Y., and Takahashi, H. (1957). Stimulation experiments on the amygdaloid nuclear complex and related structures. Effects upon the renal volume, urinary secretion, movements of the urinary bladder, blood pressure and respiratory movements. *Folia Psychiat. Neurol. Japon.* **11** : 157–206.

Komisaruk, B. R. (1968). Phasic synchrony of EEG theta rhythm, EKG and certain oscillatory EMG patterns in awake rats. Proceedings of the International Union of the Physiological Sciences, 24th International Congress, **7** : 244.

Komisaruk, B. R. (1970). Synchrony between limbic system theta activity and rhythmical behavior in rats. *Journal of Comparative and Physiological Psychology* **70** : 482–492.

Kraft, M. S., Obrist, W. D., and Pribram, H. (1960). The effect of irritative lesions of the striate cortex on learning of visual discriminations in monkeys. *Journal of Comparative and Physiological Psychology* **53** : 17–22.

Krechevsky, I. (1935). Brain mechanisms and "hypotheses." *Journal of Comparative Psychology* **19** : 425–462.

Kreindler, A., and Steriade, M. (1963). Functional differentiation within the amygdaloid complex inferred from peculiarities of epileptic afterdischarges. *Electroencephalography and Clinical Neurophysiology* **15** : 811–826.

Kreindler, A., and Steriade, M. (1964). EEG patterns of arousal and sleep induced by stimulating various amygdaloid levels in the cat. *Archieves Italienne de Biologie* **102** : 576–586.

Krieckhaus, E. E. (1962). Behavioral changes in cats following lesions of the mammillothalamic tracts. Ph.D. dissertation, University of Illinois.

Krieckhaus, E. E. (1964). Decrements in avoidance behavior following mammillothalamic tractotomy in cats. *Journal of Neurophysiology* **27** : 753–767.

Krieckhaus, E. E. (1965). Decrements in avoidance behavior following mammillothalamic tractotomy in rats and subsequent recovery with *d*-amphetamine. *Journal of Comparative and Physiological Psychology* **60** : 31–35.

Krieckhaus, E. E. (1966). Role of freezing and fear in avoidance decrements following mammillothalamic tractotomy in cat: I. Two-way avoidance behavior. *Psychonomic Science* **4** : 263–264.

Krieckhaus, E. E., and Chi, C. C. (1966). Role of freezing and fear in avoidance decrements following mammillothalamic tractotomy in cat. *Psychonomic Science* **4** : 264–266.

Krieckhaus, E. E., and Lorenz, R. (1968). Retention and relearning of lever-press avoidance following mammillothalamic tractotomy. *Physiology and Behavior* **3** : 433–438.

Krieckhaus, E. E., and Randall, D. (1968). Lesions of mammillothalamic tract in rat produce no decrements in recent memory. *Brain* **91** : 369–378.

Krieckhaus, E. E., Coons, E. E., Greenspon, T., Weiss, J., and Lorenz, R. L. (1968). Retention of choice behavior in rats following mammillothalamic tractotomy. *Physiology and Behavior* **3** : 125–131.

Laatsch, R. H., and Cowan, W. M. (1967). Electron microscopic studies of the dentata gyrus of the rat. II. Degeneration of commissural afferents. *Journal of Comparative Neurology* **130** : 241–262.

Lammers, H. J. (1972). The neural connections of the amygdaloid cortex in mammals. In Eleftheriou, B. E. (ed.), *The Neurobiology of the Amygdala*, Plenum Press, New York, pp. 123–144.

Lammers, H. J., and Lohman, A. H. M. (1957). Experimenteel anatomisch onderzoek naar de verbindingen van piriforme cortex en amygdalakernen bij de kat. *Nederlands Tijdschrift voor Geneeskunde* **101** : 1–2.

Lang, H., Tourinen, T., and Valleala, P. (1964). Amygdaloid afterdischarge and galvanic skin response. *Electroencephalography and Clinical Neurophysiology* **16** : 366–374.

Lanier, L., and Isaacson, R. L. (1974). Activity changes related to the location of lesions in the hippocampus. *Journal of Physiological and Comparative Psychology*, submitted.

Lash, L. (1964). Response discriminability and the hippocampus. *Journal of Comparative and Physiological Psychology* **57** : 251–256.

LaVaque, T. J. (1966). Conditioned avoidance response perseveration in septal rats during massed extinction trials. *Psychonomic Science* **5** : 409–410.

Leibowitz, S. (1970). A hypothalamic beta-adrenergic "satiety" system antagonizes and alpha-adrenergic "hunger" system in the rat. *Nature* **226** : 963–964.

Leonard, C. M. (1969). The prefrontal cortex of the rat. I. Cortical projection of the mediodorsal nucleus. II. Efferent connections. *Brain Research* **12** : 321–343.

LeVere, T. E., and Morlock, G. W. (1973). Nature of visual recovery following posterior neodecortication in the hooded rat. *Journal of Comparative and Physiological Psychology* **83** : 62–67.

Lidsky, T. I., Levine, M. S., Kreinick, C. J., and Schwartzbaum, J. S. (1970). Retrograde effects of amygdaloid stimulation on conditioned suppression (CER) in rats. *Journal of Comparative and Physiological Psychology* **73** : 135–149.

Liebeskind, J. C. (1962). The effect of cingulate cortex lesions on the development of resistance to stress. Ph.D. Thesis, University of Michigan.

Lints, C. E., and Harvey, J. A. (1969). Altered sensitivity to foot shock and decreased brain content of serotonin following brain lesions in the rat. *Journal of Comparative and Physiological Psychology* **67** : 23–31.

Lömo, T. (1970). Some properties of a cortical excitatory synapse. In Andersen, P., and Jansen, J., Jr. (eds.), *Excitatory Synaptic Mechanisms*, Oslo, Universitetsforlaget, pp. 207–211.

Lömo, T. (1971). Potentiation of monosynaptic EPSPs in the perforant path—dentate granule cell synapse. *Experimental Brain Research* **12** : 46–63.

Lopes DaSilva, F. H., and Kamp, A. (1969). Hippocampal theta frequency shifts and operant behaviour. *Electroencephalography and Clinical Neurophysiology* **26** : 133–143.

Lorens, S.A ., and Kondo, C. Y. (1969). Effects of septal lesions on food and water intake and operant responding for food. *Physiology and Behavior* **4** : 729–732.

Lovely, R. H., Grossen, N. E., Moot, S. A., Bauer, R. H., and Peterson, J. J. (1971). Hippocampal lesions and inhibition of avoidance behavior. *Journal of Comparative and Physiological Psychology* **77** : 345–352.

Lown, B. A., Hayes, W. N., and Schaub, R. E. (1969). The effects of bilateral septal lesions on two-way active avoidance in the guinea pig. *Psychonomic Science* **16** : 13–14.

Lubar, J. F. (1964). Effect of medial cortical lesions on the avoidance behavior of the cat. *Journal of Comparative and Physiological Psychology* **58** : 38–46.

Lubar, J. F., and Perachio, A. A. (1965). One-way and two-way learning and transfer of an active avoidance response in normal and cingulectomized cats. *Journal of Comparative and Physiological Psychology* **60** : 46–52.

Lubar, J. F., Perachio, A. A., and Kavanagh, A. J. (1966). Deficits in active avoidance behavior following lesions of the lateral and posterolateral gyrus of the cat. *Journal of Comparative and Physiological Psychology* **62** : 263–269.

Lubar, J. F., Boyce, B. A., and Shaefer, C. S. (1968). Etiology of polydipsia and polyuria in rats with septal lesions. *Physiology and Behavior* **3** : 289–292.

Lubar, J. F., Shaefer, C. S., and Wells, D. G. (1969). The role of the septal area in the regulation of water intake and associated motivational behavior. *Annals of the New York Academy of Sciences* **157** : 875–893.

Lubar, J. F., Brener, J. M., Deagle, J. H., Numan, R., and Clemens, W. J. (1970). Effect of septal lesions on detection threshold and unconditioned response to shock. *Physiology and Behavior* **5** : 459–463.

MacDonnell, M. F., and Flynn, J. P. (1966). Control of sensory fields of stimulation of hypothalamus. *Science* **152** : 1406–1408.

MacDougall, J. M., and Bevan, W. (1968). Influence of pretest shock upon rate of electrical self-stimulation of the brain. *Journal of Comparative and Physiological Psychology* **65** : 261–264.

MacDougall, J. M., Van Hoesen, G. W., and Mitchell, J. C. (1969). Development of post S^r and post non S^r DRL performance and its retention following septal lesions in rats. *Psychonomic Science* **16** : 45–46.

MacDougall, J. M., Pennebaker, J. W., and Stevenson, M. (1973). Effects of septal lesions on the social behavior of two subspecies of deer mice. *Physiology and Behavior,* Unpublished manuscript.

Mackintosh, N. J., and Mackintosh, J. (1974). Performance of octopus over a series of reversals of a simultaneous discrimination. *Animal Behavior* **12** : 321–324.

MacLean, P. D. (1949). Psychosomatic disease and the "visceral brain": Recent developments bearing on the Papez theory of emotion. *Psychosomatic Medicine* **11** : 338–353.

MacLean, P. D. (1970). The triune brain, emotion, and scientific bias. In Schmitt,

F. O. (ed.), *The Neurosciences, Second Study Program*, Rockefeller University Press, New York, pp. 336–349.

MacLean, P. D. (1972). Cerebral evolution and emotional processes. *Annals of the New York Academy of Sciences* **193** : 137–149.

McCleary, R. A. (1961). Response specificity in the behavioral effects of limbic system lesions in the cat. *Journal of Comparative and Physiological Psychology* **54** : 605–613.

McCleary, R. A. (1966). Response-modulating functions of the limbic system: Initiation and suppression. In Stellar, E., and Sprague, J. M. (eds.), *Progress in Physiological Psychology*, Vol. 1, Academic Press, New York.

McConnell, J. V., and Jacobson, A. L. (1973). Learning in invertebrates. In Dewsbury, D. A., and Rethlingshafer, D. A. (eds.), *Comparative Psychology: A Modern Survey*, McGraw-Hill, New York.

McGinty, D., Epstein, A. N., and Teitelbaum, P. (1965). The contribution of oropharyngeal sensations to hypothalamic hyperphagia. *Animal Behavior* **13** : 413–418.

McIntyre, D. C. (1970). Differential amnestic effect of cortical vs. amygdaloid elicited convulsions in rats. *Physiology and Behavior* **5** : 747–753.

McNew, J. J., and Thompson, R. (1966). Role of the limbic system in active and passive avoidance conditioning in the rat. *Journal of Comparative and Physiological Psychology* **61** : 173–180.

Maier, N. R. F. (1949). *Frustration: The Study of Behavior Without a Goal*, McGraw-Hill, New York.

Maier, N. R. F. (1964). Frustration theory: Restatement of extension. In Maier, N. R. F., and Schneirla, T. C. (eds.), *Principles of Animal Psychology*, enlarged ed., Dover, New York, pp. 595–620.

Malmo, R. (1965). Classical and instrumental conditioning with septal stimulation as reinforcement. *Journal of Comparative and Physiological Psychology* **60** : 1–8.

Margules, D. L. (1968). Noradrenergic basis of inhibition between reward and punishment in amygdala. *Journal of Comparative and Physiological Psychology* **66** : 329–334.

Margules, D. L. (1970a). Alpha-adrenergic receptors in hypothalamus for the suppression of feeding behavior by satiety. *Journal of Comparative and Physiological Psychology* **73** : 1–12.

Margules, D. L. (1970b). Beta-adrenergic receptors in hypothalamus for learned and unlearned taste-aversions. *Journal of Comparative and Physiological Psychology* **73** : 13–21.

Margules, D. L., and Stein, L. (1969). Cholinergic synapses in the ventromedial hypothalamus for the suppression of operant behavior by punishment and satiety. *Journal of Comparative and Physiological Psychology* **67** : 327–335.

Marshall, J. F., Turner, B. H., and Teitelbaum, P. (1971). Sensory neglect produced by lateral hypothalamic damage. *Science* **174** : 523–525.

Masserman, J. H., Levitt, M., McAvoy, T., Kling, A., and Pechtel, C. (1958). The amygdalae and behavior. *American Journal of Psychiatry* **115** : 14–17.

Means, L. W., Walker, D. W., and Isaacson, R. L. (1970). Facilitated single alternation go, no-go performance following hippocampectomy in the rat. *Journal of Comparative and Physiological Psychology* **22** : 278–285.

Mendelson, J. (1972). Ecological modulation of brain stimulation effects. *International Journal of Psychobiology* **2** : 285–304.

Meyer, D. R. (1972). Access to engrams. *American Psychologist* **27** : 124–133.

Meyer, P. M., Johnson, D. A., and Vaughn, D. W. (1970). The consequences of septal and neocortical ablations upon learning a two-way conditioned avoidance response. *Brain Research* **22** : 113–120.

Meyers, B., and Domino, E. F. (1964). The effect of cholinergic blocking drugs on spontaneous alternation in rats. *Archives Internationales de Pharmacodynamie* **150** : 525–529.

Milgram, N. W. (1969). Effect of hippocampal stimulation on feeding in the rat. *Physiology and Behavior* **4** : 665–670.

Miller, J. J., and Mogenson, G. J. (1971*a*). Modulatory influences of the septum on lateral hypothalamic self stimulation. *Experimental Neurology* **33** : 671 –683.

Miller, J. J., and Mogenson, G. J. (1971*b*). Effect of septal stimulation on lateral hypothalamic unit activity in the rat. *Brain Research* **32** : 125–142.

Miller, N. E. (1960). Motivational effects of brain stimulation and drugs. *Federation Proceedings* **19** : 846–854.

Miller, N. E., Bailey, C. J., and Stevenson, J. A. F. (1950). Decreased "hunger" but increased food intake resulting from hypothalamic lesions. *Science* **112** : 256–259.

Moberg, G. P., Scapagnini, U., deGroot, J., and Ganong, W. F. (1971). Effect of sectioning the fornix on diurnal fluctuation in plasma corticosterone levels in the rat. *Neuroendocrinology* **7** : 11–15.

Mogenson, G. J., and Calaresu, F. R. (1973). Cardiovascular responses to electrical stimulation of the amygdala in the rat. *Experimental Neurology* **39** : 166–180.

Mok, A. C. S., and Mogenson, G. J. (1972). An evoked potential study of the projections to the lateral habenular nucleus from the septum and the lateral preoptic area in the rat. *Brain Research* **43** : 343–360.

Molnar, P., and Grastyán, E. (1972). The significance of inhibition in motivation and reinforcement. In Boakes, R. A., and Halliday, M. S. (eds.) *Inhibition and Learning*, Academic Press, New York, pp. 403–430.

Moore, R. Y. (1964). Effects of some rhinencephalic lesions on retention of conditioned avoidance behavior in cats. *Journal of Comparative and Physiological Psychology* **53** : 540–548.

Morgan, J. M., and Mitchell, J. C. (1969). Septal lesions enhance delay of responding on a free operant avoidance schedule. *Psychonomic Science* **16** : 10–11.

Morgane, P. J. (1961). Medial forebrain bundle and "feeding centers" of the hypothalamus. *Joural of Comparative Neurology* **117** : 1–25.

Morrell, F. (1961). Effect of anodal polarization on the firing pattern of single cortical cells. *Annals of the New York Academy of Sciences* **92** : 860–876.

Morrow, J. E., and Smithson, B. L. (1969). Learning sets in an invertebrate. *Science* **164** : 850–851.

Munn, N. L. (1950). *Handbook of Psychological Research on the Rat*, Houghton-Mifflin, Boston.

Myers, R. E., and Swett, C., Jr. (1970). Social behavior deficits of free-ranging monkeys after anterior temporal cortex removal: A preliminary report. *Brain Research* **18** : 551–556.

Nadel, L. (1968). Dorsal and ventral hippocampal lesions and behavior. *Physiology and Behavior* **3** : 891–900.

Nakadate, G. M., and deGroot, J. (1963). Fornix transection and adrenocortical function in rats. *Anatomical Record* **145** : 338.

Nakajima, S. (1969). Interference with relearning in the rat after hippocampal injection of actimomycin D. *Journal of Comparative and Physiological Psychology* **67** : 457–461.

Nauta, W. J. H. (1958). Hippocampal projections and related neural pathways to the mid-brain in the cat. *Brain* **81** : 319–340.

Nauta, W. J. H. (1961). Fiber degeneration following lesions of the amygdaloid complex in the monkey. *Journal of Anatomy* **95** : 515–531.

Nauta, W. J. H. (1962). Neural associations of the amygdaloid complex in the monkey. *Brain* **85** : 505–520.

Nauta, W. J. H. (1972). In Hockman, C. H. (ed.), *Limbic System Mechanisms and Autonomic Function*, Charles C Thomas, Springfield, Ill. (see comments, p. 34).

Nonneman, A. J., and Isaacson, R. L. (1973). Task dependent recovery after early brain damage. *Behavioral Biology* **8** : 143–172.

Novick, I., and Pihl, R. (1969). Effect of amphetamine on the septal syndrome in rats. *Journal of Comparative and Physiological Psychology* **68** : 220–225.

O'Keefe, J., and Dostrovsky, J. (1971). The hippocampus as a spatial map. Preliminary evidence from unit activity in the freely-moving rat. *Brain Research* **34** : 171–175.

Olds, J. (1960). Approach–avoidance dissociations in rat brain. *American Journal of Physiology* **199** : 965–968.

Olds, J. (1972). Learning and the hippocampus. *Revue Canadienne de Psychologie* **31** : 215–238.

Olds, J., and Milner, P. (1954). Positive reinforcement produced by electrical stimulation of septal area and other regions of rat brain. *Journal of Comparative and Physiological Psychology* **47** : 419–427.

Olds, J., and Peretz, B. (1960). A motivational analysis of the reticular activitating system. *Electroencephalography and Clinical Neurophysiology* **12** : 445–454.

Olds, M. E., and Frey, J. H. (1971). Effects of hypothalamic lesions on escape behavior produced by midbrain electrical stimulation. *American Journal of Physiology* **221** : 8–18.

Olds, M. E., and Olds, J. (1962). Approach–escape interactions in the rat brain. *American Journal of Physiology* **203** : 803–810.

Olds, M. E., and Olds, J. (1963). Approach–avoidance analysis of rat diencephalon. *Journal of Comparative Neurology* **120** : 259–295.

Olton, D. S. (1970). Specific deficits in active avoidance behavior following penicillin injection into the hippocampus. *Physiology and Behavior* **5** : 957–963.

Olton, D. S. (1972). Behavioral and neuroanatomical differentiation of response suppression and response-shift mechanisms in the rat. *Journal of Comparative and Physiological Psychology* **78** : 450–456.

Olton, D. S. (1973). Shock-motivated avoidance and the analysis of behavior. *Psychological Bulletin* **79** : 243–251.

Olton, D. S., and Isaacson, R. L. (1968). Hippocampal lesions and active avoidance. *Physiology and Behavior* **3** : 719–724.

Olton, D. S., and Isaacson, R. L. (1969). Fear, hippocampal lesions, and avoidance behavior. *Communications in Behavioral Biology* **3** : 1–4.

Osterholm, J. L., and Mathews, G. J. (1972). Altered norepinephrine metabolism following experimental spinal cord injury. Part 2: Protection against traumatic spinal cord hemmorrhagic necrosis by norepinephrine synthesis blockade with alpha methyl tyrosine. *Journal of Neurosurgery* **36** : 395–401.

Pampiglione, G., and Falconer, M. A. (1956). Some observations upon stimulation of the hippocampus in man. *Electroencephalography and Clinical Neurophysiology* **8** : 718.

Papez, J. W. (1937). A proposed mechanism of emotion. *Archives of Neurology and Psychiatry* **38** : 725–744.

Papsdorf, J. D., and Woodruff, M. L. (1970). Effects of bilateral hippocampectomy on the rabbit's acquisition of shuttle-box and passive-avoidance responses. *Journal of Comparative and Physiological Psychology* **73** : 486–489.

Pellegrino, L. (1965). The effects of amygdaloid stimulation on passive avoidance. *Psychonomic Science* **2** : 189–190.

Pellegrino, L. (1968). Amygdaloid lesions and behavioral inhibition in the rat. *Journal of Comparative and Physiological Psychology* **65** : 483–491.

Pellegrino, L. J., and Clapp. D. F. (1971). Limbic lesions and externally cued DRL performance. *Physiology and Behavior* **7** : 863–868.

Pepeu, G., Bartolini, A., and Deffenu, G. (1970). In *International Symposium on the Effect of Drugs on Cholinergic Mechanisms in the C.N.S.*, Skokloster, Sweden, February.

Pepeu, G., Mulas, A., Ruffi, A., and Sotgiu, P. (1971). Brain acetylcholine levels in rats with septal lesions. *Life Sciences* **10** : 181–184.

Peretz, E. (1960). The effects of lesions of the anterior cingulate cortex on the behavior of the rat. *Journal of Comparative and Physiological Psychology* **53** : 540–548.

Pfaff, D. W., Silva, M. T. A., and Weiss, J. M. (1971). Telemetered recording of hormone effects on hippocampal neurons. *Science* **172** : 394–395.

Phillips, A. G., and Lieblich, I. (1972). Developmental and hormonal aspects of hyperemotionality produced by septal lesions in male rats. *Physiology and Behavior* **9** : 237–242.

Pinel, J. P. J., and Cooper, R. M. (1966). The relationship between incubation and ECS gradient effects. *Psychonomic Science* **6** : 125–126.

Plotnick, R. J., and Tallarico, R. B. (1966). Object-quality learning set formation in the young chicken. *Psychonomic Science* **5** : 195–196.

Poletti, C. E., Kinnard, M. A., and MacLean, P. D. (1973). Hippocampal influence on unit activity of hypothalamus, preoptic region, and basal forebrain in awake, sitting squirrel monkeys. *Journal of Neurophysiology* **36** : 308–324.

Pond, F. J., and Schwartzbaum, J. S. (1970). Hippocampal electrical activity evoked by rewarding and aversive brain stimulation in rats. *Communications in Behavioral Biology* **5** : 89–103.

Pond, F. J., Lidsky, T. I., Levine, M. S., and Schwartzbaum, J. S. (1970). Hippocampal electrical activity during hypothalamic-evoked consummatory behavior in rats. *Psychonomic Science* **21** : 21–23.

Poplawsky. A., and Johnson, D. A. (1972). Open-field social behavior of rats following lesions of medial or lateral septal nuclei or cingulate cortex. *American Zoologist* **12**:83.

Powell, E. W., and Hoelle, D. F. (1967). Septo-tectal projections in the cat. *Journal of Comparative Neurology* **18**:177–183.

Powell, E. W., Clark, W. M., and Makawa, J. (1968). An evoked potential study of limbic projections to nuclei of the cat septum. *Electroencephalography and Clinical Neurophysiology* **25**:266–273.

Powell, T. P. S., and Cowan, W. M. (1954). The origin of the mammillothalamic tract in the rat. *Journal of Anatomy* **88**:489–497.

Powley, T. L., and Keesey, R. E. (1970). Relationship of body weight to the lateral hypothalamic feeding syndrome. *Journal of Comparative and Physiological Psychology* **70**:25–36.

Pribram, K. H. (1971). *Languages of the Brain. Experimental Paradoxes and Principles in Neuropsychology*, Prentice-Hall, Englewood Cliffs, N. J., pp. 1–432.

Pribram, K. H., and Bagshaw, M. (1953). Further analysis of the temporal lobe syndrome utilizing frontotemporal ablations. *Journal of Comparative Neurology* **99**:347–375.

Pribram, K. H., and Fulton, J. F. (1954). An experimental critique of the effects of anterior cingulate ablations in monkey. *Brain* **77**:34–44.

Pribram, K. H., and MacLean, P. D. (1953). Neuronographic analysis of medial and basal cortex: II. Monkey. *Journal of Neurophysiology* **16**:323–340.

Pribram, K. H., and Weiskrantz, L. (1957). A comparison of the effects of medial and lateral cerebral resections on conditioned avoidance behavior of monkeys. *Journal of Comparative and Physiological Psychology* **50**:74–80.

Pribram, K. H., Wilson, W. H., and Connors, J. (1962). The effect of lesions of the medial forebrain on alternation behavior of rhesus monkeys. *Experimental Neurology* **6**:36–47.

Pribram, K. H., Douglas, R. J., and Pribram, B. J. (1969). The nature of nonlimbic learning. *Journal of Comparative and Physiological Psychology* **69**:765–772.

Pubols, L. M. (1966). Changes in food motivated behavior of rats as a function of septal and amygdaloid lesions. *Experimental Neurology* **15**:240–254.

Rabe, A., and Haddad, R. K. (1968). Effect of selective hippocampal lesions in the rat on acquisition, performance, and extinction of bar pressing on a fixed ratio schedule. *Experimental Brain Research* **5**:159–266.

Rabe, A., and Haddad, R. K. (1969). Acquisition of two-way shuttle-box avoidance after selective hippocampal lesions. *Physiology and Behavior* **4**:319–323.

Racine, R. J. (1972). Modification of seizure activity by electrical stimulation: I. After-discharge threshold. *Electroencephalography and Clinical Neurophysiology* **32**:269–279.

Raisman, G. (1966). The connections of the septum. *Brain* **89**:317–348.

Raisman, G. (1969). Neuronal plasticity in the septal nuclei of the adult rat. *Brain Research* **14**:25–48.

Raisman, G., Cowan, W. M., and Powell, T. P. S. (1966). An experimental analysis of the efferent projection of the hippocampus. *Brain* **89**:83–108.

Ramon y Cajal, S. (1968). *The structure of Ammon's Horn*, Charles C Thomas, Springfield, Ill.

Randrup, A., and Munkvad, I. (1972). Influence of amphetamines on animal behavior:

Stereotypy, functional impairment and possible animal—human correlations. *Neurologia, Neurochirurgia* **75** : 193—202.

Raphelson, A. C., Isaacson, R. L., and Douglas, R. J. (1965). The effect of distracting stimuli on the runway performance of the limbic damaged rats. *Psychonomic Science* **3** : 483—484.

Reeves, C. D. (1919). Discrimination of light of different wave lengths by fish. *Behavioral Monographs* **4** : 1—106.

Reis, D. J., and McHugh, P. R. (1968). Hypoxia as a cause of bradycardia during amygdala stimulation in monkey. *American Journal of Physiology* **214** : 601—610.

Reis, D. J., and Oliphant, M. C. (1964). Bradycardia and tachycardia following electrical stimulation of the amygdaloid region in monkey. *Journal of Neurophysiology* **27** : 893—912.

Riddell, W. I., Malinchoc, M., and Reimers, R. (1971). Shift and retention deficits in hippocampectomized and neodecorticate rats. Unpublished manuscript.

Riege, W. H., and Cherkin, A. (1971). One-trial learning and biphasic time course of performance in the goldfish. *Science* **172** : 966—968.

Riopelle, A. J., Alper, R. G., Strong, P. N., and Ades, H. W. (1953). Multiple discrimination and patterned string performance of normal and temporal-lobectomized monkeys. *Journal of Comparative and Physiological Psychology* **46** : 145—149.

Roberts, W. W. (1958). Both rewarding and punishing effects from stimulation of posterior hypothalamus of cat with same electrode at same intensity. *Journal of Comparative and Physiological Psychology* **51** : 400—407.

Roberts, W. W. (1962). Fear-like behavior elicited from dorsomedial thalamus of cat. *Journal of Comparative and Physiological Psychology* **55** : 191—197.

Roberts, W. W., Dember, W. N., and Brodwick, M. (1962). Alternation and exploration in rats with hippocampal lesions. *Journal of Comparative and Physiological Psychology* **55** : 695—700.

Rolls, E. T. (1971). Contrasting effects of hypothalamic and nucleus accumbens septi self-stimulation on brain stem single unit activity and cortical arousal. *Brain Research* **31** : 275—285.

Rolls, E. T., and Kelly, P. H. (1972). Neural basis of stimulus-bound locomotor activity in the rat. *Journal of Comparative and Physiological Psychology* **81** : 173—182.

Rose, M. (1929). Cytoarchitektonischer Atlas der Grosshirnrinde der Maus. *Journal of Psychology and Neurology* **40** : 1—51.

Rosvold, H. E., Fuller, J. L., and Pribram, K. H. (1951). Ablation of the pyriform, amygdala, hippocampal complex in genetically pure strain cocker spaniels. In Fulton, J. F. (ed.), *Frontal Lobotomy and Affective Behavior: A Neurophysiological Analysis*, Norton, New York, pp. 80—82.

Rosvold, H. E., Mirsky, A. F., and Pribram, K. H. (1954). Influence of amygdalectomy on social behavior in monkeys. *Journal of Comparative and Physiological Psychology* **47** : 173—178.

Routtenberg, A., and Olds, J. (1963). Attenuation of response to an aversive brain stimulus by concurrent rewarding septal stimulation. *Federation Proceedings* **22** : 515 (abst.).

Rożkowska, E., and Fonberg, E. (1971). The effects of ventromedial hypothalamic lesions on food intake and alimentary instrumental conditioned reflexes in dogs. *Acta Neurobiologiae Experimentalis* **31** : 354–364.

Sanders, F. K. (1940). Second-order olfactory and visual learning in the optic tectum of goldfish. *Journal of Experimental Biology* **30** : 412–415.

Sandwald, J. C., Porzio, N. R., Deane, G. E., and Donovick, P. J. (1970). The effects of septal and dorsal hippocampal lesions on the cardiac component of the orienting response. *Physiology and Behavior* **5** : 883–888.

Schmaltz, L. W. (1971). Deficit in active avoidance learning in rats following penicillin injection into hippocampus. *Physiology and Behavior* **6** : 667–674.

Schmaltz, L. W. and Isaacson, R. L. (1966). The effects of preliminary training conditions upon DRL 20 performance in the hippocampectomized rat. *Physiology and Behavior* **1** : 175–182.

Schmaltz, L. W., and Isaacson, R. L. (1968). Effects of caudate and frontal lesions on retention and relearning of a DRL schedule. *Journal of Comparative and Physiological Psychology* **65** : 343–348.

Schmaltz, L. W., and Theios, J. (1972). Acquisition and extinction of a classically conditioned response in hippocampectomized rabbits (*oryctolagus cuniculus*). *Journal of Comparative and Physiological Psychology* **79** : 328–333.

Schnelle, J. F., Walker, S. F., and Hurwitz, H. M. B. (1971). Concurrent performance in septally operated rats: One and two response extinction. *Physiology and Behavior* **6** : 649–654.

Schwartzbaum, J. S. (1960). Changes in reinforcing properties of stimuli following ablation of the amygdaloid complex in monkeys. *Journal of Comparative and Physiological Psychology* **53** : 388–395.

Schwartzbaum, J. S. (1961). Some characteristics of "amygdaloid hyperphagia" in monkeys. *American Journal of Psychology* **74** : 252–259.

Schwartzbaum, J. S., and Donovick, P. J. (1968). Discrimination reversal and spatial alternation associated with septal and caudate dysfunction in rats. *Journal of Comparative and Physiological Psychology* **65** : 83–92.

Schwartzbaum, J. S., and Gay, P. E. (1966). Interacting behavioral effects of septal and amygdaloid lesions in the rat. *Journal of Comparative and Physiological Psychology* **61** : 59–65.

Schwartzbaum, J. S., and Gustafson, J. W. (1970). Peripheral shock, implanted electrodes and artifactual interactions: A renewed warning. *Psychonomic Science* **20** : 49–50.

Schwartzbaum, J. S., and Poulos, D. A. (1965). Discrimination behavior after amygdalectomy in monkeys: Learning set and discrimination reversals. *Journal of Comparative and Physiological Psychology* **60** : 320–328.

Schwartzbaum, J. S., and Pribram, K. H. (1960). The effects of amygdalectomy in monkeys on transposition along a brightness continuum. *Journal of Comparative and Physiological Psychology* **53** : 396–399.

Schwartzbaum, J. S., Wilson, W. A., Jr., and Morrissette, J. R. (1961). The effect of amygdalectomy on locomotor activity in monkeys. *Journal of Comparative and Physiological Psychology* **54** : 334–336.

Schwartzbaum, J. S., Kellicutt, M. H., Spieth, L. M., and Thompson, J. D. (1964*a*). Effects of septal lesions in rats on response inhibition associated with food reinforced behavior. *Journal of Comparative and Physiological Psychology* **58** : 217–224.

Schwartzbaum, J. S., Thompson, J. D., and Kellicutt, M. H. (1964b). Auditory frequency discrimination and generalization following lesions of the amygdaloid area in rats. *Journal of Comparative and Physiological Psychology* **57**: 257–266.

Schwartzbaum, J. S., Green, R. H., Beatty, W. W., and Thompson, J. B. (1967). Acquisition of avoidance behavior following septal lesions in the rat. *Journal of Comparative and Physiological Psychology* **63** : 95–104.

Schwartzbaum, J. S., Kreinick, C. J., and Levine, M. S. (1972a). Behavioral reactivity and visual evoked potentials to photic stimuli following septal lesions in rats. *Journal of Comparative and Physiological Psychology* **80** : 123–142.

Schwartzbaum, J. S., DiLorenzo, P. M., Mello, W. F., and Kreinick, C. J. (1972b). Further evidence of dissociation between reactivity and visual evoked response following septal lesions in rats. *Journal of Comparative and Physiological Psychology* **80** : 143–149.

Sclafani, A., and Grossman, S. P. (1971). Reactivity of hyperphagic and normal rats to quinine and electric shock. *Journal of Comparative and Physiological Psychology* **74** : 157–166.

Scoville, W. B., and Milner, B. (1957). Loss of recent memory after bilateral hippocampal lesions. *Journal of Neurology, Neurosurgery and Psychiatry* **20** : 11–21.

Sears, R. (1934). Effect of optic lobe ablation on the visuomotor behavior of the goldfish. *Journal of Comparative Psychology* **17** : 233–265.

Segal, M. (1972). The hippocampus as a learning machine. Ph.D. Thesis, California Institute of Technology, unpublished.

Sereni, F., Principi, N., Perletti, L., and Sereni, L. P. (1966). Undernutrition and the developing rat brain. *Biologia Neonatorum* **10** : 254–265.

Shoemaker, W. J., and Wurtman, R. J. (1971). Perinatal undernutrition: Accumulation of catecholamines in rat brain. *Science* **171** : 1017–1019.

Showers, M. J. C. (1959). The cingulate gyrus: additional motor area and cortical autonomic regulator. *Journal of Comparative Neurology* **112** : 231–301.

Sibole, W., Miller, J. J., and Mogenson, G. J. (1971). Effects of septal stimulation on drinking elicited by electrical stimulation of the lateral hypothalamus. *Experimental Neurology* **32** : 466–477.

Sideroff, S., Schneiderman, N., and Powell, D. A. (1971). Motivational properties of septal stimulation as the US in classical conditioning of heart rate in rabbits. *Journal of Comparative and Physiological Psychology* **74** : 1–10.

Siegel, A., and Edinger, H. A. (1973). Comparative neuroanatomical analysis of the differential projections of the hippocampus to the septum. *Society of Neuroscience 3rd Annual Meeting Abstracts*, p. 284.

Siegel, A., and Tassoni, J. P. (1971a). Differential efferent projections from the ventral and dorsal hippocampus of the cat. *Brain, Behavior, and Evolution* **4** : 185–200.

Siegel, A., and Tassoni, J. P. (1971b). Differential efferent projections of the lateral and medial septal nuclei to the hippocampus in the cat. *Brain, Behavior, and Evolution* **4** : 201–219.

Singh, D. (1969). Comparison of hyperemotionality caused by lesions in the septal and ventromedial hypothalamic areas in the rat. *Psychonomic Science* **16** : 3–4.

Slangen, J. L., and Miller, N. E. (1969). Pharmacological tests for the function of hypothalamic norepinephrine in eating behavior. *Physiology and Behavior* **4** : 543–552.

Slotnick, B. M. (1967). Disturbance of maternal behaviour in the rat following lesions in the cingulate cortex. *Behaviour* **29** : 204–236.

Slotnick, B. M., and McMullen, M. F. (1972). Intraspecific fighting in albino mice with septal forebrain lesions. *Physiology and Behavior* **8** : 333–337.

Synder, D. R., and Isaacson, R. L. (1965). Effects of large and small bilateral hippocampal lesions on two types of passive-avoidance responses. *Psychological Reports* **16** : 1277–1290.

Sodetz, F. J. (1970). Septal ablation and free-operant avoidance behavior in the rat. *Physiology and Behavior* **5** : 773–777.

Sodetz, F. J., and Bunnell, B. N. (1970). Septal ablation and the social behavior of the golden hamster. *Physiology and Behavior* **6** : 79–88.

Sodetz, F. J., Matalka, E. S. and Bunnell, B. N. (1967). Septal ablation and affective behavior in the golden hamster. *Psychonomic Science* **7** : 189–190.

Sorensen, J. P., Jr., and Harvey, J. A. (1971). Decreased brain acetylcholine after septal lesions in rats: Correlation with thirst. *Physiology and Behavior* **6** : 723–725.

Stamm, J. S. (1955). The function of the median cerebral cortex in maternal behavior of rats. *Journal of Comparative and Physiological Psychology* **48** : 347–356.

Stamm, J. S., and Pribram, K. H. (1960). Effects of epileptogenic lesions in frontal cortex on learning and retention in monkeys. *Journal of Neurophysiology* **23** : 552–563.

Stark, P., and Totty, C. W. (1967). Effects of amphetamines on eating elicited by hypothalamic stimulation. *Journal of Pharmacology and Experimental Therapeutics* **158** : 272.

Stein, D. G., and Kirkby, R. J. (1967), The effects of training on passive avoidance deficits in rats with hippocampal lesions: A reply to Isaacson, Olton, Bauer, and Swart. *Psychonomic Science* **7** : 7–8.

Stein, L. (1969). Chemistry of purposive behavior. In Tapp, J. T. (ed.), *Reinforcement and Behavior*, Academic Press, New York and London, pp. 329–352.

Stein, L., and Wise, C. D. (1969). Release of norepinephrine from hypothalamus and amygdala by rewarding medial forebrain bundle stimulation and amphetamine. *Journal of Comparative and Physiological Psychology* **67** : 189–198.

Stein, L., Wise, C. D., and Berger, B. D. (1972). Noradrenergic reward mechanisms, recovery of function, and schizophrenia. In McGaugh, J. L. (ed.), *The Chemistry of Mood, Motivation, and Memory*, Plenum Press, New York, pp. 81–103.

Stumpf, C. (1965). Drug action on the electrical activity of the hippocampus. *International Review of Neurobiology* **8** : 77–138.

Suits, E., and Isaacson, R. L. (1968). The effects of scopolamine hydrobromide on one-way and two-way avoidance learning in rats. *International Journal of Neuropharmacology* **7** : 441–446.

Szerb, J. C. (1967). Cortical acetycholine release and electroencephalographic arousal. *Journal of Physiology (London)* **192** : 329–343.

Teitelbaum, H., and Milner, P. M. (1963). Activity changes following partial hippocampal lesions in rats. *Journal of Comparative and Physiological Psychology* **56** : 284–289.

Teitelbaum, P. (1955). Sensory control of hypothalamic hyperphagia. *Journal of Comparative and Physiological Psychology* **48** : 158–163.

Teitelbaum, P. (1957). Random and food-directed activity in hyperphagic and normal rats. *Journal of Comparative and Physiological Psychology* **50** : 486–490.

Teitelbaum, P., and Campbell, B. A. (1958). Injection patterns in hyperphagic and normal rats. *Journal of Comparative and Physiological Psychology* **51** : 135–141.

Teitelbaum, P. and Epstein, A. N. (1962). The lateral hypothalamic syndrome: Recovery of feeding and drinking after lateral hypothalamic lesions. *Psychological Review* **69** : 74–90.

Teitelbaum, P., Cheng, M. F., and Rozin, P. (1969). Development of feeding parallels its recovery after hypothalamic damage. *Journal of Comparative and Physiological Psychology* **67** : 430–441.

Thode, W. F., and Carlisle, H. J. (1968). Effect of lateral hypothalamic stimulation on amphetamine-induced anorexia. *Journal of Comparative and Physiological Psychology* **66** : 547–548.

Thomas, G. J. (1971). Maze retention by rats with hippocampal lesions and with fornicotomies. *Journal of Comparative and Physiological Psychology* **75** : 41–49.

Thomas, G. J. and Slotnick, B. M. (1962). Effect of lesions in the cingulum on maze learning and avoidance conditioning in the rat. *Journal of Comparative and Physiological Psychology* **55** : 1085–1091.

Thomas, G. J., and Slotnick, B. M. (1963). Impairment of avoidance responding by lesions in the cingulate cortex in rats depends on food drive. *Journal of Comparative and Physiological Psychology* **56** : 959–964.

Thomas, G. J., Frey, W. J., Slotnick, B. M., and Kreickhaus, E. E. (1963). Behavioral effects of mammillothalamic tractotomy in cats. *Journal of Neurophysiology* **26** : 857–876.

Thompson, J. B., and Schwartzbaum, J. S. (1964). Discrimination behavior and conditioned suppression (CER) following localized lesions in the amygdala and putamen. *Psychological Reports, Monograph Supplement*, No. 4-VI5.

Thompson, R. (1964). In Warren, J. M., and Akert, K. (eds.), *The frontal Granular Cortex and Behavior: A Symposium*, McGraw-Hill, New York.

Thompson, R., Langer, S. K., and Rich, I. (1964). Lesion studies on the functional significance of the posterior thalamomesencephalic tract. *Journal of Comparative Neurology* **123** : 29–44.

Torii, S. (1961). Two types of pattern of hippocampal electrical activity induced by stimulation of hypothalamus and surrounding parts of rabbit's brain. *Japanese Journal of Physiology* **11** : 147–157.

Trafton, C. L., and Marques, P. R. (1971). Effects of septal area and cingulate cortex lesions on opiate addiction behavior in rats. *Journal of Comparative and Physiological Psychology* **75** : 277–285.

Trafton, C. L., Fibley, R. A., and Johnson, R. W. (1969). Avoidance behavior in rats as a function of the size and location of anterior cingulate cortex lesions. *Psychonomic Science* **14** : 100–102.

Turner, B. H. (1970). Neural structures involved in the rage syndrome of the rat. *Journal of Comparative and Physiological Psychology* **71** : 103–113.

Turner, B. H. (1973). Sensorimotor syndrome produced by lesions of the amygdala and lateral hypothalamus. *Journal of Comparative and Physiological Psychology* **82** : 37–47.

Ursin, H. (1965). The effect of amygdaloid lesions on flight and defense behavior in cats. *Experimental Neurology* **11** : 61–79.

Ursin, H., and Kaada, B. R. (1960). Functional localization within the amygdaloid complex in the cat. *Electroencephalography and Clinical Neurophysiology* **12** : 1–20.

Ursin, H., Wester, K., and Ursin, R. (1967). Habituation to electrical stimulation of the brain in unanesthetized cats. *Electroencephalography and Clinical Neurophysiology* **23** : 41–49.

Ursin, H., Sundberg, H., and Menaker, S. I. (1969). Habituation of the orienting response elicited by stimulation of the caudate nucleus in the cat. *Neuropsychologia* **7** : 313–318.

Valenstein, E. S. (1969). Behavior elicited by hypothalamic stimulation: A prepotency hypothesis. *Brain, Behavior, and Evolution* **2** : 295–316.

Valenstein, E. S., and Campbell, J. F. (1966). Medial forebrain bundle–lateral hypothalamic area and reinforcing brain stimulation. *American Journal of Physiology* **210** : 270–274.

Valenstein, E. S., and Cox, V. C. (1970). The influence of hunger, thirst and previous experience in the test chamber on stimulus-bound eating and drinking. *Journal of Comparative and Physiological Psychology* **70** : 189–199.

Valenstein, E. S., Cox, V. C., and Kakolewski, J. W. (1969). The hypothalamus and motivated behavior. In Tapp, J. T. (ed.), *Reinforcement and Behavior*, Academic Press, New York, pp. 242–285.

Valverde, F. (1963). Amygdaloid projection field. In Bargmann, W., and Schade, J. P. (eds.), *Progress in Brain Research*, Vol. 3: *The Rhinencephalon and Related Structures*, Elsevier, Amsterdam.

Valverde, F. (1965). *Studies on the Pyriform Lobe*, Harvard University Press, Cambridge, Mass.

Van Atta, L., and Sutin, J. (1971). The response of single lateral hypothalamic neurons to ventromedial nucleus and limbic stimulation. *Physiology and Behavior* **6** : 523–536.

Vanderwolf, C. H. (1964). Effect of combined medial thalamic and septal lesions on active-avoidance behavior. *Journal of Comparative and Physiological Psychology* **58** : 31–37.

Vanderwolf, C. H. (1969). Hippocampal electrical activity and voluntary movement in the rat. *Electroencephalography and Clinical Neurophysiology* **26** : 407–418.

Vanderwolf, C. H. (1971). Limbic–diencephalic mechanisms of voluntary movement. *Psychological Review* **78** : 83–113.

Van Hartesveldt, C. (1974). Effect of drugs on DRL performance by rats with hippocampal lesions. Submitted.

Van Hartesveldt, C., and Vernadakis, A. (1972). Convulsive responses in rats with hippocampal and neocortical lesions. *Experimental Neurology* **36** : 563–571.

Van Hartesveldt, C., and Walker, D. (1974). Effect of external stimuli on DRL performance in animals with hippocampal lesions. In preparation.

Van Hoesen, G. W., MacDougall, J. M., Wilson, J. R., and Mitchell, J. C. (1971). Septal lesions and the acquisition and maintenance of a discrete-trial DRL task. *Physiology and Behavior* **7** : 471–475.

Van Hoesen, G. W., Wilson, L. M., MacDougall, J. M., and Mitchell, J. C. (1972). Selective hippocampal complex deafferentation and avoidance behavior in rats. Unpublished manuscript.

Van Wimersma-Greidanus, Tj. B., and DeWied, D. (1969). Effects of intracerebral implantation of corticosteroids on extinction of an avoidance response in rats. *Physiology and Behavior* **4** : 365–370.

Van Wimersma-Greidanus, Tj. B., and DeWied, D. (1971). Effects of systemic and intracerebral administration of two opposite acting ACTH-related peptides on on extinction of conditioned avoidance behavior. *Neuroendocrinology* **7** : 291–301.

Van Wimersma-Greidanus, Tj.B., Bohus, B., and DeWied, D.(1973). Effects of peptide hormones on behaviour. In Scow, R. (Ed.) *Endocrinology. The Proceedings of the Fourth International Congress of Endocrinology.* Amsterdam: *Excerpta Medica,* pp. 197–201.

Votaw, C. L. (1959). Certain functional and anatomical relations of the cornu ammonis of the macaque monkey. I. Functional relations. *Journal of Comparative Neurology* **112** : 353–382.

Votaw, C. L. (1960). Certain functional and anatomical relations of the cornu ammonis is of the macaque monkey. II. Anatomical relations. *Journal of Comparative Neurology* **114** : 283–293.

Votaw, C. L., and Lauer, E. W. (1963). Blood pressure, pulse and respiratory changes produced by stimulation of the hippocampus of the monkey. *Experimental Neurology* **7** : 502–517.

Warburton, D. M. (1969*a*). Effects of atropine sulfate on single alternation in hippocampectomized rats. *Physiology and Behavior* **4** : 641–644.

Warburton, D. M. (1969*b*). Behavioral effects of central and peripheral changes in acetylcholine systems. *Journal of Comparative and Physiological Psychology* **68** : 56–64.

Warburton, D. M., and Russell, R. W. (1969). Some behavioral effects of cholinergic stimulation in the hippocampus. *Life Sciences* **8** : 617–627.

Warren, J. M. (1973). Learning in vertebrates. In Dewsbury, D. A., and Rethlingshafer, D.A. (eds.), *Comparative Psychology:A Modern Survey,* McGraw-Hill, New York.

Warrington, E. K., and Weiskrantz, L. (1973). An analysis of short-term and long-term memory defects in man. In Deutsch, J. A. (ed.), *Physiological Basis of Memory,* Academic Press, New York.

Waxler, M., and Rosvold, H. E. (1970). Delayed alternation in monkeys after removal of the hippocampus. *Neuropsychologia* **8** : 137–146.

Weiskrantz, L. (1956). Behavioral change associated with ablation of the amygdaloid complex in monkeys. *Journal of Comparative and Physiological Psychology* **49** : 381–391.

Weiskrantz, L. (1971). Comparison of amnesic states in monkey and man. In Jarrard, L. (ed.), *Cognitive Processes in Non-human Primates,* Academic Press, New York, pp. 25–46.

Weiskrantz, L., and Wilson, W. A., Jr. (1955). The effects of reserpine (serpasil) on emotional behavior of normal and brain-operated monkeys. *Annals of the New York Academy of Sciences* **61** : 36–55.

Weiskrantz, L., and Wilson, W. A. (1958). The effect of ventral rhinencephalic lesions on avoidance thresholds in monkeys. *Journal of Comparative and Physiological Psychology* **51** : 167–171.

Wetzel, A. B., Conner, R. L., and Levine, S. (1967). Shock-induced fighting in septal-lesioned rats. *Psychonomic Science* **9** : 133–134.

Whishaw, I. Q., and Vanderwolf, C. H. (1971). Hippocampal EEG and behavior: Effects of variation in body temperature and relation of EEG to vibrassae movement, swimming and shivering. *Physiology and Behavior* **6** : 391–397.

White, L. E., Jr. (1959). Ipsilateral afferents to the hippocampal formation in the albino rat. I. Cingulum projections. *Journal of Comparative Neurology* **113** : 1–32.

White, N. (1971). Perseveration by rats with amygdaloid lesions. *Journal of Comparative and Physiological Psychology* **77** : 416–426.

Whitlock, D. G., and Nauta, W. J. H. (1956). Subcortical projections from the temporal neocortex in *Macaca mulatta*. *Journal of Comparative Neurology* **112** : 353–382.

Wickelgren, W. O., and Isaacson, R. L. (1963). Effect of the introduction of an irrelevant stimulus in runway performance of the hippocampectomized rat. *Nature* **200** : 48–50.

Wikler, A., Norrell, H., and Miller, D. (1972). Limbic system and opioid addicition in the rat. *Experimental Neurology* **34** : 543–557.

Wilson, M., Kaufman, H. M., Zieler, R. E., and Lieb, J. P. (1972). Visual identification and memory in monkeys with circumscribed inferotemporal lesions. *Journal of Comparative and Physiological Psychology* **78** : 173–183.

Wilson, W. A., and Mishkin, M. (1959). Comparison of the effects of inferotemporal and lateral occipital lesions on visually guided behavior in monkeys. *Journal of Comparative and Physiological Psychology* **52** : 10–17.

Wilsoncroft, W. E. (1963). Effects of medial cortex lesions on the maternal behavior of the rat. *Psychological Reports* **13** : 835–838.

Wimer, C. C., Wimer, R. E., and Roderick, T. H. (1971). Some behavioral differences associated with relative size of hippocampus in the mouse. *Journal of Comparative and Physiological Psychology* **76** : 57–65.

Winocur, G., and Mills, J. A. (1970). Transfer between related and unrelated problems following hippocampal lesions in rats. *Journal of Comparative and Physiological Psychology* **73** : 162–169.

Winson, J. (1972). Interspecies differences in the occurrence of theta. *Behavioral Biology* **7** : 479–487.

Winson, J. (1974). The theta mode of hippocampal function. In Isaacson, R. L., and Pribram, K. H. (eds.) *The Hippocampus: A Comprehensive Treatise,* Plenum Press, New York, in press.

Wishart, T. B., and Mogenson, G. J. (1970a). Reduction of water intake by electrical stimulation of the septal region of the rat brain. *Physiology and Behavior* **5** : 1399–1404.

Wishart, T. B., and Mogenson, G. J. (1970b). Effects of lesions of the hippocampus and septum before and after passive avoidance training. *Physiology and Behavior* **5** : 31–34.

Wodinsky, J., and Bitterman, M. E. (1959). Partial reinforcement in the fish. *American Journal of Psychology* **72** : 184–199.

Wodinsky, J., and Bitterman, M. E. (1960). Resistance to extinction in the fish after extensive training with partial reinforcement. *American Journal of Psychology* **73** : 429–434.

Woodruff, M. L., and Isaacson, R. L. (1972). Discrimination learning in animals with lesions of hippocampus. *Behavioral Biology* **7** : 489–501.

Woodruff, M. L., Schneiderman, B., and Isaacson, R. L. (1972). Impaired acquisition of a simultaneous brightness discrimination by cortically and hippocampally lesioned rats. *Psychonomic Science* **27** : 269–271.

Woodruff, M. L., Gage, F. H., and Isaacson, R. L. (1973*a*). Changes in focal epileptic activity produced by brain stem sections in the rabbit. *Electroencephalography and Clinical Neurophysiology* **35** : 475–486.

Woodruff, M. L., Kearley, R., and Isaacson, R. L. (1973*b*). The effects of daily injections of an epileptogenic agent (penicillin) into neocortex and hippocampus on a visual discrimination task. *Behavioral Biology,* submitted.

Yunger, L. M., and Harvey, J. A. (1973). Effect of lesions in the medial forebrain bundle on three measures of pain sensitivity and noise-elicited startle. *Journal of Comparative and Physiological Psychology* **83** : 173–183.

Zucker, I., and McCleary, R. A. (1964). Perseveration in septal cats. *Psychonomic Science* **1** : 387–388.

AUTHOR INDEX

Ackil, J. E. 174
Ades, H. W. 231
Adey, W. R. 54, 201
Adler, M. W. 208
Ahmad, S. S. 139
Allen, J. D. 126
Allen, R. P. 101
Allen, W. F. 172
Alper, R. G. 231
Anchel, H. 204
Anden, N. -E. 17
Andersen, P. 40
Anderson, C. 151
Angevine, J. B., Jr. 34
Aronson, F. F. 223
Aronson, L. R. 223

Bagshaw, M. H. 109, 110, 111, 117, 126, 128, 129, 130
Bailey, C. J. 82
Baisden, R. H., 156, 168
Baldwin, M. 210
Ball, G. G. 65, 205
Bandler, R. J., Jr. 81
Barker, D. J. 101
Barrett, R. J. 216
Barrett, T. W. 125, 127, 194

Bartolini, A. 155
Batenchuk, C. 206
Bauer, B. 174
Bauer, J. H. 241
Bauer, R. H. 140
Baumann, I. R. 229
Beatty, W. W. 136, 144, 198
Beckman, G. J. 117, 120, 207
Beharry, E. 193
Behrend, E. R. 223
Bennett, T. L. 201, 202, 203
Benzies, S. 109
Berger, B. D. 56, 77, 86, 88, 92, 93
Beritoff, J. S. 224, 227, 228, 237
Best, P. 238
Bevan, W. 73
Bieliauskas, L. 138
Bishop, M. P. 62
Bitterman, M. E. 223, 224, 225, 226
Black, A. H. 202, 206, 207
Blackstad, T. W. 37, 38, 40, 44
Blanchard, D. C. 162
Blanchard, R. J. 140, 162
Blass, E. M. 137
Bliss, T. V. P. 40
Bobo, E. G. 109
Bonvallet, M. 109

Borbély, A. A. 228–229
Bower, G. H. 63
Boyce, B. A. 137
Boyd, E. S. 63
Brady, J. V. 133, 197
Breglio, V. 151
Brener, J. M. 135
Bresnahan, E. 123
Broca, A. 1, 2
Brodwick, M. 166
Brown, G. E. 142, 147
Brutkowski, S. 98, 118
Bucy, P. C. 124
Buddington, R. W. 133, 145
Buerger, A. A. 168
Bull, H. 223
Bunnell, B. N. 115, 133, 137, 144, 164
Burkett, E. E. 145
Burright, R. G. 136, 137, 142
Butler, C. M. 125
Butters, N. 147

Caggiula, A. R. 64
Calaresu, F. R. 109
Campbell, B. A. 82, 165
Campbell, C. B. G. 9
Campbell, J. F. 63
Campenot, R. B. 120
Capobianco, S. 142
Carder, B. 153
Cardo, B. 96
Carey, R. J. 136, 137, 177, 142
Carlisle, J. H. 92
Carlson, N. R. 143, 148, 149
Carlton, P. 88, 94, 134
Carter, E. N. 148
Casey, K. L. 65, 66, 73
Cerny, M. C. 194
Chalmers, B. M. 153
Chang, H. K. 162
Chang, M. F. 76
Cherkin, A. 226
Chi, C. C. 83, 86, 96
Choi, H. 162
Chow, K. L. 211
Clapp, D. F. 177
Clark, C. V. H. 176, 216
Clark, W. M. 48
Clemens, W. J. 135

Clody, D. E. 134
Cohen, J. S. 193
Cole, J. R. 149
Conner, H. S. 213
Connor, R. L. 139
Connors, J. 127
Coons, E. E. 97
Cooper, R. M. 227, 241
Coover, G. D. 166
Corman, C. D. 140
Corsellis, J. A. N. 210
Cowan, W. M. 16, 27, 44
Cox, V. C. 64, 67, 70, 71
Coyle, P. 49
Cragg, B. G. 49
Crawford, F. T. 223
Crosby, E. C. 55, 107
Crowne, D. P. 166

Dahlström, A. 17, 90
Dalby, D. A. 143
Dalland, T. 147, 168
Davison, C. 126
Deagle, J. H. 135, 142, 143, 144
Deane, G. E. 170
Deffenu, G. 155
De Fries, J. C. 163
DeGroot, J. 20, 170
Delgado, J. M. R. 63, 65, 111
Deloache, J. 167
Dember, W. N. 166
De Olmos, J. S. 18, 21, 22
Desiraju, T. 44
De Toledo, L. 207
Deutsch, J. A. 72
De Wied, D. 172
Diamond, I. T. 196, 239
DiCara, L. V. 119
DiLorenzo, P. M. 136
Dodo, T. 108, 169
Domesick, V. B. 52, 53, 54
Domino, E. F. 168
Donovick, P. J. 121, 135, 136, 137, 142,
    147, 153, 170
Dostrovsky, O. 169
Douglas, R. J. 110, 129, 130, 140, 166,
    167, 168, 172, 193, 194, 195
Duncan, N. C. 144, 173
Duncan, P. M. 140, 144, 173

Dunsmore, R. 151
Dupree, M. 125

Eager, R. P. 83
Earle, K. M. 210
Eclancher, F. S. 85
Egger, M. D. 112
Eichelman, B. S. Jr. 139, 163
Elazar, Z. 201
Elder, S. T. 62
Eleftheriou, B. E. 125
Elias, M. F. 125
Ellen, P. 145, 146, 167
Elliot Smith, G. 3
Ellison, G. D. 78, 83
Elul, R. 208
Enlow, L. J. 115
Epstein, A. N. 75, 82, 83

Faillace, L. A. 101
Falconer, M. A. 169, 210
Fallon, D. 147
Fedio, P. 101
Feindel, W. 116
Feldman, R. S. 169
Fial, R. A. 140
Fibley, R. A. 99
Finch, D. M. 115
Fisher, A. E. 89
Flaherty, C. F. 142
Flynn, J. P. 71, 78, 81, 86, 112
Foltz, E. L. 101
Fonberg, E. 87, 111, 112, 114, 118
Freeman, W. J. 48
French, J. D. 51
Frey, J. H. 79
Frey, W. J. 95
Fried, P. A. 198, 199
Froloff, J. 223
Frommer, G. P. 174
Fuller, J. L. 115, 124
Fulton, J. F. 98
Fuse, S. 169
Fuxe, K. 17, 54, 90, 94

Gage, F. W. 208
Galef, B. C. 115
Gallistel, C. R. 70, 72, 73
Ganong, W. F. 170

Gardner, L. C. 63, 151
Gay, P. E. 140
Gellerman, L. W. 179
Gellhorn, E. 74
Genthon, C. 44
Gerbrandt, L. K. 239
Giris, M. 107
Gittelson, P. L. 137–142, 147
Giurgea, Cornelius 172
Glass, D. H., 101
Glick, S. D. 78
Glickman, S. E. 163–230
Gloor, P. 40, 116
Goddard, G. V. 114, 121, 122, 123, 124
Gold, R. M. 83, 84, 85
Gollender, M. 101
Gonzalez, R. C. 224, 225
Gostnell, D. 99
Gotsick, J. E. 134, 139
Gottfried, J. 203
Grant, L. E. 199
Grastyán, E. 66, 105
Gray, J. A. 202–205
Green, R. H. 136–144
Greene, E. G. 156, 165
Greenspon, T. 97
Greenstein, S. 78
Gregoire, K. 137
Grossen, N. E. 140
Grossman, L. 83, 84, 86
Grossman, S. P. 77, 83–86, 88, 146, 155
Gurowitz, E. M. 100
Gustafson, J. W. 121

Haddad, R. K. 197
Halgren, C. 174
Hamberger, B. 54
Hamilton, G. 213, 214
Hamilton, L. W. 142, 144, 145
Han, P. W. 83
Hanson, D. G. 137
Hara, K. 115
Harlow, H. F. 224
Harrell, E. 142
Harrison, J. M. 135
Harvey, J. A. 80, 135, 136, 137, 139, 146,
        155, 197
Hattori, Y. 171
Hayes, W. N. 143

Heath, R. G. 62, 64
Heatherington, A. W. 82
Hegman, J. P. 163
Heimer, L. 24, 85
Heller, A. 17, 57, 81, 90
Hendrickson, C. W. 166
Henke, P. G. 126
Henry, C. E. 211
Hernandez-Peón, R. 51
Herrick, C. J. 6, 9, 31
Hess, W. R. 74
Higgins, T. 163, 230
Hiram, T. 238
Hirsh, R. 193
Hjorth-Simonsen, A. 32, 39, 45
Hodos, W. 9
Hoebel, B. G. 66, 77, 83, 88
Hoelle, D. F. 49
Hökfelt, T. 17, 54, 94
Holdstock, T. L. 153, 154, 198
Holloway, F. A. 155
Holmes, J. E. 207
Hotersall, D. 146
Howarth, C. I. 72
Hull, C. 60
Humphrey, N. K. 239
Humphrey, T. 55, 107
Hunt, H. F. 136, 137, 146, 197
Hurwitz, H. M. B. 147
Huston, J. P. 72, 228, 229
Hutt, M. L. 222

Ihata, Y. 44
Inman, D. P. 201
Ireland, L. 166
Isaacson, R. L. 75, 101, 118, 140, 143,
        145, 163, 164, 166, 168, 171,
        172, 173, 174, 175, 176, 177,
        178, 179, 187, 189, 191, 192,
        195, 196, 208, 209, 213, 214,
        216, 222, 230, 234, 235
Ison, J. R. 101
Ito, M. 205

Jackson, W. J. 168, 234
Jacobs, B. L. 78
Jacobs, H. L. 91
Jacobson, A. L. 222
Jarrard, L. E. 162, 163, 164, 170, 176,
        199

Jeune, B. 39
Johnson, D. A. 138, 145, 146
Johnson, R. R. 115
Johnson, R. W. 100
Johnston, J. B. 18, 23
Jonason, K. R. 115

Killefer, F. A. 82
Kim, C. 162
Kim, C. C. 162
Kim, J. K. 162
Kim, J. Y. 162
Kim, M. S. 162
Kimble, D. P. 99, 109, 110, 163, 165,
        166, 173, 178 182, 183, 187, 191,
        192, 195
Kimble, R. J. 166, 182, 183, 234
King, F. A. 99, 112, 118, 133, 141, 142
        143, 145
Kings, R. B. 114, 117
Kinnard, M. A. 209, 238
Kirby, R. J. 173, 174
Klein, S. B. 227
Klemm, W. R. 202
Klüver, H. 124
Koepp, K. 137
Koikegami, H. 19, 108, 169
Komisaruk, B. R. 202
Kondo, C. Y. 146
Korn, J. H. 170
Krechevcky, I. 183
Kreinick, C. J. 121, 136
Krieckhaus, E. E. 95, 96, 97, 143
Kreindler, A. 116
Kveim, O. 85, 142

Laatch, R. H. 44
Lammers, H. J. 22, 23, 54
Lang, H. 109
Langdon, J. W. 223
Langer, S. K. 97
Langfeldt, T. 169
Lanier, L. 164, 171, 196
Laroche, J. P. 193
Larsson, K. 17, 85
Lash, L. 168
Lashley, K. 240
LaVaque, T. J. 143, 147
Laver, E. W. 55, 107
Law, O. T. 101

Lee, I. G. 162
Leech, C. K. 122
Leibowitz, S. 77, 89, 90, 91, 92
Leith, N. J. 216
Lennox, R. 51
Leonard, C. M. 52
LeVere, T. E. 241
Levine, M. S. 122, 136, 137, 203
Levine, S. 139, 166
Levitt, M. 124
Lidsky, T. I. 122, 203
Lieb, J. P. 240
Lieblich, I. 134
Lindsley, D. B. 204
Livingston, R. B. 51
Lohman, A. H. M. 54
Lopez de Silva, F. H. 202
Lömo, T. 40
Lorente de Nò, R. 34
Lorenz, R. 96
Lorenz, S. A. 146
Lovely, R. H. 140
Lown, B. A. 143
Lubar, J. F. 98, 99, 135, 137, 142, 143,
    144
Lynch, G. 165
Lyon, M. 135

MacDonnell, M. F. 81
MacDougall, J. M. 73, 138, 146, 165, 197,
    198
Mackintosh, N. J. 224
Mackworth, N. H. 130
MacLean, P. D. 51, 209, 220, 221, 223,
    238
Maier, N. R. F. 188, 189, 190
Malinchoc, M. 233
Malmo, R. B. 151, 154
Margules, D. L. 87, 90, 91, 92
Marques, R. R. 140
Marshall, J. F. 81
Marshall, R. C. 134
Masserman, J. H. 101, 124
Matalka, E. S. 133
Matthews, G. J. 78
McAvoy, T. 124
McCleary, R. A. 99, 141, 142, 145, 146
    153, 155
McConnell, J. V. 222
McGinty, D. 83

McHugh, P. R. 108
McIntyre, D. C. 122, 123
McMullen, M. F. 138
McNew, J. J. 85, 119
McQueen, J. D. 102
Means, L. W. 168, 234
Mellgren, R. L. 174
Mello, W. F. 136
Mempel, E. 98, 118
Menaker, S. J. 109
Mendelson, J. 104
Merrill, H. K. 151
Meyer, D. R. 140, 241
Meyer, M. 54
Meyer, P. M. 114, 140, 145
Meyers, B. 168
Meyers, R. E. 115, 116
Mickle, W. A. 64
Milgram, N. W. 72
Miller, D. 102
Miller, J. J. 154
Miller, N. E. 63, 64, 65, 82, 88, 149, 150,
    152
Mills, J. A. 234
Milner, B. 210
Milner, P. M. 60, 61, 62, 63, 149, 166
Mirsky, A. F. 115
Mishkin, M. 125, 211
Mitchell, J. C. 144, 146, 165, 197, 198
Miyamoto, T. 171
Moberg, G. P. 170
Mochida, Y. 108, 169
Mogenson, G. J. 8, 109, 149, 150, 152,
    154, 174, 198
Mok, A. C. S. 8
Molnár, P. 106
Moon, Y. B. 162
Moore, R. Y. 134, 172, 197
Moot, S. A. 140
Morgan, J. M. 144
Morgane, P. J. 105
Morlock, G. W. 241
Morrell, F. 201
Morrow, J. F. 223
Munkvad, I. 156
Munn, N. L. 180

Nadel, L. 195, 197
Nakadate, G. M. 170
Nakajima, S. 212

Nakamura, Y. 203
Nauta, W. J. H. 21, 24, 26, 43, 49, 54,
    112, 204
Neff, W. D. 239
Nonneman, A. J. 173, 177, 189, 235
Norman, R. J. 149
Norman, R. L. 125
Norrel, H. 102
Northrup, B. 102
Novick, I. 156
Numan, R. 135
Nunn, P. J. 201

Obrist, W. D. 211
O'Keefe, J. 169
Olds, J. 60, 61, 62, 63, 64, 65, 79, 80,
    149, 150, 151, 205, 237, 238
Olds, M. E. 62, 64, 65, 80
O'Leary, J. L. 117
Oliphant, M. C. 109
Olson, L. 17
Olton, D. S. 145–172, 174, 175–187, 190,
    212
Ommaya, A. K. 102
Orbach, J. 118
Osterholm, J. L. 78

Pampiglione, G. 169
Papez, J. W. 50
Pappas, G. D. 44
Papsdorf, J. D. 173
Patel, H. H. 48
Pechtel, C. 124
Pellegrino, L. J. 121, 127, 177
Penfield, W. 210
Pennebaker, J. W. 138
Pepeu, G. 155
Perachio, A. A. 99
Peretz, B. 64
Peretz, E. 99
Perletti, L. 78
Peterson, J. J. 140
Pfaff, D. W. 171
Phillips, A. G. 134
Pihl, R. 156
Pinel, J. P. J. 227
Plotnick, R. J. 225
Poletti, C. E. 238
Pond, F. J. 118, 203, 205

Poplawski, A. 138
Porzio, N. R. 170
Poulos, D. A. 125, 231
Powell, D. A. 154
Powell, E. W. 48, 49, 145, 146
Powell, T. P. S. 16, 27, 44
Powley, T. L. 76
Pribram, J. D. 126
Pribram, K. H. 51, 98, 109–111, 115, 117,
    119, 124, 127–130, 166, 193,
    194, 195, 211–239
Principi, N. 78
Proulx, D. M. 85
Pubols, L. M. 147

Rabe, A. 197
Racine, R. J. 123
Raisman, G. 16, 27, 44, 47, 49
Ramón y Cajal, S. 29, 30, 31, 33, 34, 36
Randall, D. 97
Randrup, A. 156
Ranson, S. W. 82
Raphelson, A. C. 166
Rasmussen, E. W. 85, 142
Ray, O. S. 216
Reeves, C. D. 223
Reimers, R. 233
Reis, D. J. 108, 109
Remley, N. R. 142, 147
Rich, I. 97
Riddell, W. I. 166, 233
Riege, W. H. 226
Riopelle, A. J. 231
Roberts, L. 133, 145
Roberts, W. W. 63–67, 166, 233
Roderick, T. H. 165
Rolls, E. T. 72–73
Rose, M. 52
Rosen, A. J. 100
Rosvold, H. E. 115, 124, 125, 147
Routtenberg, A. 64, 123, 150, 151
Rozin, P. 76
Rożkowska, E. 88
Russell, R. W. 155

Sanders, F. K. 223
Sandwald, J. C. 170
Sapagnini, U. 170
Schaffer, K. 31–32

Schaub, R. E. 143
Schmaltz, L. W. 176, 211, 212, 230
Schneiderman, B. 178
Schneiderman, N. 154
Schnelle, J. F. 147
Schricker, J. L. 117
Schwartzbaum, J. S. 110, 111, 120, 121,
        122, 124, 125, 128, 136, 140,
        144, 147, 153, 198, 203, 205, 231
Schwarz, N. 118
Sclafani, A. 85
Scoville, W. B. 210
Sears, R. 223
Sekiguchi, M. 171
Serafetinides, E. A. 210
Sereni, F. 78
Sereni, L. P. 78
Seto, K. 170
Shaefer, C. S. 137
Sharma, K. N. 91
Shoemaker, W. J. 78
Showers, M. J. 52
Sibole, W. 154
Sideroff, S. 154
Siegel, A. 41, 43, 44, 48, 49
Silva, M. T. A. 171
Singh, D. 134
Skinner, B. F. 60
Slotnick, B. M. 96, 98, 99, 100, 138
Smithson, B. L. 223
Snyder, D. R. 173
Sodetz, F. J. 133, 139, 144
Sorenson, C. A. 78
Sorenson, J. P., Jr. 155
Spear, N. E. 227
Spence, K. 60
Sperti, L. 40
Spieth, L. M. 121, 125, 147
Spinelli, D. N. 239
Stamm, J. S. 100, 211
Stark, P. 88
Stein, D. G. 173, 174
Stein, L. 56, 77, 86, 87, 88, 92, 93
Steriade, M. 116
Stern, W. E. 82
Stevenson, J. A. F. 82
Stevenson, M. 138
Storm Van Leeuwen, W. 202
Strong, P. N., Jr. 168, 231–234

Stumpf, C. 203
Suits, E. 216
Sundberg, H. 109
Surwit, R. S. 115
Swart, P. 174
Swett, C. 116
Szerb, J. C. 155

Takahashi, H. 108, 169
Tallarico, R. B. 225
Tassoni, J. P. 41, 43, 44, 48, 49
Teitelbaum, P. 75, 76, 77, 81, 82, 83, 166
Terasawa, E. 171
Tessel, R. E. 101
Thatcher, K. 146
Thode, W. F. 92
Thomas, G. J. 95, 96, 98, 99, 100, 192
Thomas, T. T. 137
Thompson, J. B. 120, 121, 125, 144, 147
Thompson, R. 85, 97, 119
Thompson, R. D. 66
Totty, C. W. 88
Tokizane, T. 203
Torii, S. 203–204
Tourinen, I. 109
Towne, J. 118
Trafton, C. L. 100, 102, 140
Turner, B. H. 81, 134

Ungerstedt, U. 17, 94
Ursin, H. 109, 112, 113, 114, 119
Ursin, R. 109
Valenstein, E. S. 63, 64, 67, 70, 71
Vallante, M. 148
Valleale, P. 109
Vallentine, P., II 165
Valverde, F. 7, 18
Vanderwolf, C. H. 143, 201, 202
Van Hartesveldt, C. 168, 176, 177, 208,
        217, 235
Van Hoesen, G. W. 146, 165, 197, 198
Van Wimersma-Greidanus, Tj B. 171
Vaughn, D. W. 145
Vera, L. C. 40
Vernadakis, A. 208
Votaw, C. L. 45

Walberg, F. 44
Walker, D. W. 168, 177, 234

Walker, S. F. 147
Warburton, D. M. 155, 216
Warren, J. M. 225
Warrington, E. K. 232–233
Weiskrantz, L. 98, 114, 119, 232, 233, 239
Weiss, J. M. 97, 171
Wells, D. G. 137
Wester, K. 109
Wetzel, A. B. 139
Whishaw, I. Q. 202
White, L. E., Jr. 37, 44, 101
White, N. 126
Whitlock, D. G. 49
Wickelgren, W. O. 166, 173
Wikler, A. 102
Wilson, A. S. 145
Wilson, J. R. 146, 197–198
Wilson, L. M. 165
Wilson, M. 240

Wilson, W. A. 111, 119, 211
Wilsoncroft, W. E. 100, 146
Wimer, C. C. 165
Wimer, R. E. 165
Winocur, G. 234
Winson, J. 206
Wise, C. D. 56, 77, 86, 87, 88, 92, 93
Wishart, T. B. 154, 174, 198
Wodinsky, J. 224
Wolf, G. 83
Woodruff, M. L. 168, 173, 178, 208–214
Wurtman, R. J. 78

Yoshida, K. 171
Young, G. A. 206
Yunger, L. M. 80

Zieler, R. E. 240
Zucker, I. 146

SUBJECT INDEX

Allocortex 1

Amphetamine 88, 92, 93, 96, 216

Amphibian, brain of 2, 3, 6

Amygdala (see also stria terminalis)
  anatomical groups 6, 18, 107, 127, 131
  effect of norepinephrine injection 92
  fiber systems of 16, 19–27
  "kindling effect" 122, 123
  learning sets 231
  lesion, effects of
    and GSR 127
    behavioral effects 16, 117–121, 125,
      131, 132
    compared with hippocampal lesions
      125, 129
    compared with orbitofrontal lesions
      125
    emotional changes 114, 115, 126,
      131
    enhanced novelty reactions 129,
      130
    food intake 110, 124
    incentive motivation 124, 132
    learning sets 125
    locomotor activity 110
    orienting reflex 109
    perseveration of responses 124, 125
    social behavior 115, 116, 132

Amygdala (cont.)
    stimulus generalization 129
    strain differences 125, 126
    visual attention 110
  stimulation of 114
    arousal 116, 131
    behavioral changes 121, 123, 124
    dorsal–ventral differences 116, 131
    flight and aggression 112, 113, 121
    "state dependent" effects 122, 124

Anterior limbic field 123

Arousal 64, 65, 72, 73

Behaviorism 61

Brain stem reticular formation 56

Brain stimulation
  affective quality of 64, 65
  and rewards 104
  discovery of self-stimulation 60
  "dual effect" 66, 104
  effect of brain lesions on 62, 63
  effects on thalamic neurons 66
  "elicited behaviors" 67–72
    forms of 67
    relation to biological motives 67
    relation to support objects 69
    variability of 68–69
  mapping of brain 62, 63

Brain stimulation (*cont.*)
　medial forebrain bundle 62, 73
　pain 65, 66
　parameters of stimulation 63
　punishing effects 63
　reaction reversal 63, 64
　reinforcing and motivational qualities 72
　ventromedial nucleus of hypothalamus
　　65

Catecholamines 54
Central gray, fiber connections of 56
Cholinergic effects 86, 94
Command areas, of brain stem 67, 68, 104
Cortex
　auditory areas 239
　cingulate 51, 52, 54
　　arousal and stress 100–102
　　behavioral effects of lesions 97–100
　　drug addiction and withdrawal 102
　　fear responses 99
　　freezing responses 99
　　hyperactivity and hyperirritability 111
　　pain 101
　　relation to septal area 98–99
　　relation to visual cortex 99
　　species typical behaviors 100
　entorhinal 35, 37, 38, 165, 197, 198
　inferotemporal 110, 239–241
　juxtaallocortex 1
　parasubiculum 35, 37, 38
　prefrontal 27, 116, 165
　presubiculum 35, 37, 38
　subiculum 35, 37, 38
　temporal 209, 210
　transitional zones 37–40, 165
　visual areas 239

Dentate gyrus 35, 36, 39, 40
Diagonal band of Broca 48
Dopamine 57

Eating, adrenergic systems 77, 78, 88
Emotion 50

Forel's field H of 43
Fornix 40–42, 170
　postcommissural 40
　precommissural 40
　species differences in fiber distribution
　　41, 42

Frustration
　genetic differences in tolerance 193
　hippocampal lesions and 189
　Maier's theory of 188, 189
　perseveration and 188, 193

Habituation 94
Hippocampus (see also dentate gyrus,
　　fornix)
　anatomy of 5, 6
　　alveus 33
　　cellular layers 29–34
　　perforant path 37, 39, 40
　　psalterium 37
　anterior hippocampal rudiment 45
　autonomic regulation 169, 170
　behavioral inhibition 214
　cholinergic stimulation of 199
　definition of 27
　effects of lesions
　　active avoidance 177, 172
　　activity 163, 164, 165, 235
　　"all–or–none" effects 192
　　brightness discrimination performance
　　　178, 179, 183, 231, 234
　　comparison with septal lesions 172
　　DRL performance 175, 178
　　drugs 216, 217
　　emotional changes 162
　　extinction 197
　　genetic contributions 163, 164, 187
　　go, no–go performance 168
　　hypothesis behavior 183, 184, 185,
　　　187, 193, 194, 195
　　interaction with motivational states
　　　174
　　operant avoidance learning 173
　　passive avoidance 171, 173, 175
　　regional differences 195–200
　　response perseveration 168, 187, 188,
　　　193, 194, 195
　　sleep 162, 163
　　"spontaneous alternation" 167
　　visual discriminations 173
　　water consumption 198
　electrical rhythms 203, 204, 206
　　behavior, and 200–206
　　desynchronization 207
　　locomotion, and 207
　　orienting response, and 201

Hippocampus (*cont.*)
    paradoxical sleep, and 206
    relation to neocortical activity 207
    species differences 206
    voluntary movements, and 201, 202
  epileptic activity, effects of 208, 210,
      211, 212, 213, 214
  "failure of forgetting" 231
  hippocampal–septal connections 43, 44,
    45
  hormones, and 170, 171
  regional differences 199
  Schaffer collaterals 32, 40
  single unit activity 205, 237, 238
  spatial maps 169
Homologous areas of brain 8, 9, 10
Hypothalamus (see also mammillary bodies)
    10
  anatomy of 11, 12, 13–17
  autonomic regulation 10
  circumscription of 78
  cuts made through regions 83, 84, 85
  effects of ventromedial lesions 82, 84, 85
  ergotropic and trophotropic systems 74,
    75
  far lateral area 92, 105, 106
  homeostatic regulation 59, 60
  lesions of
    escape behavior 79
    food intake 76, 77, 82, 90
    recovery after lateral damage 75–77
    stimulation of lateral 80
    ventromedial nucleus 84
Hypothesis behavior 183, 231, 234

Images 224, 227, 228, 237
Induseum griseum 45
Inhibition
  behavioral 87
  medial and lateral hypothalamus 90
Interference, proactive 232–235

Language 241, 242
Learning sets 224, 225
"Limbic lobe" 1

Mammillary bodies 54, 94
Mass action, law of 240
Medial forebrain bundle 6, 15, 16, 17, 40,
    46, 47, 55–57
α-methyl-*p*-tyrosine 77, 78

Neomammalian brain (of MacLean) 220,
    221, 239, 243
Nucleus
  accumbens septi 46, 49, 135
  Darkschewitsch's 41
  dorsomedial, of thalamus
  interpeduncular 56
  of diagonal band of Broca 41, 44, 46
  of stria terminalis 46
  triangularis septi 46

Olfactory bulb, lesions of 154
Orienting reflex 110, 127
Oxytocin 47

Paleomammalian brain of MacLean 220,
    229, 239
Papez' theory of limbic system 50
Parolfactory area 46
Physostigmine 217
"Pleasure centers" of the brain 103–104
Protoreptilian brain (of MacLean) 220–229

Response suppression 93–95, 120, 124
    125
Reversal learning 225, 226
Reward system, noradrenergic theory of 86,
    87
Rhinencephalon 2

Scopolamine 216
Sensory neglect 81
Septal area
  anatomy of 5, 6, 15, 45, 48
  effects of lesions
    active avoidance 98
    activity 139
    emotional changes 133, 134, 157
    evoked potentials 136
    freezing responses, and 140
    hormones, and 137
    predominant behavioral tendencies
      138, 158
    regional differences 15, 134, 135,
      138, 157, 158
    sociability 138, 139
    species differences 134, 138
    taste aversion 137
    thirst and water consumption 136,
      137, 138, 158

Septal area (*cont.*)
  lateral septal nucleus 5, 6, 41–44
  medial septal nucleus 5, 6, 46, 47
  neuronal plasticity in 47
  response initiation 250
  "septal syndrome" 134, 135, 157
  septo-habenular connections 47, 48
  septo-hippocampal connections 41, 43,
    44
  septo-hypothalamic connections 47
Sexual behavior 75
Spontaneous alternation 167, 168
Stria terminalis 16, 21
  bed nucleus of 46
  effect on hypothalamus 131
  septal rage syndrome and 135
Strychnine neuronography 51

Tracts
  alveus 37

Tracts (*cont.*)
  cingulate fasciculus 54
  cingulum, brain stem connections of
    54
  fornix 16, 40
  habenulointerpeduncular (retroflexus) 7,
    8, 55
  hypothalamotegmental 15, 16
  mammillopeduncular 55
  mammillotegmental 55
  mammillothalamic 55, 95–98, 102
  medial forebrain bundle 6, 15, 16, 17,
    40, 46, 47, 55–57, 80
  nigrostriatal 57
  ventral amygdalofugal 16
  Zuckerkandl's bundle 41
Transfer of training 128, 229, 232
Transposition 128, 129
Triune brain (of MacLean) 220
Tsai, ventrotegmental area of 56